MEDICAL ETHICS

Jones and Bartlett Series in Philosophy
Robert Ginsberg, General Editor

A. J. Ayer, 1994 reissue with new introduction
by Thomas Magnell, Drew University
Metaphysics and Common Sense

Francis J. Beckwith,
University of Nevada, Las Vegas, Editor
*Do the Right Thing: A Philosophical Dialogue
on the Moral and Social Issues of Our Time*

Anne H. Bishop and John R. Scudder, Jr.,
Lynchburg College
Nursing Ethics: Therapeutic Caring Presence

Peter Caws, The George Washington University
Ethics from Experience

Joseph P. DeMarco, Cleveland State University
Moral Theory: A Contemporary Overview

Bernard Gert et al., Dartmouth College
Morality and the New Genetics

Michael Gorr, Illinois State University, and
Sterling Harwood, San Jose State University,
Editors
Crime and Punishment: Philosophic Explorations

Joram Graf Haber,
Bergen Community College, Interviewer
Ethics in the 90's, a 26-part Video Series

Sterling Harwood,
San Jose State University, Editor
*Business as Ethical and Business as Usual:
Text, Readings, and Cases*

John Heil, Davidson College
First Order Logic: A Concise Introduction

Gary Jason, San Diego State University
Introduction to Logic

Brendan Minogue, Youngstown State University
Bioethics: A Committee Approach

Marilyn Moriarty, Hollins College
Writing Science through Critical Thinking

Linus Pauling, and Ikeda Daisaku,
Richard L. Gage, Translator and Editor
A Lifelong Quest for Peace, A Dialogue

Louis P. Pojman,
The University of Mississippi, and
Francis Beckwith,
University of Nevada Las Vegas, Editors
The Abortion Controversy: A Reader

Louis P. Pojman,
The University of Mississippi
*Life and Death: Grappling with the
Moral Dilemmas of Our Time*

Louis P. Pojman,
The University of Mississippi, Editor
Life and Death: A Reader in Moral Problems

Louis P. Pojman,
The University of Mississippi, Editor
*Environmental Ethics:
Readings in Theory and Application*

Holmes Rolston III,
Colorado State University, Editor
Biology, Ethics, and the Origins of Life

Melville Stewart, Bethel College
*Philosophy of Religion: An Anthology of
Contemporary Views*

Dabney Townsend,
The University of Texas at Arlington, Editor
*Aesthetics: Classic Readings from the
Western Tradition*

Robert M. Veatch,
Georgetown University, Editor
Cross-Cultural Perspectives in Medical Ethics

D.P. Verene, Emory University, Editor
*Sexual Love and Western Morality, A Philo-
sophical Anthology, Second Edition*

MEDICAL ETHICS

SECOND EDITION

Edited by

Robert M. Veatch

Kennedy Institute of Ethics
Georgetown University

Jones and Bartlett Publishers
Sudbury, Massachusetts

Boston • London • Singapore

Editorial, Sales, and Customer Service Offices

Jones and Bartlett Publishers
40 Tall Pine Drive
Sudbury, MA 01776
508-443-5000
800-832-0034
info@jbpub.com
http://www.jbpub.com

Jones and Bartlett Publishers International
Barb House, Barb Mews
London W6 7PA
UK

Library of Congress Cataloging-in-Publication Data

Medical ethics / edited by Robert M. Veatch. — 2nd ed.
    p.   cm.
  Includes bibliographical references and index.
  ISBN 0-86720-974-7 (alk. paper)
  1. Medical ethics.   I. Veatch, Robert M.
R724.M2927 1997
174'.2--dc20   96-24292
                                       CIP

Vice President/Editor: Joseph E. Burns
Production Editor: Marilyn E. Rash
Manufacturing Manager: Dana L. Cerrito
Typesetting: UltraGraphics
Cover Design: Hannus Design Associates
Printing and Binding: Edwards Brothers, Inc.
Cover Printing: Coral Graphic Services, Inc.

Printed in the United States of America
00 99 98 97 96   10 9 8 7 6 5 4 3 2

Contents

4   The Physician–Patient Relationship   75
Howard Brody

5   Limiting Procreation   103
Judith Areen

6   Human Experimentation   135
A. M. Capron

7   Informed Consent   185

Tom L. Beauchamp

8   Reproductive Technologies and Genetics   209

LeRoy Walters

9   Ethical Issues in Organ Transplantation   239

Albert R. Jonsen

Contributors

CHAPTER 1

Robert M. Veatch is Director and Professor of Medical Ethics at Georgetown University's Kennedy Institute of Ethics; Professor of Philosophy at Georgetown University; and Adjunct Professor, Departments of Community and Family Medicine, and Obstetrics and Gynecology at the Georgetown University School of Medicine.

CHAPTER 2

James F. Childress is Edwin B. Kyle Professor of Religious Studies and Professor of Medical Education at the University of Virginia, where he is also Chairman of the Department of Religious Studies.

CHAPTER 3

Arthur L. Caplan is the Director of the Center for Bioethics at the University of Pennsylvania Medical Center, and Trustee Professor of Bioethics.

CHAPTER 4

Howard Brody is Director, Center for Ethics and Humanities in the Life Sciences, Associate Professor of Family Practice and Philosophy, and Coordinator of the Medical Humanities Program at Michigan State University, East Lansing.

CHAPTER 5

Judith Areen is Dean, Georgetown University Law Center, and Professor of Community and Family Medicine, Georgetown University School of Medicine.

CHAPTER 6

Alexander M. Capron holds the Norman Topping Chair in Law, Medicine and Public Policy at the University of Southern California. He gratefully acknowledges the support of the USC Law Center faculty summer research fund and the assistance of Tamara Byram, class of 1989.

CHAPTER 7

Tom L. Beauchamp is Professor of Philosophy at Georgetown University, and Senior Research Scholar at Georgetown University's Kennedy Institute of Ethics.

CHAPTER 8

LeRoy Walters is Joseph P. Kennedy, Sr., Professor of Christian Ethics, and Senior Research Scholar at Georgetown University's Kennedy Institute of Ethics.

CHAPTER 9

Albert R. Jonsen is Professor of Ethics in Medicine and Chairman of the Department of Medical History and Ethics at the University of Washington School of Medicine.

CHAPTER 10

Loretta M. Kopelman is Professor of Humanities and Chair of the Department of Medical Humanities at the East Carolina University School of Medicine.

CHAPTER 11

Allen Buchanan is Grainger Professor of Business Ethics, School of Business, University of Wisconsin.

CHAPTER 12

Dan W. Brock is University Professor and Professor of Philosophy, Department of Philosophy, and Director of the Center for Bioethics, Brown University.

CHAPTER 13

Ronald Bayer is a Professor at the School of Public Health, Columbia University.

CHAPTER 14

Norman Daniels is Goldthwaite Professor of Rhetoric, and Professor of Medical Ethics, Department of Community Health, Tufts University School of Medicine.

Preface

In the eight years that have passed since the appearance of the first edition of *Medical Ethics*, our expectation of continued growth and richness of moral issues in medical decisions has come to pass. For a field that is growing so rapidly, a revision became necessary after what, for the timeless field of ethics, seems like a very brief interlude.

But, since 1989, important changes have occurred that affect every chapter in this book. With the collapse of the Soviet Union, the Marxist Oath for Soviet Physicians disappeared as quickly as it had appeared some 20 years earlier, and it has been replaced in Russia by a new oath for Russian physicians, an oath that has a radically different, more traditional, Hippocratic character.

Although in 1989 an approach relying on principles clearly dominated contemporary medical ethics, in the years since then, the entire "principlist" approach has been challenged by those committed to more case-oriented "casuistry," virtue ethics, care theory, and feminist bioethics. New limits on abortion have been debated and tested in the courts; a massive project to map every gene in the human genome is well underway; organ transplantation has become a much more routine practice, generating far from routine costs and moral controversies about how to procure adequate supplies of organs.

We have been fortunate to retain all 12 of the original chapter authors from the first edition—each a preeminent scholar on the subject of his or her chapter. But two developments have so dominated medical ethics of the past eight years that they simply had to have chapters of their own. Ronald Bayer, a leading author on social and ethical issues related to AIDS, has contributed a new chapter on ethics and HIV, and Norman Daniels, a former member of the ethics advisory group for President Clinton's Health Care Task Force, has adapted some of the work originally done for that effort to provide a more explicit moral analysis of the options for health-care reform in the United States. His chapter, combined with the chapter on health-care delivery and resource allocation by Allen Buchanan, is designed to provide the background necessary for an understanding of the moral issues of health-care reform as it is debated as we move into the twenty-first century. Whatever policy options command attention over the next years,

Daniels' systematic review of the issues will provide a framework for understanding the ethical dimension of the policy debate.

I want to thank the authors and their staffs for their extensive work on revising this volume. Joe Burns, the Executive Editor at Jones and Bartlett, has continued to be a loyal and enthusiastic supporter of this project and of bioethics publishing in general. His long-term commitment to this project is very much appreciated. I also want to thank Irene McDonald, the Executive Assistant to the Director of the Kennedy Institute of Ethics, for continuing support, and Kier Olsen, William Stempsey, S.J., M.D., and Laura Baker for their research and editorial assistance.

Preface to the First Edition

Ethical problems in medicine and the biological sciences have, in the past few years, exploded into the public consciousness at an exponential rate. Partly this is a result of new, increasingly complex technologies: ventilators, artificial kidney machines, new lifesaving medications, and transplant technologies. Partly it is a result of increasing access to existing medical services brought on by better insurance. Partly it comes from increased public awareness of medical decisions that have always been made in the privacy of the health professional's conscience.

Underlying all these developments is an increasingly complex set of ethical and other value choices that must be made by patients and their agents, by public officials, such as judges and legislators, as well as by health professionals. We now recognize that someone must decide whether to stop a ventilator on a patient who has suffered a stroke and will never again regain consciousness. A choice must be made whether it is morally appropriate to abort a pregnancy when a genetic test reveals a disease incompatible with life. A decision must be made about who will get a scarce piece of biomedical equipment like a bed in an intensive care unit when there are more persons in need than there are beds.

It was once thought that these were "medical" choices in the sense that they should be made by people with medical expertise, perhaps on the assumption that we should, as a society, do everything we can to prolong life as long as possible and that people with medical expertise were the ones best equipped to determine how life could be prolonged. The prolongation of the life of the permanently unconscious octogenarian and the controversy over the justification of abortion make clear, however, that not everyone believes it is automatically morally correct to prolong life in all circumstances.

Moreover, many continuing ethical problems in health care have nothing to do with prolonging life. They involve problems of privacy and confidentiality, consent, disclosure of critical illness or contagious disease, or problems in psychiatry. It is becoming increasingly clear that different ethical positions will lead to different conclusions about what is morally appropriate in these circumstances. Someone committed to an ethic emphasizing liberty may well come to a different conclusion than someone committed to maximizing patient welfare or someone committed to the priority of equality in allocating resources. There is no reason to assume that being skilled in medical science will make one an expert in choosing among these basic philosophical and ethical positions.

Medical ethics is now, as never before, for everyone: for patients, parents and other family members, public officials, and educators as well as for health professionals. Among health professionals it is for nurses, pharmacists, dentists, social workers, and chaplains as well as for physicians.

As these issues emerged in the 1970s, articles on specific issues began appearing with increasing frequency. Some adventuresome critics began writing whole volumes on the issues of medical ethics. Others, recognizing the enormity of the field, began collecting together essays by others or excerpts of such essays to publish as anthologies and readers.

In a way medical ethics has paralleled the development of medicine more generally. Now only the most ambitious, some would say immodest, author would attempt to write a textbook of medicine, surgery, or the other clinical sciences. The most authoritative volumes are now produced by large teams of authors, each a specialist in some aspect of medicine. Even books in the basic medical sciences are now routinely authored by large groups with each author writing on an area in which he or she has specialized.

The time has come when medical ethics must be approached in the same way if we are to have authoritative, critical examination of the issues in the various subspecialties of medical ethics. This volume, for the first time, brings together the leading authorities in medical ethics, giving each an opportunity to develop a text surveying the most critical issues in one of the major subareas of the field. For each chapter a leading scholar has been asked to develop a discussion of the critical concepts, arguments, and positions in an aspect of medical ethics and, without arguing for one position or another, to present the state of the art of his or her area. The combined result is a discussion at a level that is at once meant to be readable by the undergraduate or graduate student and to present the current state of the debate in medical ethics.

Each chapter begins with a summary and concludes with a set of questions for further exploration of the issues. A glossary of terms is included at the back of the book.

This has been a cooperative project, with many of the authors not only writing their own chapters but reading and commenting on other chapters. A number of reviewers and colleagues have read and provided helpful comments on single chapters of the entire volume. Several people deserve special mention for their help in the preparation of the manuscript. Joseph Burns, the editor at Jones and Bartlett, has been very supportive and patient throughout. Carol Mason and Karen Roberts have provided research and editing assistance, and Denise Brooks, Michelle Lewis, and Nancy Martin have helped in manuscript preparation. To them I and the other authors owe our gratitude.

Every reader, whether committed to a professional health career or being a responsible decision maker about his or her own health is encouraged to explore the importance of different ethical positions in deciding what counts as responsible medical choices.

1

Medical Ethics
An Introduction

ROBERT M. VEATCH

SUMMARY

Ethics is the enterprise of disciplined reflection on the moral intuitions and moral choices that people make. Medical ethics is the analysis of choices in medicine. As used in this volume, medicine refers to the entire range of choices made in the medical sphere. Medical ethics covers choices made not only by physicians, but also by other health profession-als—nurses, pharmacists, hospital chaplains, and so forth. More important, it covers choices made by medical lay people—patients, parents, legislators, public officials, and judges.

Chapter 1 provides an introduction to the more or less well-thought-out views about the ethics of medical choices, what could be called basic theories or systems in medical ethics. The chapter also surveys the history of medical ethical systems and the traditions of medical professionals that have gained prominence in the West. The most well-known of these is the Hippocratic Oath; the medical tradition based on the Hippo-cratic Oath has given rise to several professional ethical codes in modern times and they are discussed in the chapter. Also, the origin and development of Percival's eighteenth-century medical ethics, the ethical codes of the American Medical Association, and the codes of other health professionals are traced, and the chapter explores the influ-ences they have had on medicine and health care.

The second section of this chapter shifts emphasis away from professional codes and examines the development and impact of ethical positions developed in the Western reli-gious and political traditions outside of organized professional groups. These include the Jewish, Roman Catholic, and Protestant traditions and secular philosophical thought. Each of these schools of ethics has a distinct history and a special impact on health care. Ethical systems also exist beyond those of the Anglo-American West. The chapter explores the medical ethical positions prevalent in Eastern Europe, Islam, China, India, and Japan.

In studying medical ethical traditions it is important to examine the role codes of ethics should play in ethical decision making. The chapter considers the debate about whether ethical codes should be treated as rules, guidelines, covenants, or contracts, and the implications for each. Finally, the chapter explores the different bases for adopt-ing an articulation of an ethical code as one's own.

Ethical problems increasingly command the attention of medical decision makers, health professionals, and lay persons alike. They arise not only in the ethically obvious decisions—abortion, euthanasia, heart transplants, and research on human subjects—but also in everyday medical decisions—what physicians should tell patients about their diseases, what treatments patients should consent to (or refuse), and how much of society's funds should be spent on health care, and on which patients. In fact, it is the very nature of medical decisions that value choices must be made constantly. To decide to pursue a particular course is to decide that it is better or more right than alternatives available, and deciding something is better or more right means making evaluative judgments. Many of those evaluative judgments, many of those decisions about what is right or fitting, involve ethical choices. Thus, for people to make choices about their health is at its core an exercise in ethics. For patients interacting with health-care professionals to propose, accept, or reject a treatment plan is necessarily a value choice.

Many ethical and other value choices can be made instinctively, drawing on one's long-standing beliefs, commitments, and habits. Not every ethical or value choice in life requires conscious reflection. Medical choices are no different. In some cases, however, our intuitions fail. They do not give us a clear answer. In other cases they may deceive us, giving clear signals that may, nevertheless, be erroneous. We may be confronted by others who have equally clear intuitions that disagree with our own.

A person who has just experienced the long, painful death of a loved one may be convinced that merciful hastening of death is the only thing that makes sense. That person may be confronted by someone else who, believing that life is sacred, is equally certain that great wrong would come from policies permitting euthanasia. Consider Case 1.1 involving a patient with AIDS, a medical problem that is ethically controversial in part because it raises so many different problems about which intuitions differ.

CASE 1.1   The HIV-Positive Patient Who Is Dying

Twenty-seven-year-old Billy Harnack had been admitted to the intensive care unit (ICU) for the fourth time in the past 9 months. He had experienced severe difficulty breathing through the night. Dr. Karen Gladnow, the chief of the intensive care unit, was convinced even without the lab work that it was another episode of *Pneumocystis carinii* pneumonia, one of the most common AIDS-related infections. Each time the disease was more difficult to treat. Mr. Harnack also had Kaposi's sarcoma, a tumor of the blood vessel cells. Mr. Harnack's prognosis was very bleak. He was virtually certain to be dead in a matter of months. In fact, his quality of life had deteriorated to the point where Dr. Gladnow was convinced that were she the patient, she would refuse further treatment. She thought the time had come where death should no longer be opposed.

Her first problem was whether to write an order not to resuscitate the patient in case of a cardiopulmonary arrest. She believed that not resuscitating was realistically what was in the patient's interest, and her traditional Hippocratic duty would be to serve her patient by doing what she thought was in his interest. She was also sure, however, that Mr. Harnack did not seem ready to end his struggle against the disease. If the pneumonia was arrested, he could have several more months of life. Some of that time might be miserable, but parts of it might be good. He hoped to return to his work as a part-time clerk in a liquor store. Is Dr. Gladnow to do what she thinks is best or is she to respect his autonomous choice, even though she thinks it is wrong?

Since Mr. Harnack was too sick and too feeble to discuss the matter at this time, she could turn to his family for their opinion. There were several problems with doing that, however. First, she wasn't sure whether the family's opinion should count more than hers if it differed from the patient's views. Second, she was fairly sure the family really didn't know Mr. Harnack's diagnosis. They knew he had been sick for some time and had been told he had pneumonia and a type of cancer, but apparently they did not know he had AIDS. Could she really discuss the case with them without breaking the confidential relation she had with her patient?

Another dimension to the case that troubled Dr. Gladnow was that she had learned from Mr. Harnack during a previous admission that he had never really adjusted to his illness. He had become angry that he had been struck down, and had been almost irrational in striking out at others for the hand that fate had dealt him. She strongly suspected that he had remained sexually active, exposing his sexual partners to the HIV virus. In fact, he apparently believed that, since he had been treated so unkindly by fate, he would take as many others with him as he could. Dr. Gladnow realized that were she to successfully treat this episode, he would likely purposely expose others to a terrible illness. Could she purposely let her patient die as a way to protect others or should she remain true to her traditional ethical obligation to serve only the welfare of the patient, and exclude from moral consideration the welfare of others? Does the irresponsible behavior by her patient justify sacrificing his interests to protect others? If Dr. Gladnow should not let her patient's pneumonia go untreated because of this, should she at least report Mr. Harnack's behavior to authorities or would that also be a violation of confidentiality?

Even if Dr. Gladnow ought morally to have avoided sacrificing her patient's medical interests as a way to protect others in the society, she faced still another problem. The ICU was a very busy place. Beds were scarce. Treating Mr. Harnack aggressively in the ICU this time would only mean he would live to return again for further treatment. Other patients currently could be served by the unit. Although one patient was recovering from a heart attack and probably would do well if moved to the step-down unit, another was clearly terminal with muscular dystrophy and probably was not going to live through the night in any case. Other patients were competing for ICU beds. Dr. Gladnow had to make a choice about how Mr. Harnack compared with the other patients.

One moral approach in allocating scarce medical resources such as ICU beds is to ask how the beds can do the most good. That can include assessment not only of the medical benefits, but of the social benefits as well. Dr. Gladnow had real doubts about the benefits that would accrue from aggressive treatment of Mr. Harnack. He was not going to do well medically in the long run, but more than that, his temporary improvement was not going to do anyone much good. In fact, to be realistic about it, Dr. Gladnow thought his treatment would probably result in substantial net harm to others. Is that a relevant consideration in deciding whether he should be treated?

Another complicating dimension in Dr. Gladnow's decision about treatment in the ICU was that Dr. Gladnow believed that Mr. Harnack became exposed to AIDS through behaviors he voluntarily chose. He was both an active homosexual and an intravenous drug abuser. Dr. Gladnow believed that even if she should not generally take into account social factors in deciding which patients receive treatment, this patient had, in a certain way, brought on his own illness. Can it be, she asked herself, that medicine has to patch up the problems that people bring on themselves with the same priority as the patient with muscular dystrophy or some other genetic disease clearly unrelated to personal choice?

Here, in just one case, is a wide range of serious and controversial medical ethical issues: autonomy and paternalism; confidentiality; conflict between the individual patient's interests and those of society; the ethics of the allocation of resources; and the role voluntary behavior ought to play, if any, in allocating resources. In other settings, AIDS introduces questions of compulsory testing, reporting, and treatment.

Public health has traditionally been seen as a justification for overriding both the right to refuse treatment and the privacy of the confidential relation. AIDS, however, is a public health problem of a special sort. Its mode of transmission is different from many of the traditional infectious diseases. Public health ethics is being challenged by the AIDS epidemic. So is the ethics of medical research. Researchers are being asked to give special priority to a disease with which many of them would rather not become involved. Both researchers and clinicians are asking whether they have the right to refuse to participate in the care of AIDS patients because of the risks, no matter how small, the disease might pose to them.

In short, AIDS presents an amazing mix of extremely complicated ethical issues. Although no one of them is very new, the urgency with which they are presented and the combination of them in one complex disease phenomenon is new. What is needed is a discipline for teasing out the issues and reflecting on our moral intuitions about them.

Ethics is the enterprise of disciplined reflection on the moral intuitions and moral choices that people make, and often begins with our intuitions and long-held convictions. Ethics attempts to compare our choices for consistency, formulate rules of conduct accounting for our considered judgments, and articulate general principles that might underlie these judgments and rules. Ethics confronts questions such as how more general rules and principles relate to one another and to our judgments. Finally, it deals with basic questions of what we mean when we say something is ethical or unethical, and how we can know what is right and wrong.

As such, ethics is a branch of the disciplines that deal with basic questions of meaning and value: philosophy and theology. Some philosophers and theologians spend entire lifetimes dealing with these issues at a rather abstract or theoretical level. Increasingly, however, ethics is becoming a discipline that is applied to real problems of the real world, such as issues in medicine. Applied ethics takes various rules and principles and integrates them with detailed knowledge of the relevant facts and customs of a particular sphere of life, such as politics, race relations, or the work place. This book explores the application of ethics to the sphere of medicine.

Medicine is a more ambiguous term than many people realize. Sometimes medical ethics is assumed to be the ethics of decisions made by physicians. Medicine is taken to be the work of doctors. Many other health professionals are engaged in the medical enterprise, however. Nurses, pharmacists, dentists, hospital chaplains, and health-care administrators are all part of what is sometimes called the *health-care team*. They are an integral part of the decision-making process. Sometimes they face unique problems, such as what a nurse should do when she is given an "order" from a physician not to resuscitate a patient in the event of a cardiac arrest, when the nurse feels that failing to resuscitate is unethical. These decisions, faced by each member of the health-care team, are also part of the ethics of medicine.

More important, many of the choices made by lay people are also decisions in the medical sphere. The woman who decides to be sterilized, the parent who decides not to seek psychiatric counsel for a disturbed child, the legislator who votes for a "natural death act," or the judge who decides that a patient's consent was not adequately informed are all making decisions that naturally fall within the scope of medical ethics. Medicine, then, is a term that applies to all decisions having to do with health and disease. Most of those are made by lay people. Medical ethics, as used in this book, covers all such choices, not only those made by health care professionals and certainly not only those made by physicians. Some people prefer to use the term *health care* for the broader area of decisions having to do with health and disease, and reserve the term *medicine* for the behavior of physicians. We use *medicine* to refer to the sphere of life having to do with the well-being of the body. Just as education is a term not reserved for the work of teachers, so medicine as used in this volume will not be limited to the work of physicians.

Sometimes the term *bioethics* is used instead of medical ethics. The terms are now used almost interchangeably. Sometimes bioethics has a slightly broader meaning, including ethical problems of the biological sciences outside of medicine—research on animals, efforts to manipulate the genetic makeup of nonhuman species, and so forth. We shall not make a sharp distinction between the two terms. This book examines systematically the major ethical issues arising in medicine and, to some extent, those in the biological sciences.

THE HISTORY OF MEDICAL ETHICAL SYSTEMS

While individual health-care professionals and lay persons may have collections of more or less well-thought-out views about the ethics of medical choices, a number of major positions have gained enough prominence that they can be considered "systems" or "traditions" in medical ethics. The most well known, at least in the West, is the Hippocratic tradition.

Professional Codes in the West

The Hippocratic Tradition

The Hippocratic Oath is often acknowledged by both physicians and lay people to be the foundation of medical ethics for physicians in the West. Although the ethics of physician behavior is only one part of medical ethics, it has historically been the part receiving the greatest attention. Until very recently, medical choices were thought to be the province of trained professionals. Sometimes choices were thought to be too complex for uneducated, untrained lay persons. Sometimes they were thought to rest directly on esoteric, scientific knowledge that was only accessible to those socialized into the profession of medicine. Sometimes physicians were seen as a "profession" in the sense that in addition to having a body of specialized knowledge, they were committed to a special ethic that bound the members of the profession to special norms, duties, and virtues. For whatever reason, physicians have had a special ethical tradition and that tradition is best summarized in the Hippocratic Oath.

The Hippocratic Oath is of uncertain origin. It is traced to a group of physicians in ancient Greece. At the time there was no single school of medical orthodoxy. Different "schools" of physicians reflected different medical and philosophical beliefs. One of these schools had its center on the island of Cos. It emerged in the fifth century B.C. and produced a large body of scientific and ethical writings. Its acknowledged head was Hippocrates, but surely not all of the writings were, in fact, authored by him. These writings were later gathered together into various collections and referred to as the *Hippocratic corpus*. Since as early as the time of Galen (ca. 130–200 A.D.), there are well-documented disputes over the authorship of many of these writings (Edelstein 1967; Smith 1979; Carrick 1985). Although some of the writings describe human anatomy or deal with scientific problems, others are decidedly ethical in tone. These include *Precepts, Aphorisms, Law,* and *On Decorum.* Of these the *Hippocratic Oath* is the shortest and, by far, the most important historically. It is to the Hippocratic Oath that Western physicians in the Hippocratic tradition trace the foundations of their ethics.

The date of the Hippocratic Oath is not certain. There is good evidence that it dates from the late fourth century B.C. (Edelstein 1967, 55–61). This is based in part on linguistic considerations and in part on its content. The doctrines it contains are not consistent with much of Greek thought, but are characteristic of the Pythagorean school of that time.

The Hippocratic Oath is divided into two parts. The first, an oath of allegiance, pledges the Hippocratic physician to consider his teacher as equal to his parents and to regard his teacher's offspring as equal to his brothers. It is as if the student is being initiated into a Greek cult. He pledges to share the precepts or instruction only with those who have "signed the covenant," a notion strangely at odds with modern commitments to share medical knowledge, but understandable in the context of Greek society famous for its secretive cultic groups. The arrangement whereby the student honors his teacher as a father by adoption is distinctively a pattern of fourth-century Pythagoreans. The new initiate even pledges to help his teacher financially in time of need.

The covenant, which makes up the first part of the oath, is separated from the second part, often referred to as the code of ethics. The requirements of the code are also quite unusual for Greek ethics (or any other ethical system). Medicine is divided into three parts: dietetics, pharmacology, and surgery. The Hippocratic physician pledges in the section on dietetics to apply measures "for the benefit of the sick according to my ability and judgment."

This is probably the most important line in the Hippocratic Oath. It is the thought that many modern physicians carry with them as the essence of the Hippocratic ethic. They expand it beyond its original literal dietetic application to apply to all medical treatment, in fact, to all behavior affecting the patient.

In the section on pharmacology, the physician pledges not to give a deadly drug or to give a woman an abortive remedy, both distinctively Pythagorean ethical positions. That section also extols the virtues of "purity and holiness," both characteristically religious terms.

In the section on surgery, a strange prohibition is included. The Hippocratic physician will not use the knife (that is, perform surgery) "even on sufferers from stone [presumably bladder stones], but will withdraw in favor of such men as are engaged in this work." There is thus a division of labor with Hippocratic physicians eschewing surgery. It is not that they consider surgery itself immoral, but rather that it should be left for others. One explanation is that Pythagoreans viewed surgery as defiling their divine purity

(Edelstein 1967, 32). They could, thus, leave surgery for those who did not need to worry about ritual contamination.

The remaining sentences proscribe sexual relations with patients and enjoin confidentiality (by ambiguously prohibiting disclosure of "those things that ought not to be spread abroad"). The Hippocratic Oath closes by having the physician ask that if he keeps the oath he be granted enjoyment of life and fame for all time to come, but that if he breaks it, the opposite should be his lot.

The Hippocratic Oath is thus a mixture of apparently uncontroversial maxims (such as benefiting the patient and confidentiality) and injunctions that are hard for the modern to understand (such as the prohibition on surgery and a pledge not to disclose medical knowledge). In fact, even the apparently uncontroversial maxims have generated debate recently. Sometimes the maxim that the physician should benefit the patient according to his ability and judgment has been cited as an authorization for treating patients against their wishes or for deceiving patients by withholding a diagnosis of terminal illness.

Critics have accused the Hippocratic Oath of condoning paternalism. They have also questioned the confidentiality clause, pointing out that prohibiting disclosure of that which should not be spread abroad appears to condone disclosures of those things that should be spread abroad, thus opening the door for toleration of disclosures for either paternalistic or social reasons. In any case, at least since the time of Galen, the Hippocratic Oath has been elevated to premier status among physicians as the summary of their sense of ethical obligation. What was once a code of a minority medical group became the dominant ethical document for all professional medicine in the West.

The Hippocratic Oath Insofar as a Christian May Swear It

Some people have suggested that the reason the Hippocratic Oath emerged as dominant was that, after Constantine and the Christianization of Europe, other Greek ethical systems lost favor, but the Hippocratic ethic was elevated because of its similarities to Christian ethics. There are, in fact, points of similarity. A new version, called *The Oath According to Hippocrates insofar as a Christian May Swear It* (Jones 1924), emerged for Christian physicians. Some obvious changes were made such as the removal of references to the Greek gods and goddesses. There were also more subtle changes. The entire covenant including the pledge not to disclose medical knowledge and the ritualistic adoption of the teacher as father were dropped. The abortion prohibition was strengthened and the prohibition against surgery was dropped.

From the title of the Christian version it is clear that even in the Middle Ages there was a sense among Christians of tension between Hippocratic and Christian ethics. In fact, there is virtually no evidence that early Christian writers were aware of the Hippocratic Oath, much less endorsed it or adopted it as their own (Veatch and Mason 1987). It was not until about the tenth century, when many Greek writings including the Hippocratic writings were recovered from Arabic sources, that renewed interest in the Hippocratic ethic began.

Percival and Eighteenth-Century Medical Ethics

In modern times, the first major interest in medical ethics in the Anglo-Saxon world appeared in the eighteenth century. The most important example of a comprehensive medical ethics is John Gregory's (1724–1773) *Lectures on the Duties and Qualifications of a Physician*, which depends not so much on the Hippocratic tradition as on the broader philosophical thought then prevalent, such as that of Scottish moralists David Hume and Francis Hutcheson.

The most influential development of the time, however, was the byproduct of a local dispute at the Manchester Infirmary. In 1789, an epidemic taxed the infirmary staff and created a feud among the physicians, surgeons, and apothecaries. The trustees approached a distinguished physician, Thomas Percival, who had been on the staff before a physical disability forced him to resign. They asked him to draw up a "scheme of professional conduct" to prevent such disputes in the future. The result was Percival's *Medical Ethics*, which became the foundation of modern Anglo-American professional physician ethics. It has many features in common with the Hippocratic Oath but also some differences. It focuses much more on the institutional ethics of health care, dealing with physician's relations with hospitals and with other health professionals. It is a document that is much more socially aware than the Hippocratic Oath.

To the extent that Percival's work is in communication with ethics from outside the medical profession, it seems to represent the ethic of a British gentleman. The religious virtues of purity and holiness of the Hippocratic Oath are replaced with the virtues of the gentleman: physicians should "unite *tenderness* with *steadiness*, and *condescension* with *authority* (Percival 1927, 71)." In the introduction, Percival commends the study of professional ethics, saying it will "soften your manners, expand your affections, and form you to that propriety and dignity of conduct, which are essential to the character of a GENTLEMAN (Percival 1927, 63)."

The Ethical Codes of the American Medical Association

A half-century later, American medicine was involved in a dispute among several schools of medicine. The group that eventually became known as the orthodox practitioners formed the American Medical Association (AMA) in 1847. It is clear from the founding documents that "self-constituted doctors and doctresses" and other so-called quack practitioners were a great concern.

One of the documents growing out of the founding convention in Philadelphia was the *Code of Medical Ethics*. It followed the pattern of Percival's *Medical Ethics*. It contained three sections beginning with "Of the Duties of Physicians to Their Patients, and the Obligations of Patients to Their Physicians" and "Of the Duties of Physicians to Each Other, and to the Profession at Large." The influence of Percival is unmistakable. Whole paragraphs had been taken verbatim from Percival's work, including the explicit reference to tenderness, firmness, condescension, and authority.

Revisions occurred in 1903, 1912, and 1947, and in 1957 an entirely new format was adopted ("Principles of Medical Ethics"). In place of the lengthy document, ten succinct principles were adopted. These were supplemented by more lengthy opinions of the AMA's Judicial Council, the body responsible for interpreting the AMA's principles. The principles were general and sometimes platitudinous. They committed the AMA physician to "render service to humanity." The language condemning other practitioners as unscientific was toned down and, in contrast to the Hippocratic Oath, there was a clearly acknowledged responsibility to the society as well as to the individual. Nevertheless, there still remained an unmistakable paternalistic quality. In the opinion of the AMA, for instance, confidences could be broken when it became necessary to protect the welfare of the individual or the community.

In 1980 the most recent revision was adopted (American Medical Association, 1981). It probably represented the most substantive ethical change in the history of codes of ethics for physicians written by the profession. The result was a set of seven general principles, but with a tone quite different from anything previously written by a professional organization of physicians. AMA physicians are now expected to be dedicated to service with compassion and respect for human dignity. They are to respect the law and to deal honestly with patients, a radical change from the previously widely held view that physicians had the right (if not the duty) to deceive patients whenever they thought it was in the interest of the patient to do so. For instance, if the truth about a cancer diagnosis was likely to disturb the patient, physicians routinely withheld the truth or lied to patients and defended their actions by appeal to the Hippocratic maxim to act so as to benefit the patient.

For the first time in any codification written by physicians, the 1980 code contains an explicit commitment to the rights of patients. Although previous codes had given attention to the welfare of patients, patients' rights had never been acknowledged. In place of a confidentiality principle that permitted exceptions in the interest of the welfare of the patient or the community, the new provision committed the AMA physician to safeguard patient confidences within the constraints of the law. Although the law requires some disclosures for the protection of the community, it does not require or even permit disclosures to protect the individual patient. Thus, the paternalism has been dropped.

As in all of the editions of the AMA "Principles" since 1957, the 1980 version is supplemented with the current opinions of the AMA Judicial Council. The name of that group is now changed to the Council on Ethical and Judicial Affairs, to reflect the greater emphasis on ethics.

Sometimes the opinions still reveal more traditional thinking and its Hippocratic influences in spite of the changes in the more general principles from which the opinions are supposed to be derived. For example, with regard to confidentiality, at one point the opinion of the Council on Ethical and Judicial Affairs repeated the position in the *Principles*: "The physician should not reveal confidential communications or information without the express consent of the patient, unless required to do so by law" (American Medical Association 1994, 71). However, for the past several editions, the older, more paternalistic formulation is also revived in the text, with exceptions permitted for the welfare of the individual or community (American Medical Association 1994, 96). In June 1994, the main confidentiality opinion was modified to restore the paternalistic exception. The opinion now permits breaking of confidence if the patient threatens to inflict serious bodily harm to him- or herself or to another person (American Medical Association 1994, 71). At another point, after making a strong commitment to the notion of informed consent (a notion totally absent from the Hippocratic tradition), the Council states its opinion that consent need not be obtained "when risk-disclosure poses such a serious psychological threat of detriment to the patient as to be medically contraindicated" (American Medical Association 1994, 114). The older Hippocratic notion that information could be "medically contraindicated" if it would upset the patient takes precedence once again over the more liberal philosophical notion of respect for the individual autonomy of the patient. Thus, the AMA now has more modern, liberal antipaternalism stated in its official principles, but reverts to more traditional thinking in its Council opinions. The contradiction between the two has not been addressed.

Other Contemporary Physician Codes

To make matters more confusing, there are many other professionally written codes of ethics purporting to specify proper ethical conduct for physicians, and many other national medical associations have their own codes. Moreover, the World Medical Association, a federation of national medical associations, has adopted two codes of ethics, The Declaration of Geneva in 1948 and the International Code of Medical Ethics in 1949. The Declaration of Geneva is consciously patterned after the Hippocratic Oath. It is meant to be an updating. It retains a pledge to give teachers "respect and gratitude" (but no money). Reminiscent of the Hippocratic pledge that physicians will work for the benefit of the patient according to their ability and judgment, the Declaration of Geneva has the physician pledge "The health of my patient will be my first consideration." In contrast to the ambiguous provision in the Hippocratic Oath, it contains an apparently exceptionless confidentiality clause: "I will respect the secrets confided in me." It has the physician treat colleagues as brothers and "maintain . . . the honor and the noble traditions of the medical profession." (For discussion of the characteristics of these codes see Veatch [1995]. For the texts of a great number of these codes and further analysis see Spicer [1995]).

Other Codifications in Western Thought

There are thus many different formulations of the physician's duty written by professional groups in different times and places. They do not always agree with one another. The matter becomes even more complicated when one realizes that professional groups are not the only ones writing codes of ethics governing medical practice. Ethics has long been a matter of importance to religious groups, and most religious groups have codified positions on the ethics of medical decision making.

Religious Groups

Judaism   Jewish scholars have long recognized that Judaism has a set of laws that provides uniquely Jewish views on such matters as autopsy, circumcision, and abortion. Orthodox scholars of the Talmud hold that life is sacred and to be preserved until the time when the patient is *gesisah* or moribund (Bleich 1979, 33–35).

A Hebrew physician's oath is preserved from the seventh century. Referred to as the Oath of Asaf, it was administered by a teacher to his students (Etziony 1973, 24–26). It contains prohibitions on causing death, performing an abortion (for the adulterous wife), and revealing confidences. In contrast with the almost complete lack of concern about the needy in the Hippocratic tradition, there is also a specific injunction to show mercy to the poor and the needy, a provision one would expect in Jewish ethics, but not in Greek thought in the Hippocratic tradition. Also consistent with Jewish thought, there is a warning to avoid sorcery, magic, and witchcraft.

Another Jewish text is a prayer of Yehuda Halevi, an eleventh- to twelfth-century Judeo-Spanish philosopher and physician. Like the Oath of Asaf, the prayer emphasizes that it is God who heals, not the physician. The most well-known Jewish document is a prayer attributed to the twelfth-century Jewish physician, Moses Maimonides. It, in fact, probably dates from eighteenth-century Germany. This prayer condemns "thirst for profit" and "ambition for renown and admiration." These, together with more recent writing on Jewish medical ethics (Jakobovits 1959; Franck 1980; Rosner and Bleich 1979; Tendler 1975), provide a framework for medical ethics quite different from the professionally articulated codes.

Roman Catholicism   Roman Catholic scholars have, since the Middle Ages, written on medical ethical problems from the perspective of Christian theological ethics. Papal statements on abortion, contraception, and sexual ethics are well known. Of equal importance, however, are well-developed positions on many other medical issues including the care of the critically and terminally ill patient. The opposition to active killing of terminally ill patients on grounds of mercy is counterbalanced with a nuanced doctrine of the justifiability of withholding treatments that are considered "extraordinary" in the sense that they involve disproportionate burden (Pope Pius XII 1958; Congregation for The Doctrine of the Faith 1980).

Catholic thought also has developed what is referred to as the doctrine of double effect, whereby indirect evil effects of an action, provided they are not intended, can be tolerated under certain conditions. The doctrine is applied in medical ethics to justify the unavoidable killing of a fetus in a woman with a cancerous uterus by removal of the organ. It also justifies the unintended killing of a cancer patient with a narcotic given to relieve pain.

The document of greatest importance to medical ethics in the American context is the *Ethical and Religious Directives for Catholic Health Care Services* of the United States Catholic Conference (1995). It is a succinct compendium of the positions of Catholic thought on the full range of medical ethical issues.

Protestant Thought   Virtually every major Protestant denomination has endorsed official positions on the full range of medical ethical issues. The variety of their positions is great, but certain patterns can be recognized. Although many more conservative Protestant groups still have serious reservations, since 1930 there has been an opening of Protestant thinkers to the ideas of contraception, and eventually to sterilization and abortion. There has generally been an openness to decisions to refuse life-prolonging treatments, although only occasionally has that encompassed an acceptance of the ethics of active killing. In this matter, the Protestants have followed closely Catholic thinkers.

Perhaps the most important contribution of Protestant thinkers to medical ethics has not been on specific substantive issues, but more in their approach to knowing what is ethical in a medical context. Protestants are, by tradition, committed to giving the lay person an increased role in ethical and theological matters. Protestants believe that the text ought to be in the hands of the lay person. This has manifested itself in medical ethics with a heavy emphasis on the role of the lay person having access to medical information and in making medical decisions about his or her own care. The patients' rights movement has had great affinity with Protestant thought. In fact, many of the persons working in the current generation of medical ethics are trained in Protestant theology. Their antipaternalism can be accounted for, in part, by their Protestant heritage.

Secular Philosophical Thought

Although the patients' rights movement has considerable support from religious, especially Protestant, ethics, it also resonates well with many secular philosophical trends, especially those grounded in liberal political philosophy. In fact, the concept of rights, totally alien to the Hippocratic ethical tradition, has its roots in liberal political philosophy. Many secular ethical thinkers standing in this tradition have developed medical ethical positions that, taken together, can be thought of as a "school of medical ethics." They draw on the historical concepts and documents of the liberal tradition including Locke, Jefferson, and the Bill of Rights. That tradition, far more than the tradition of Hippocratic medicine, has been manifested in the legal decisions that have become such a prominent part of the American medical ethics scene since about 1960.

The first important expression of this is somewhat earlier, in the Nuremberg trials of the late 1940s. In those trials, in which those who conducted horrifying research on prisoners were condemned, a Nuremberg Code was produced. This code became the first major publicly produced code of ethics for a branch of medical practice. It has a legal and moral status quite different from earlier codes generated by the professional groups themselves. It abandons the older notion that subjects of research should be protected solely by the commitment of the professional to the subject and replaces it with a notion of self-determination for potential subjects that gives rise to a requirement for informed consent.

At the national level, a similar legal commitment to patient self-determination was emerging in case law. A doctrine of informed consent, rooted in a right to self-determination that is quite different from anything in the Hippocratic tradition, has emerged in the courts and jurisprudential scholarship.

Similar trends were manifest in two national governmental commissions. The first, the National Commission for the Protection of Human Subjects of Biomedical and Behavioral Research, was established in 1973. Stimulated by a recent exposure of research that had for decades withheld treatment from patients with syphilis, its mandate was to provide a public review of the ethical and legal problems of human subjects research. In the process it developed the first formal governmental analysis of the ethical principles that underlie medical ethical decisions from the point of view of a secular, nonprofessional body. That commission was the first secular body working in medical ethics that, by law, had a majority of members from outside the health professions (National Commission for the Protection of Human Subjects of Biomedical and Behavioral Research 1978).

The successor to this commission devoted to medical research was the President's Commission on the Study of Ethical Problems in Medicine and Biomedical and Behavioral Research. Its mandate was broader; it dealt with the full range of medical ethical issues including the care of the dying, genetics, issues of health-care decisions such as informed consent, and allocation of health resources. Its reports, produced in a number of volumes, have become definitive treatises on medical ethics in a secular, public context (President's Commission 1983).

Although the Commission represents the consensus mainstream thought of the American secular public on these topics, subcultural groups, religious or secular, also have special, more or less well-developed positions on important medical ethical issues. These positions are not limited to groups such as Jehovah's Witnesses and Christian Scientists, who have special views on blood transfusions or medical interventions. They also include groups with special ethnic, cultural, and ideological perspectives. There is not yet a full analysis of the medical ethics of black or Hispanic or feminist culture, but they exist, at least in the thinking of members of these groups. Some writings are being produced (Flack and Pellegrino 1992; Holmes and Purdy 1992; Sherwin 1992; Mahowald 1993; Dula and Goering 1994) that sometimes provide a radical contrast to more orthodox thinking, whether it be from health-care professionals or lay people. Patients coming from any of these groups, whether from the mainstream of liberal thought or minority groups, can provide a real challenge to the ethical thinking of health-care professionals who encounter them in hospital emergency rooms, clinics, and physicians' offices.

Medical Ethics in Other Cultures

The diversity of medical ethical positions is great even within Anglo-American Western culture. It is even greater if the net is cast more broadly. Patients or health-care workers coming from cultures outside the Anglo-American West may bring with them belief systems with medical ethical implications difficult for Westerners to comprehend. People concerned about problems in medical ethics are wise to examine these positions as well as those from more familiar traditions if they want to grasp the full range of possible positions on a medical ethical issue.

Eastern Europe

The former Soviet block in Eastern Europe had a medical ethic that differed in some respects from the traditions described thus far. The medical ethics of socialist societies of countries such as those of Eastern Europe, Cuba, and China can be expected to reflect their basic value commitments. The USSR had a medical ethic summarized in The Oath of Soviet Physicians. It was fundamentally different from the Hippocratic Oath and the codes of the Western professional associations in that it was passed by the Presidium of the Supreme Soviet, not by a professional organization. All graduating Soviet medical students took this oath. There was a stronger emphasis on preventive medicine than in the Western codes. There was also a much stronger commitment to the interests of society. The Soviet physician pledged "to work conscientiously wherever the interests of the society will require it"; "to conduct all my actions according to the principles of the Communistic [morality]"; and to always keep in mind the ". . . high responsibility I have to my people and to the Soviet government." At the same time, many of the traditional themes of Western professional oaths were included: a pledge to keep professional secrets, to improve knowledge, to consult colleagues, and never refuse to give advice or help.

Since the breakup of the Soviet block, the countries of Eastern Europe have adopted medical ethical codes that reflect more traditionally Western professional perspectives. Poland's new code condemned abortion, reflecting the reemergence of Catholic influences in that country (General Medical Council 1992; Baker 1992).

Russia replaced its Soviet code with a post-Soviet one clearly based on the Hippocratic Oath (Solemn Oath of a Physician of Russia). In a reaction against the social orientation of the Soviet Oath, the new code focuses exclusively on the individual patient. In so doing, it moves to a more individualistic position than that of the American Medical Association, which emphasizes that the physician has a duty to the society as well as the individual.

Islam

The people of the Islamic tradition also have a history of views on medical ethics. As might be anticipated, the ethics are based on Quranic teaching. The Oath of the Islamic Medical Association of the United States and Canada (Rahman, Amine, and Elkadi 1981) contains a strong prohibition on killing, similar to that seen in Jewish thought. Islamic physicians are committed to the virtues of strength, fortitude, wisdom, and understanding. They are to be honest, modest, merciful, and objective. There is a strong commitment to serving mankind "poor or rich, wise or illiterate, Muslim or non-Muslim, black or white."

Sometimes Muslims express an almost fatalistic reliance on the will of Allah. This has been expressed in reluctance to authorize nontreatment decisions for comatose patients and opposition to birth control, although Muslim scholars offer no formal opposition to the practice of contraception.

China

The cultures of the East also have long historical traditions of interest in medical ethics. In China, records exist of medical ethical writings as early as Sun Szu-miao's writings in the seventh century (Unschuld 1979, 24–33). These writings, in contrast to many key documents in Hippocratic medical ethics, closely depend on the major philosophical/ethical systems of the broader culture. Sun Szu-miao was identified with Taoism, but also reflected significant Buddhist influences. Confucian thought provides the background of many other early Chinese medical ethical texts.

Several themes that are alien to Western professional medical ethics repeatedly occur in these Chinese writings. The Confucian writings have long shown an acceptance of the limits of the human capacity to struggle against death. There is a constant concern for the care given to the poor. Injunctions to treat the poor and the rich without regard for financial status are repeated many times.

The three classic virtues are humaneness, compassion, and filial piety. The last is linked to a notion completely foreign to Hippocratic ethics. Loyalty to one's family has always been important in Chinese culture. Originally in Confucian society, someone in the family was responsible for medical knowledge. Loyalty to one's brother became the moral basis for rendering health care. As knowledge became more complex, professionalization emerged. When people could not get care from the designated family member, they had to be satisfied with a mere professional physician—one acting on a professional basis rather than out of a sense of familial loyalty. This is considerably different from the exalted status of the professional in Western medicine, in which it is considered unethical, or at least irresponsible, for a physician to treat a personal family member.

India

Indian medical ethics also depends closely on the ethical traditions of the broader culture. The most important texts in ancient Indian medical ethics are the *Caraka Samhita*, which is part of a Vedic religious writing on medicine, and the *Susruta Samhita*. The *Caraka Samhita*, written about the first century A.D., contains maxims appropriate for the elite of Indian culture—the physician should lead the life of a celibate, grow his hair and beard, speak only the truth, eat no meat, eat only pure particles of food, be free from envy, and carry no arms. The physician should endeavor to relieve patients and should not desert or injure them and should not cause another's death. The physician is committed to being helpful to the patient, which leads, as in Hippocratic ethics, to benevolent decisions not to tell patients of their terminal illnesses. "Even knowing that the patient's span of life has come to its close, it shall not be mentioned by thee there, where if so done, it would cause shock to the patient or to others."

The most provocative paragraph is one that can only be understood in the context of the Indian doctrine of karma, the doctrine that links one's present status in life with the way one has led previous incarnations. One of the earliest codes to address the problem of allocating health resources, the *Caraka Samhita* says, "No persons, who are hated by the king or who are haters of the king or who are hated by the public or who are haters of the public, shall receive treatment. Similarly, those who are extremely abnormal, wicked, and of miserable character and conduct, those who have not vindicated their honor, those who are on the point of death, and similarly women who are unattended by their husbands or guardians shall not receive treatment." That text contrasts with the strong commitment to the needy in Judeo-Christian and Chinese medical ethics and the silence on these matters in the Hippocratic tradition.

Japan

Like the other Eastern cultures, Japan's medical ethics has also been influenced by broader cultural traditions, in this case indigenous Shinto thought and Buddhist and Confucian thought from China. In the modern culture, in Japan as in the other cultures mentioned, many Western themes from the Hippocratic and liberal traditions have had their influence. One example of a traditional Japanese code of medical ethics comes from the Ri-shu school of medical practice dating from about the sixteenth century. The code, the Seventeen Rules of Enjuin, has many similarities with the Hippocratic Oath including a strong commitment to serving the patient and to secrecy. The physician is to protect against disclosing any secrets he learns during his medical education. He is even given instructions to make sure that his books are returned to the school on the physician's death.

Other Cultures

Other cultures also have their own medical ethical systems. Most national medical groups have codes of ethics that reflect the unique character of the culture as well as the physicians in that culture. Much remains to be learned about some cultures. The medical ethics of African cultures, for example, are virtually unknown in the West. In studying medical ethics, it is important to keep in mind that the number of medical ethical codes (and the systems they reflect) is great and that cultural traditions vary tremendously in the ethical practices they expect of health professionals and lay people.

THE ROLE OF CODES

The existence of this wide variety of codes of ethics in medicine raises some interesting questions about the way codes ought to be used. Presumably, the codes represent the collective wisdom of the group that authored and endorsed them. As such, they at times may sound platitudinous. Nevertheless, they manage to express some very controversial notions that are at least controversial if not offensive to those outside the group endorsing the code.

Rules versus Guidelines

Even among those who endorse codes, there is some question about the role they ought to play. Some people attempt to interpret them as a set of rules spelling out exactly what conduct is appropriate for medical decision makers.

In extreme cases, they are viewed essentially as law, in which violation is cause for legal or quasilegal action. Some disciplinary proceedings of medical professional organizations come complete with legal counsel, due process, and juries. Sometimes codes are introduced into public judicial proceedings as if they were legally binding on members of professional groups.

On the other hand, some people view codes as mere guidelines, general principles of appropriate conduct that should guide the individual as he or she makes moral choices. That seems to be the view in the minds of the drafters of the 1980 revision of the AMA's Principles of Medical Ethics. The Preface says the principles "are not laws, but standards of conduct which define the essentials of honorable behavior for the physician." They are "intended as guides to responsible professional behavior, but they are not presented as the sole or only route to medical morality." At the same time, failure to conform can result in disciplinary proceedings within the association. This ambivalence probably reflects a gradual historical evolution in the concept of a code of ethics from one in which the professional group is authoritative to one in which differing religious and philosophical world views contribute perspectives from which ethical conduct may be judged.

Although professional codes are viewed, even by their authors, as guidelines from which the individual clinician must make responsible moral decisions, there is another view of a code that is much more stringent. As we have seen, some codes of medical ethics have a status far different from expressions of professional consensus. The Nuremberg Code, for example, has the status of international law. The positions of the President's Commission on the Study of Ethical Problems in Medicine and Biomedical and Behavioral Research are not legally binding, but they are increasingly taken to represent the collective wisdom of the American population. In both cases, it is hard to discount the positions expressed as "mere opinion" without legitimate authority. The status of the Nuremberg Code is least ambiguous. Anyone violating this code is presumably guilty not only of unethical conduct but of violation of international law. But someone who went against the wisdom of the President's Commission would not necessarily be violating the law, but would have a moral burden of proof. In legal cases in which the "reasonable person" standard is used, such as in informed-consent cases, the views of the Commission could be (and have been) introduced as evidence of national policy.

A similar tension between codes as guidelines and as rigid rules occurs within various religious traditions. Some traditions, for example, Protestantism, tend to view church pronouncements as matters for guidance of members and anyone else in the general public who cares to listen. In other cases, pronouncements have a more binding quality, at least to the extent that violation can lead to expulsion from membership in the group.

Thus, codes sometimes have legal standing and function to determine what the law requires, but in other cases, they are moral documents articulating the moral positions of members of various groups. Among those codes that are viewed as moral codes, some groups expect their members to treat the codes as guides for individual moral judgment; others assume that members will follow them as moral rules of conduct.

Codes, Covenants, and Contracts

The dispute over whether ethical codes are rules of conduct or are guidelines is not the only disagreement. Not all medical ethics writings are, by any means, in the form of codes. Some are essays, written by individuals attempting to defend a particular moral point of view or offer an analysis of several points of view. Others are what could be termed "covenants" or "contracts."

William May, currently a professor at Southern Methodist University, has written a provocative analysis entitled "Code, Covenant, Contract, or Philanthropy?" In it, May examines the general form of the code as an ethical document. A code, he suggests, is a compilation of patterns of behavior for particular groups of people, particularly relevant to "inner circles within certain societies," among friends or professionals within a guild. They tend to make conduct matters of aesthetics. Morality becomes a matter of conforming elegantly to an ideal of character envisioned in the code. More important, to May a code does not encourage or necessitate personal involvement with other persons; a code is created unilaterally. May cites the Hemingway hero—the bull fighter or the soldier—as an example. They live by a code that eschews involvement. The ideal is created entirely by the group itself without participation by others.

May contrasts the *code* as a mode of articulating an ethic with a *covenant*. A covenant has its roots in specific historical events. "It always has reference to specific historical exchange between partners leading to a promissory event" (May 1975). The pledge that the young physician makes to his teacher in the Hippocratic Oath is a covenant. The obligations he takes on vis-à-vis patients constitute a code. Patients play no role in the articulation of the moral duties of either party. According to May, the same thing has happened in the creation of other professional codes—those of Percival, the AMA, and the World Medical Association. The AMA meeting in 1847 articulated the obligations of patients to physicians as well as of physicians to patients, but patients played no part in the specification of these obligations. The covenant, whether in its prototypical religious form or in the form establishing mutual promises among professionals and lay people, involves a mutuality, a promise that shapes both partners and binds them in the future. The code, on the other hand, has philanthropy as its ideal. The commitment is unilateral; the commitment is bestowed gratuitously on the other party rather than being responsive and reciprocal.

May and others have further questioned the relationship between a covenant model and one referred to as a *contract*. Both involve mutual participation of the parties. But May defines *contract* quite specifically to involve agreements in which "two parties calculate their own best interests and agree upon some joint project in which both derive roughly equivalent benefits for goods contributed by each." He seems to have in mind the contemporary idea of a legal or business contract, with the overtones of legalism, self-interest, and individual "deal-making."

Although that meaning is one use of the term contract, there are others that do not have these overtones. In particular, modern liberal thought is based on what philosophers refer to as a *social contract*. In some cases, the concept of the social contract is a highly qualified, metaphorical image in which members of the society agree on what the basic principles of the society should be. Sometimes they are even seen as agreeing on what a set of preexisting principles are. In this broader usage, contract is a general term implying mutuality and promising, but is not necessarily limited to arrangements between individuals, and has no legal implications. The term *marriage contract* is only one example of this broader usage in which the parties may not have in mind exclusive self-interest and legal obligations. Some people use the term contract to include what May calls covenants as well as other types of mutual promises. May, in response, considers the term contract too infiltrated with negative connotation and prefers to stay with the term covenant. Regardless of the term used, the idea that ethical obligations between professionals and lay people may be based on mutual promises provides an alternative to the ethics of codes.

Codes raise a particularly interesting problem when the other party does not acknowledge or even desire the commitment made by the philanthropic gesture. For example, physicians pledge to act to benefit their patients according to their ability and judgment. This has given rise to well-meaning disclosures of confidential information to third parties even in cases in which the patient might not want it disclosed. It has given rise to medical treatments believed by the physician to be for the benefit of the patient even in cases where patients may not want the treatments. Most recently, physicians have suggested paternalistic, unilateral withdrawal of life support of patients who are suffering, sometimes in cases in which the patient is not yet ready to die. There is the possibility with a unilaterally generated code that a group of persons may promise to engage in what they think are benevolent actions toward outsiders when, in reality, some of those outsiders do not want the purported benefits. May and others prefer that the mode of mutual participation be the basis for articulating sets of duties in professional relationships such as between health professionals and patients. This would have the impact of viewing the patient as well as the professional as an active participant with the potential for obligations as well as claims against the other party (Veatch 1991).

The AMA is apparently aware of the tension between unilaterally articulated codes and mutually agreed upon sets of moral obligations. In the report of the committee of the AMA that revised the Principles of Medical Ethics, it states that "The profession does not exist for itself; it exists for a purpose, and increasingly that purpose will be defined by society." Nevertheless, the 1980 revision was a project written by and approved by only members of the AMA.

CHOOSING AMONG PROFESSIONAL AND OTHER CODIFICATIONS

Once one recognizes that there are many different codifications of the duties of health professionals and lay people for decisions in a medical context, the question of choosing among them becomes critical. We must ask why persons would feel obligated to follow one particular codification or another.

One basis for adopting an articulation of an ethical code as one's own is that one has voluntarily become a member of a group and, in doing so, has subscribed to its moral formulation. Thus, the Hippocratic medical student on the Isle of Cos could be viewed as having voluntarily committed himself to the obligations to teachers, colleagues, and patients called for by the Hippocratic guild.

This is a peculiarly modern notion of the origin of moral obligation, however. It rests on the idea that moral duties arise only when people voluntarily commit themselves to them. That may work for the twentieth-century physician who seeks to join the AMA, but it hardly applies to the ancient physician. It probably does not work very well in other cultures, even in the modern period. For example, were Soviet physicians thought to be bound to the Soviet Oath because they voluntarily decided to join the guild of Soviet physicians? Are Jewish physicians committed to Talmudic morality simply because they have voluntarily chosen to be Jews?

This concept presents larger problems for physicians and other health professionals who are not members of their professional organization. Approximately half the physicians licensed to practice medicine in the United States are not members of the AMA. Does that mean they are exempt from the professional duties articulated by the AMA? If so, are they bound by some other ethic? Which one?

An even more complicated problem arises for persons who voluntarily join (or accept themselves as members of) two groups, each of which has a set of medical ethical standards that it considers authoritative. This situation might arise if a physician specializing in a branch of medicine such as obstetrics or neurology is simultaneously a member of both the specialty association and the state or national medical organization. It could arise if a physician considers himself or herself bound by both a national association and the World Medical Association codes when the two conflict. Most commonly, it can arise when a person is simultaneously a member of a medical professional organization and some other group purporting to speak on matters of medical ethics. A Jewish physician, for example, may feel simultaneously bound by the Talmudic obligation to preserve life and by the AMA's commitment to accept treatment refusal decisions from competent patients, even though the result will be a quicker death.

The Jewish physician is forced to decide which group he or she considers to be authoritative morally (or how he or she will combine the moral insights of each with his or her moral judgments). Eventually the physician must face the question of the nature of the claims of each of these groups to be morally authoritative. Religious groups have traditionally claimed to be legitimate sources of moral insight for their members. They may claim to have knowledge of revelation or be capable of using reason to discern moral laws. Some groups have established patterns of moral authority—persons identified as authoritative teachers, such as priests or rabbis. Others may give substantial latitude for individual members to discern moral requirements based on their individual interpretation of Scripture and doctrine, as is the case in Protestant thought and in secular liberal philosophy.

Those who approach ethics secularly also must make decisions about how moral knowledge is acquired. Some might yield to the state authority to establish ethical requirements. Others may turn to reason and intuition or the authority of individuals or groups. The question critical for those who make use of professionally articulated codes is to what extent the professional groups are legitimately recognized as authoritative in identifying moral obligations for members of their profession.

Professional groups have long written codes of ethics and assumed they were binding on their members, but the exact nature of their claim to authority has never been fully analyzed. Some groups have claimed that the group is authoritative because the group literally creates the ethic. One official of a major professional organization once referred to his organization's code of ethics as one that the members have "imposed upon themselves." This would easily explain why members ought to feel bound, but it gives the agreement no weight for nonmembers, professional or lay. It also seems to fly in the face of what most people believe to be the nature of ethics. Ethical obligations are not merely self-imposed duties. Rather, they are perceived as coming from outside the individual.

In other cases, somewhat more sophisticated professional organizations claim that they do not literally create the obligations, they only articulate them. They argue that being socialized into the profession and understanding the complex and esoteric nature of the professional role is the only way one possibly can understand the moral duties that the member of the profession must bear. The professional group, it is claimed, is responsible for articulating the professional duty, which is not something the group invents.

That is a view of ethics that has been held by certain groups in certain periods of history, that only people with special skills or knowledge or training can know ethical truths. In fact, that seems to be the position of the Hippocratic group of ancient Greece. It is a controversial position in modern society, however, one that many people have rejected in favor of a position acknowledging that all may have moral insight. This position is usually based on the belief that morality is universal in the sense that some common set of principles, some common system of ethics, applies universally and can be known without special esoteric skills.

These ideas in no way imply that all persons have exactly the same duties. Surely, parents or police or physicians have duties that are unique to their roles. But holders of the latter view maintain that, in principle, anyone can recognize and understand the special duties of the parent or policeman or physician. In addition, anyone, according to this view, can understand the duties of the lay person. It is this framework that appears to underlie the position of those who are striving to make medical ethics a matter of mutuality in which professionals and lay persons have a shared understanding of their rights and duties.

DISCUSSION QUESTIONS

1. How has the Hippocratic system of medical ethics changed over the years? Is it possible for an ethical code or oath produced for a particular group of physicians in the culture of ancient Greece to be meaningful today for physicians in a different culture?

2. What are the key differences between the ethics of the Hippocratic tradition and the ethics of the nursing profession? Ought nursing to be governed by the ethics articulated by physicians? If not, how ought ethical conflicts between physicians and nurses be resolved?

3. Is it reasonable for patients, legislators, judges, and other medical lay people to assume that the ethics for professional–lay relationships should be governed by professionally articulated ethical positions?

4. If a physician is a member of a professional group and also of a religious group that in some way differs from the professional group on some key ethical issue, by which ethical tradition ought the physician be guided?

5. Should physicians who come from non-Western ethical traditions be guided by their own ethical traditions or by that of Western medicine? What should a physician do who encounters a patient standing in an ethical tradition that is in conflict with the ethics of the physician? Should people from other parts of the world or from different ethical traditions in the West be exempt from the ethics of Western medicine?

REFERENCES

American Medical Association. *Code of Medical Ethics: Adopted by the American Medical Association at Philadelphia, May, 1847, and by the New York Academy of Medicine in October, 1847.* New York: H. Ludwig and Company, 1848.

American Medical Association, Council on Ethical and Judicial Affairs. *Code of Medical Ethics: Current Opinions with Annotations.* Chicago: American Medical Association, 1994.

American Medical Association. *Current Opinions of the Judicial Council of the American Medical Association.* Chicago: American Medical Association, 1981.

Baker, Robert. "Medical Ethics in a Time of De-Communization." *Kennedy Inst Ethics J* 2(4) (1992): 363–370.

Bleich, J. David. "The Obligation to Heal in the Judaic Tradition: A Comparative Analysis." In Fred Rosner and J. David Bleich, Eds., *Jewish Bioethics.* New York: Sanhedrin Press, 1979: 1–44.

British Medical Association. *The Handbook of Medical Ethics.* Luton and London: The Leagrave Press, Ltd., 1984.

Carrick, Paul. *Medical Ethics in Antiquity: Philosophical Perspectives on Abortion and Euthanasia.* Dordrecht, Holland: D. Reidel Publishing Company, 1985.

Congregation for The Doctrine of The Faith. *Declaration On Euthanasia.* Rome: The Sacred Congregation for the Doctrine of the Faith, May 5, 1980.

Dula, Annette, Goering, Sara, Eds. *It Just Ain't Fair: The Ethics of Healthcare for African Americans.* Westport, CN: Greenwood Publishing, 1994.

Edelstein, Ludwig. "The Hippocratic Oath: Text, Translation and Interpretation." In Owsei Temkin and C. Lilian Temkin, Eds., *Ancient Medicine: Selected Papers of Ludwig Edelstein.* Baltimore: The Johns Hopkins University Press, 1967: 3–64.

Etziony, M. B. *The Physician's Creed: An Anthology of Medical Prayers, Oaths and Codes of Ethics Written and Recited by Medical Practitioners Through the Ages.* Springfield, IL: Charles C Thomas, 1973.

Flack, Harley E., Pellegrino, Edmund D., Eds. *African American Perspectives on Biomedical Ethics.* Washington, DC: Georgetown University Press, 1992.

Franck, Isaac, Ed. *Biomedical Ethics In Perspective of Jewish Teaching and Tradition: Proceedings of an Academic Conference.* Washington, DC: College of Jewish Studies of Greater Washington, DC, 1980.

General Medical Council, [Polish] National Congress of Physicians. "The Code of Medical Ethics." *Kennedy Inst Ethics J* 2(4) (1992): 371–384.

Gregory, John. *Lectures on the Duties and Qualifications of a Physician.* Philadelphia: M. Carey & Son, 1817.

Holmes, Helen Bequaert, Purdy, Laura M., Eds. *Feminist Perspectives in Medical Ethics.* Bloomington: Indiana University Press, 1992.

Jakobovits, Immanuel. *Jewish Medical Ethics.* New York: Bloch Publishing Co., 1959.

Jones, W. H. S. *The Doctor's Oath: An Essay in The History of Medicine.* Cambridge: Cambridge University Press, 1924.

Judicial Council, American Medical Association. *Current Opinions of the Judicial Council of the American Medical Association—1984: Including the Principles of Medical Ethics and Rules of the Judicial Council.* Chicago: American Medical Association, 1984.

Mahowald, Mary Briody. *Women and Children in Health Care: An Unequal Majority.* New York: Oxford University Press, 1993.

May, William F. "Code, Covenant, Contract, or Philanthropy?" *Hastings Cent Rep* 5 (December 1975): 29–38.

National Commission for the Protection of Human Subjects of Biomedical and Behavioral Research. *The Belmont Report: Ethical Principles and Guidelines for the Protection of Human Subjects of Research.* Washington, DC: Government Printing Office, 1978.

"Oath of Initiation (Caraka Samhita)." In Warren T. Reich, Ed., *Encyclopedia of Bioethics*, Vol. 4. New York: The Free Press, 1978: 1732–1733.

"The Oath of Soviet Physicians" (Zenonas Danilevicius, trans.). *JAMA* 217 (1971): 834.

Percival, Thomas. *Percival's Medical Ethics, 1803.* (Reprint, Chauncey D. Leake, Ed.) Baltimore: Williams & Wilkins, 1927.

Pope Pius XII. "The Prolongation of Life: An Address of Pope Pius XII to an International Congress of Anesthesiologists." *The Pope Speaks* 4 (1958): 393–398.

President's Commission for the Study of Ethical Problems in Medicine and Biomedical and Behavioral Research. *Summing Up: Final Report on Studies of the Ethical and Legal Problems in Medicine and Biomedical and Behavioral Research.* Washington, DC: Government Printing Office, 1983.

"Principles of Medical Ethics of the American Medical Association." *JAMA* 164 (1957): 11119–11120.

Rahman, Abdul, Amine, C., Elkadi, Ahmed. "Islamic Code of Medical Professional Ethics." Papers presented to the First International Conference on Islamic Medicine Celebrating the Advent of the Fifteenth Century Hijri. Kuwait Ministry of Health: Kuwait, 1981.

Rosner, Fred, Bleich, J. David, Eds. *Jewish Bioethics.* New York: Sanhedrin Press, 1979.

Sherwin, Susan. *No Longer Patient: Feminist Ethics and Health Care.* Philadelphia: Temple University Press, 1992.

Smith, Wesley D. *The Hippocratic Tradition.* Ithaca: Cornell University Press, 1979.

"Solemn Oath of a Physician of Russia." *Kennedy Inst Ethics J* 3(4) (1993): 419.

Spicer, Carol Mason, Ed. "Codes, Oaths, and Directives Related to Bioethics." In Warren T. Reich, Ed., Appendix to *Encyclopedia of Bioethics*, revised ed. New York: The Free Press (1995): vol. 5, 2601–2842.

Tendler, M. D., Ed. *Medical Ethics: A Compendium of Jewish Moral, Ethical and Religious Principles in Medical Practice*, 5th ed. New York: Committee of Religious Affairs, Federation of Jewish Philanthropies of New York, Inc., 1975.

United States Catholic Conference, Department of Health Affairs. *Ethical and Religious Directives for Catholic Health Care Services.* Washington, DC: United States Catholic Conference, 1995.

Unschuld, Paul U. *Medical Ethics in Imperial China: A Study in Historical Anthropology,* Berkeley: University of California Press, 1979.

Veatch, Robert M. "Codes of Medical Ethics: Ethical Analysis." In Warren T. Reich, Ed., *Encyclopedia of Bioethics,* revised ed. New York: The Free Press (1995): vol. 3, 1419–1434.

Veatch, Robert M., Mason, Carol G. "Hippocratic vs. Judeo-Christian Medical Ethics: Principles in Conflict." *J Relig Ethics* 15 (1987): 86–105.

Veatch, Robert M. *The Patient-Physician Relation: The Patient as Partner, Part 2.* Bloomington: Indiana University Press, 1991.

World Medical Association. "Declaration of Geneva." *World Med J* 3 (suppl.) (1956): 12.

World Medical Association. "International Code of Medical Ethics." *World Med J* 3 (suppl.) (1956): 12.

2

The Normative Principles of Medical Ethics

JAMES F. CHILDRESS

SUMMARY

Moral dilemmas are often generated by conflicts among moral principles. As general action guides, moral principles describe the characteristics of actions that make them morally right or wrong: for example, beneficence (doing good), nonmaleficence (avoiding evil), respect for autonomy, and justice. This chapter analyzes the debate about normative principles in biomedical ethics, indicating the major issues and lines of argument. The first section of the chapter addresses the issues of moral justification, moral theories, and dilemmas that derive from conflicts among moral principles. It is possible to assess an action by considering several different aspects: the agent, the act itself, the end, and the consequences. Ethical theories differ in part according to which aspect is primary in evaluation.

The chapter concentrates on the role of ethical principles in these evaluations. Even proponents of the same principles and rules often disagree widely about what those principles and rules imply for particular cases, largely because of disputes about their meaning and their weight. The chapter also explores several different views about the interpretation of the meaning and weights of moral principles and rules and how they are connected to particular moral judgments.

The final section surveys and assesses major recent criticisms of appeals to ethical principles and rules in biomedical ethics. Throughout this chapter, the author suggests that the difficult question is not whether to invoke or apply principles and rules but rather which principles and rules should be adopted, how they should be interpreted, how much weight and strength they should be accorded, which have priority in a conflict, and in what relations and situations they apply.

MORAL JUSTIFICATION AND MORAL THEORIES

Many debates in biomedical ethics reflect disputes about normative principles—which principles, if any, are applicable, how much weight they have, especially if they conflict, and what they imply for particular cases. This chapter analyzes the debate about normative principles in biomedical ethics, indicating the major issues and lines of argument. When referring to principles-based approaches to biomedical ethics, I will sometimes use the label "principlism" even though the term was coined by opponents of one particular principles-based approach (Clouser and Gert 1990).

Case 2.1 raises some major issues in moral justification and ethical reflection.

CASE 2.1

> For the last 3 years a 5-year-old girl has suffered from progressive renal failure as a result of glomerulonephritis. She was not doing well on chronic renal dialysis and the staff proposed transplantation after determining that there was "a clear possibility" that a transplanted kidney would not undergo the same disease process. The parents accepted this proposal. It was clear from tissue typing that the patient would be difficult to match. Her two siblings, ages 2 and 4, were too young to be organ donors, and her mother was not histocompatible, but her father was quite compatible. When the nephrologist met with the father and informed him of the test results, as well as the uncertain prognosis for his daughter even with a kidney transplant, the father decided not to donate one of his kidneys to his daughter. He gave several reasons for his decision: In addition to the uncertain prognosis for his daughter, there was a possibility of a cadaver kidney, his daughter had already undergone a great deal of suffering, and he lacked the courage to make this donation.
>
> However, the father was afraid that if the family knew the truth they would blame him for allowing his daughter to die and then the family itself would be wrecked. Therefore, he asked the physician to tell the members of the family that he was not histocompatible, when in fact he was. The physician did not feel comfortable about carrying out this request, but he finally agreed to tell the man's wife that the father could not donate a kidney "for medical reasons" (Levine et al. 1977, 205).

The physician felt uncomfortable in carrying out the father's request because of what he experienced as a moral conflict, quandary, or dilemma. Moral dilemmas are often generated by conflicts between moral principles. As a character in Tom Stoppard's play *Professional Foul* (1978, 99) notes, "there would be no moral dilemmas if moral principles worked in straight lines and never crossed each other." However, in science, medicine, and health care, as well as elsewhere, agents experience such conflicts. Resolving these conflicts often requires further examination of the relevant principles and their meaning and their weight to see what ought to be done in the situation. In this case, the physician had to attend to such moral considerations as truthfulness, acting in the daughter's interest, confidentiality, protecting the father, and preserving the family.

Some of these moral considerations may be viewed as principles, others as rules. Both principles and rules are "general action guides specifying that some type of action is prohibited, required, or permitted in certain circumstances" (Solomon 1978, 408). Even though the term "principles" often encompasses rules, it is useful to distinguish principles from rules for this discussion. Principles are more general and frequently serve as sources or foundations of rules, which specify more concretely the type of prohibited, required, or permitted action. With this distinction, it is possible to think about the process of moral justification in an appellate fashion, with the justification of particular moral judgments often (but not always) involving more general moral appeals. This process can be sketched in terms of tiers or levels of moral justification (Beauchamp and Childress 1994, Chapters 1 and 2):

1. Principles
2. Rules
3. Particular Judgments

Apparently, the physician in Case 2.1 believed that it was wrong to lie and thus refrained from saying directly that the father was not histocompatible. If asked why he thought it was wrong to lie to the mother, he might have appealed to a moral rule that prohibits lying, and he might have justified this moral rule by appealing to various principles such as respect for persons and utility (maximizing welfare)—for example, a rule against lying is important to maintain trust between professionals and patients.

If the moral rule against lying had been the only moral consideration in this case, the physician would not have experienced a dilemma. However, there were other relevant moral considerations, including protecting confidentiality (the physician had gained information about the father in the course of an examination and the rule of confidentiality limits the disclosure of such information to other parties without the examinee's consent) and not wrecking the family (which reflects the principle of utility). The physician found what he deemed a satisfactory moral compromise: He did not directly lie because "medical reasons" may include psychological reasons, but he also did not disclose the full truth as a way to protect the confidentiality of the information he had gained and to avoid wrecking the family.

The physician's action could be assessed from several standpoints.

Aspects of Human Action

(1) Agent   (2) Acts   (3) Ends   and   (4) Consequences

Ethical theories differ in part according to which aspect of human action they emphasize. *Virtue* theories emphasize (1), holding that actions are right or wrong depending on what they express about the agent. Actions are right if they express virtue, wrong if they express vice. Although it may be difficult to come to a conclusive judgment in Case 2.1, the actions could be assessed according to what they express about the agents. For example, both the father's cowardice in not wanting to donate or to face blame from the family and his concern for his daughter and his family are relevant. And the physician attempted to protect his integrity by choosing an ambiguous explanation rather than a direct lie.

Deontological theories emphasize (2), acts in and of themselves, holding that some inherent or intrinsic features of actions make them right or wrong, not simply their ends and their consequences. For example, deontological arguments could consider whether the father violated an implicit commitment to his daughter when he refused to accept the risk of organ donation on her behalf, or whether the physician violated the rule against deception, even if he did not directly lie. As a deontologist, the physician could have argued that the rule of confidentiality outweighed the rule of truthfulness, but deontological critics could respond that he did not have to disclose any information, much less deceptive information. In contrast to some interpretations, deontological theories do not have to hold that some actions are absolutely right or wrong—though they may do so—but only that some of their intrinsic or inherent features are always right-making or wrong-making characteristics.

Teleological theories emphasize (3), the ends of action, while *consequentialist* theories emphasize (4), the consequences or effects of action. Both these theories downplay or deny the importance of intrinsic or inherent features of actions, such as whether actions are in accord with a moral rule against lying, in order to concentrate on what actions are intended to produce, what they actually produce, or both. For example, the physician's actions might be assessed as means to his goal of not wrecking the family. Then it would be necessary to determine whether the means would probably be effective (e.g., the family might not be salvageable or the mother might press questions about "medical reasons") and also whether, if effective, the actions would produce other bad consequences that might outweigh the good ones (e.g., the father might later experience guilt that would destroy the family).

This chapter concentrates on the debate about the adequacy of teleological-consequentialist theories, which affirm principles regarding the production of good and avoidance of bad consequences, and deontological theories, which affirm principles regarding the inherent or intrinsic rightness or wrongness of actions. Then the chapter returns at the end to the virtue theories' critiques of principles-based theories. Many theories of biomedical ethics attempt to include both consequentialist and nonconsequentialist considerations—they seek to determine the rightness or wrongness of actions according to whether the actions conform to principles and rules and also maximize good consequences.

MORAL PRINCIPLES AND RULES

The literature in biomedical ethics in the last 25 years has identified several moral principles, often but not always the same ones. For example, the National Commission for the Protection of Human Subjects of Biomedical and Behavioral Research (1978) justified its recommendations for policies by appealing to three major principles: respect for persons, beneficence (which includes what some have called nonmaleficence), and justice. However they are labeled, principles in biomedical ethics represent the following sorts of general moral considerations: obligations to respect the wishes of competent persons (respect for persons or autonomy); obligations not to harm others, including not killing them or treating them cruelly (nonmaleficence); obligations to benefit others (beneficence); obligations to produce a net balance of benefits over harms (utility); obligations to distribute benefits and harms fairly (justice); obligations to keep promises and contracts (fidelity); obligations of truthfulness; obligations to disclose information; and obligations to respect privacy and to protect confidential information (confidentiality).

Sometimes the obligations are stated as principles, sometimes as rules. Some obligations are viewed as primary and fundamental; others as secondary and derivative. For example, Beauchamp and Childress (1994) recognize primary principles of autonomy, nonmaleficence, beneficence (including utility), and justice, and derivative principles or rules of veracity, fidelity, privacy, and confidentiality. Robert Veatch's (1981) list of primary principles overlaps in important respects but differs in others: beneficence; contract-keeping; autonomy; honesty; avoiding killing; and justice. Veatch also recognizes several moral rules or intermediate moral formulations, such as informed consent. In a much shorter list, Tristram Engelhardt (1986) accepts only the principles of autonomy and beneficence and reduces justice to these two considerations, but he then recognizes several derivative obligations. Thus, ethical theories often differ according to how they sort out different obligations. Some theories may encompass several obligations under a few general headings, while others may view them as distinct and even separable obligations.

Other principles and rules have been proposed in addition to those already identified. For example, universalizability is widely accepted as a principle of and in morality. It is often viewed as a formal principle of morality, that is, as a necessary condition for any moral judgment. It is also widely viewed as a formal principle of justice within morality: Treat similar cases in a similar way. This principle has affinities with the Golden Rule—do unto others as you would have them do unto you.

Sometimes the Golden Rule is invoked in biomedical ethics as though it is all that agents need to make their decisions. It is easy to dismiss the Golden Rule if it is viewed as a sufficient principle but much harder to dismiss it if it is viewed only as a necessary principle. It is probably best viewed as a test of reasons for action, especially to determine if one is making an unjustified exception of oneself. It thus functions best, as Marcus Singer (1963) indicates, when it is conceived in terms of general rather than specific desires or general rules rather than particular actions.

If the "Golden Rule" (perhaps more properly construed as a principle than as a rule) is applied to specific desires or particular actions it may be plausibly viewed as "morally dangerous" (Veatch 1981, 313)—for example, using the Golden Rule in this way, physicians may decide whether to tell the patient the truth about a diagnosis of cancer and a prognosis of death by asking themselves whether the bad news would upset them if they were in the patient's situation. However, the Golden Rule or the principle of universalizability is more properly applied in the following way: The physician should ask by what rule he or she would want to be treated in such circumstances: Would he or she prefer to be treated under a rule that permitted or one that prohibited nondisclosure? Properly understood, the principle of universalizability or the Golden Rule is not dangerous, even though unsophisticated applications may be dangerous, and it is both necessary and helpful.

Ethical theories differ not only on the aspects of human action they emphasize and the moral principles and rules they propose, but also on the grounds or foundations they offer for the principles and rules. Sometimes the debate between utilitarians and deontologists has been misplaced because some utilitarians suppose that deontologists have a more difficult time than they in laying foundations for their ethical principles and rules. This misplaced debate may stem from the tendency to view deontological theories as mere reflections of common morality. However, the problems deontologists encounter in justifying several distinct principles and rules of obligation do not differ fundamentally from those faced by utilitarians when they attempt to justify the ultimate principle of utility. Deontologists and utilitarians may appeal to the same foundations: revelation (e.g., the divine will); intuition; reason (e.g., the nature of practical reason); human nature (e.g., natural law); a hypothetical contract; tradition; and so on. Debates about the acceptability or superiority of any ethical theory hinge on such obvious formal criteria as consistency, coherence, simplicity, and comprehensiveness, and, more controversially, on such substantive criteria as the theory's capacity to account for and to direct moral experience. (For further debates about justification, see Beauchamp and Childress 1994; Veatch 1981; Engelhardt 1986; Clouser and Gert 1990).

THE MEANING AND WEIGHT OF PRINCIPLES AND RULES

Even among proponents of the same principles and rules, there is wide disagreement about what the principles and rules imply for particular cases because of disputes about their meaning and weight. It is important to consider meaning and weight together. For example, in Case 2.1, the physician might have held that the rule of confidentiality outweighed the rule of truthfulness or that the avoidance of bad consequences (wrecking the family) outweighed the rule of truthfulness. However, there are different interpretations of the meaning of the rules of confidentiality and truthfulness, as well as of their weight and stringency.

On the one hand, if "lying" is defined as an intentionally deceptive statement, it might be held that the physician told a lie when he said that for "medical reasons" the father should not donate a kidney. In view of this definition, the moral debate would focus on whether the rule against lying could be overridden in this case by another rule (the rule of confidentiality) or by the consequences (avoiding the destruction of the family). Whatever is held about this particular case, few if any ethical theories consistently hold that lying so defined is absolutely wrong.

On the other hand, if "lying" is defined as intentionally withholding information from or deceiving someone who has a right to the truth, the moral debate about this case would focus on whether the physician actually lied and ultimately on whether the man's wife had a right to the information that had emerged in the relationship between her husband and the nephrologist. If this second definition of lying is accepted, it would be possible to hold that the rule against lying is absolute because all the difficult moral questions would be answered by determining who has a right to the truth.

The necessity of considering the meaning and the weight of a rule together is evident in a recent study. Dennis Novack and his colleagues attempted to determine physicians' attitudes toward the use of deception by means of a questionnaire with hypothetical cases. One case concerned Mrs. Lewis, a 52–year-old patient who is undergoing her annual examination (Novack et al. 1989). "You tell her that everything looks normal and that you are going to order routine blood tests and her annual screening mammography, which you feel is important for women of her age. She is against the mammography, saying that the last time you ordered it, she had to pay for it herself. You know she is of modest means and cannot easily afford it. You are surprised that her health insurance did not cover it. Upon asking your secretary, you learn that the insurance covers the cost of mammography only if there is a breast mass or objective clinical evidence of the possibility of cancer. The secretary tells you that the way to get around this is to put down 'rule out cancer' instead of 'screening mammography' on the form."

The physicians surveyed were asked what they would do. Nearly 70 percent indicated that they would write "rule out cancer," and 85 percent of that group stated that they would not be deceiving the insurance company by doing so. They could have conceded that they were deceiving the insurance company but then argued that their deception was justified as a way to help the patient. But most simply denied that their act would be deceptive. Thus, they could consistently view deception as absolutely wrong and still write "rule out cancer" on the form.

The following chart suggests the continuum of the weight or stringency of moral principles and rules:

Legalism   Antinomianism
              Absolute / Prima Facie / Relative

Joseph Fletcher (1966) offered his method of "situation ethics" as a third way between the extremes of legalism and antinomianism. He insisted that there is only one absolute principle of neighbor-love or utility and that all other principles and rules are mere maxims or rules of thumb (parallel to the one in baseball that says "don't bunt on third strike"). The other principles and rules suggest actions that people have been found to produce or subvert good consequences. They only illuminate courses of action; they do not prescribe what ought to be done. Reducing all principles and rules to mere maxims regarding utility, Fletcher came perilously close to antinomianism. His position failed to recognize that principles and rules can be prescriptive without being absolute. They can be prima facie binding, that is, binding if other things are equal. As prima facie, they direct courses of action but they can be overridden or outweighed by other prima facie principles and rules when they come into conflict in a situation.

Beauchamp and Childress (1994 and earlier) argue that the principles they identify—respect for autonomy, nonmaleficence, beneficence (including utility or proportionality), and justice, along with such derivative principles or rules as veracity, fidelity, privacy, and confidentiality—are only prima facie binding. None can be considered as absolute. And these principles and rules have to be weighed and balanced in situations of decision.

This perspective might appear to be very close to Fletcher's maxims or rules of thumb, but there is an important difference. For Beauchamp and Childress, the principles and rules are prima facie binding and thus prescriptive; for Fletcher the principles and rules only illuminate the application of the one ultimate principle of neighbor-love (or utility). Hence for Beauchamp and Childress, the moral agent has to justify departures from moral principles and rules by showing that in the situation some other principles and rules have more weight. However, the assignment of weight or priority depends on the situation rather than on an abstract, a priori, ranking. The approach of Beauchamp and Childress suffers from the limitations of any pluralistic approach that does not assign weights or priorities to various principles in advance. Much rests on what has been variously called prudence, practical moral reasoning, or discernment in the situation.

A rule utilitarian may find the pluralistic approach to moral principles and rules less troubling than a rule deontologist because the former has the ultimate principle of utility, which justifies various other principles and rules and also adjudicates conflicts among them. Some deontologists have explored priority rules, contending, for example, that the principle of autonomy always trumps or overrides the principle of beneficence when the only beneficiary is the competent person whose wishes, choices, or actions are overridden.

A major effort to find a lexical or serial ordering of principles appears in Robert Veatch's *A Theory of Medical Ethics* (1981), in which all the deontological or nonconsequentialist principles "are together given lexical priority over the principle of beneficence" (326). However, in cases of conflict, the deontological or nonconsequentialist principles are themselves balanced against each other in what Veatch labels a "balancing strategy." Veatch thus finds "a solution to the inevitable unacceptable tension between Hippocratic individualism and the utilitarian drive toward aggregate net benefit" (326). This solution "comes from the articulation of other nonconsequentialist principles that will necessarily have a bearing on medical ethical decisions: contract keeping, autonomy, honesty, avoiding killing, and justice" (326) and from assigning them collective priority over the production of good consequences for individuals (Hippocratic individualism) or society (utilitarianism). Nonconsequentialist principles are thus given "coequal ranking" in relation to each other and "lexical ranking" over the principle of beneficence. Similarly, Engelhardt (1986) gives the principle of autonomy priority over the principle of beneficence. Further problems of ranking and ordering principles will appear in my analysis of efforts to connect principles to concrete cases.

CONNECTING GENERAL PRINCIPLES TO PARTICULAR JUDGMENTS ABOUT CASES

Principles-oriented ethics still requires interpretation and even bridges to concrete, particular judgments. Suppose a family considers whether to terminate artificial nutrition and hydration for an elderly, incompetent relative. The family may be uncertain whether such an action would fall under a principle that prohibits harming the patient or under a principle that requires benefiting the patient. The same principle may point in different directions—for example, the principle of benefiting the patient may offer ambiguous directives. Furthermore, any relevant principle may conflict with other relevant principles, such as respecting the patient's previously expressed wishes. In addition, different parties may have moral disagreements with each other about the appropriateness of withdrawing artificial nutrition and hydration.

Proponents of principles have various ways to connect their principles to particular judgments. According to Henry Richardson (1990), there are three major models of connection between principles and case judgments: (1) application, which involves the deductive application of principles and rules; (2) balancing, which depends on intuitive weighing of conflicting principles; and (3) specification, which proceeds by "qualitatively tailoring our norms to cases" (283).

Many principlists have used the metaphor of *application*, as in *applied ethics*, but most would concede that this metaphor is misleading if taken too literally. Few principlists take a mechanical or deductive view of application, as critics sometimes suggest. Perhaps some absolutist interpreters of principles and rules take this approach, but, as the discussion of lying and deception suggested, others (e.g., Ramsey 1970) incorporate exceptional cases through deepening the meaning of the principles or rules by a process that is very close to specification. Even though some principles may genuinely apply to concrete cases, this metaphor cannot helpfully cover all the significant relations between principles and particular judgments about those cases. Not all such relations involve rational deduction from principles to particular judgments. And many principlists recognize that particular case judgments may modify our interpretation of principles and rules.

The process of *balancing* is common in principlist approaches—for example, it appears extensively in Beauchamp and Childress, *Principles of Biomedical Ethics* (1994 and earlier), and significantly (but within limits) in Veatch, *A Theory of Medical Ethics* (1981). Balancing fits best with a view of principles as prima facie or presumptively binding but also as potentially in conflict in particular cases. The main criticism of the process of balancing is its intuitive assignment of weights to conflicting principles or rules, since an a priori assignment would involve something like application or specification. One effort to structure the process of balancing to reduce (but not eliminate) the reliance on intuition identifies several conditions that need to be met before one prima facie principle can outweigh or override another in a conflict situation.

This structure of practical reasoning focuses on several questions (Beauchamp and Childress 1994). For example, when a patient who has HIV infection indicates that he does not inform his lovers of his condition and does not practice safer sex, the physician has to consider whether the duty to respect confidentiality outweighs the duty to protect third parties. In addition to pondering the specific weights of these duties in the situation, the physician should ask whether breaching confidentiality would offer a reasonable chance of preventing harm to others, whether there are morally acceptable alternatives to the breach of confidentiality (e.g., could the physician persuade the patient to inform sexual partners?), and whether the contemplated breach of the rule of confidentiality is the least infringement of the rule consistent with protecting others.

Specification is the third model for connecting general principles to cases. Principles are frequently specified through rules that are more specific, concrete, and detailed. For example, rules that require physicians to seek voluntary informed consent before undertaking certain procedures on patients specify the requirements of the principle of respect for autonomy. And rules of confidentiality specify the requirements of several principles, including respect for autonomy and utility, the latter because of the value of confidential relations for the provision of effective health care.

Efforts have been undertaken to broaden the role of specification in bioethics. For example, DeGrazia (1991) favors "specified principlism," and Beauchamp and Childress (1994) combine specification with balancing. Even though specification has been offered as a way to reduce the role of intuition, there is debate about whether it actually succeeds, and some charge that it falls prey to the same problems as balancing (Arras 1994).

Although the process of specification usually focuses on the meaning, range, and scope of general moral principles in an effort to make them more determinate, a similar process can occur regarding their weight or stringency. For instance, Robert Veatch's (1981) efforts, noted above, to assign priority to some principles over others can be viewed as a procedure of specification that involves their weight and stringency rather than their range and scope. Again, debates about the strength and the meaning of moral principles cannot be completely separated.

Following are three examples of principles-oriented approaches to major problem areas in bioethics. These three examples do not illustrate all the complexities involved in connecting principles to cases. The first example indicates how the connection may occur through a process of specification of rules and conditions for justified research involving human subjects, but with ongoing debates about both balancing and deductive application. The second example focuses on a conflict between utility and justice or equity in health policy, and the third example focuses on a conflict between benefiting a patient and respecting his wishes.

A straightforward consequentialist approach to research involving human subjects, particularly one based on utilitarian calculation and unfettered by deontological constraints (or rule-utilitarian constraints), might justify research that is deceptive or coercive as a way to produce significant benefits for a large number of people. Such an approach, further tainted by a racist ideology, was adopted in Nazi Germany. However, utilitarianism may avoid such a conclusion by being truly universalistic (rather than denying the relevance of harms to some human beings) and by considering a broad range of goods over time (rather than simply immediate scientific progress). By contrast, a rule deontologist, such as Paul Ramsey (1970) would hold that the ends justify only the means that pass an independent moral audit or inspection. For the deontologist, actions have features other than their effectiveness and efficiency as means; they should also be assessed in relation to such independent principles as respect for autonomy and justice.

Most ethical assessments of research involving human subjects appeal to both consequentialist and deontological considerations and to a wide range of moral principles and rules, as is evident in the following conditions or criteria of ethically justified research that are already embedded in codes, regulations, and practices and that can be justified by the general moral principles already identified (Childress 1981; Walters 1977). (1) The end of the research—the knowledge sought—should be important. (2) There should be a reasonable prospect that the research will generate the knowledge that is sought. (3) The use of human subjects in a research project should be a matter of last resort. Their use should be preceded by other studies, including animal experimentation, and should be necessary. The Nuremberg Code holds that "the experiment should be such as to yield fruitful results for the good of society, unprocurable by other methods or means of study." (4) The risks to the subjects should be minimized. (5) The research should meet the principle of utility or proportionality in the balance of probable benefits to the society, including the subjects, and risks, burdens, and costs to subjects.

The first five conditions focus on the probable consequences of the research for the society and the subjects, as viewed in relation to the principles of beneficence, nonmaleficence, and utility. Although these conditions are necessary, they are not sufficient from most ethical perspectives. Even though it can be argued that these conditions should be considered first, some other conditions are also necessary and may morally invalidate research that satisfies the first five conditions. (6) The selection of research subjects should be fair and equitable (the principle of justice), and (7) the researchers must have the subjects' (or the proxies' where appropriate) voluntary and informed consent to participate (the principle of respect for persons and their autonomy). In addition, (8) the principles or rules of privacy, confidentiality, and promise-keeping set limits on the conduct of the research.

There is no moral right to seek research subjects unless the first five conditions have been met (usually determined by an Institutional Review Board); there is no moral right to proceed with these research subjects unless conditions six and seven have been met; and the research is wrongly conducted unless the eighth condition is met. If all these conditions are necessary for ethically justified research with human subjects, research that meets the principles of beneficence, nonmaleficence, and utility, but not the principles of justice, autonomy, privacy, confidentiality, and promise-keeping, is unjustified.

For most ethical theories, the conflict between producing good for the society through research and not wronging research subjects should be resolved through assigning priority to the nonconsequentialist principles in cases of conflict. It is unjustified to violate those nonconsequentialist standards, even to increase the number of participants so as to conduct more valid research, as apparently occurred in the U.S. radiation experiments on unconsenting subjects, who were allegedly often unaware of what was being done to them or of the risk/benefit calculus involved. Defenders of a "lexical order" of nonconsequentialist principles over consequentialist ones, such as Veatch (1981) and Engelhardt (1986), doubt that a theory that balances prima facie various prima facie principles can always yield the right conclusion in such a conflict. It remains to be seen whether the use of specification, in conjunction with balancing, will be satisfactory (Beauchamp and Childress 1994).

A conflict between utility and justice (or equity) can be seen in the debate about policies to control hypertension in the American population.

CASE 2.2

It has been estimated that 17% of adults in the United States (approximately 24 million persons) have hypertension, which can lead to major health problems. According to Milton Weinstein and William B. Stason (1977), minimally adequate treatment for all of these people would cost over $5 billion annually. Treatment is difficult because almost half of the people with hypertension are not aware of their problem and only one-sixth of those who know about their problem are receiving proper treatment. Weinstein and Stason tried to determine the most cost-effective way to control hypertension; as an expression of the principle of utility, cost-effectiveness analysis is an attempt to determine which policy would produce the greatest aggregate benefits such as quality-adjusted life years for the money. (Cost-effectiveness analysis differs from cost-benefit analysis in that it does not convert the benefits along with the costs into a common denominator of money.) Several factors were important in the analysis, including the difficulty of convincing people identified as hypertensives through mass screening and education programs to seek medical treatment and to comply with the recommended treatment. The analysis led Weinstein and Stason to conclude that a "community with limited resources would probably do better to concentrate its efforts on improving adherence of known hypertensives, even at a sacrifice in terms of the numbers screened. This conclusion holds even if such proadherence interventions are rather expensive and only moderately effective, and even if screening is very inexpensive" (Weinstein and Stason 1977, 28). Furthermore, they concluded, screening patients already under the care of a physician is more cost effective than public screening.

Although a policy to control hypertension as a concern of public health may be justified on grounds of its cost effectiveness, it may be problematic from the standpoint of distributive justice or equity. Many poor people and blacks would not know of their hypertension because they are not under medical care. For example, blacks, who comprise 18 percent of hypertensives but only 9 percent of the total U.S. population, have not had equal access to good medical care. In addition, if hypertension as a disease of modern industrial society is exacerbated by the unequal distribution of power, there may be other claims of injustice (Guttmacher 1981). It might also be argued that the society has a stronger moral obligation to inform everyone of his or her hypertension through public screening than "to cajole people to take care of themselves when others might be denied the basic information about their condition that would allow them to make a choice." (Weinstein and Stason 1977).

A final example to illustrate the connection between principles and cases involves an apparent conflict between the principle of beneficence and the principles of respect for autonomy and truthfulness in the deceptive use of a placebo.

CASE 2.3

Mr. X, a 65-year-old retired army officer who had been very successful in the military and in teaching and research, had had several abdominal operations for gallstones, postoperative adhesions, and bowel obstructions. Because of chronic pain, he was somewhat depressed, had lost weight, had poor hygiene, and had withdrawn socially because he had to assume awkward or embarrassing postures to control his pain. He had used parenteral pentazocine six times a day for more than 2 years to control pain, but now had so much tissue and muscle damage that he had trouble finding injection sites. (Pentazocine may be addictive.)

Stating that his goal was "to get more out of life in spite of my pain," Mr. X voluntarily entered a psychiatric ward, which included individual behavior therapy programs, daily group therapy, and so forth. Mr. X reduced his use of pentazocine to four times a day and insisted that this level was necessary to control his pain. After considerable discussion with their colleagues, the therapists decided to withdraw the pentazocine over time without the patient's knowledge by diluting it with increasing proportions of normal saline.

Mr. X experienced nausea, diarrhea, and cramps, but he thought these withdrawal symptoms were the result of amitriptyline, which the therapist had introduced to relieve the withdrawal symptoms. Self-control techniques were continued, and the intervals between injections were increased. Although the patient was aware of the changes in intervals, he was not aware that he was receiving only saline. After 3 weeks, his therapists disclosed that he was receiving a placebo, not pentazocine. After initial anger, Mr. X asked that the saline be discontinued and the self-control techniques continued. When he was discharged 3 weeks later, Mr. X reported that he could control his abdominal pain more effectively with the self-control techniques than he could earlier with pentazocine. A follow-up 6 months later showed that he was still using the relaxation techniques and had resumed social activities and part-time teaching.

The therapists justified their deceptive use of a placebo on grounds of its effectiveness: "We felt ethically obliged to use a treatment that had a high probability of success. To withhold the procedure may have protected some standard of openness but may not have been in his [the patient's] best interests. We saw no option without ethical problems. Although it is precarious to justify the means by the end, we felt most obliged to use a procedure designed to help the patient achieve a personally and medically desirable goal" (Levendusky and Pankratz 1975, 165–168).

On one level, this case appears to involve a straightforward conflict between the principle of beneficence—benefiting the patient—and the principles of respect for autonomy and veracity. The therapists saw "no option without ethical problems," and concluded that the ends justified the means in this case. Thus, ranking consequentialist principles over nonconsequentialist ones, at least in this sort of case, they justified paternalistic actions in apparent violation of the principles of respect for autonomy and veracity. There is considerable debate about whether paternalistic actions—refusals to acquiesce in a person's wishes, choices, and actions for that person's own benefit—can be justified. Both a conceptual point and a normative point are involved.

Normatively, some consequentialists argue that beneficence (as well as nonmaleficence and utility) toward a patient can justify overriding that patient's autonomy. By contrast, some nonconsequentialists contend that the principle of autonomy always trumps the principle of beneficence when only the patient's welfare is involved (i.e., when there is no harm to other parties). In this case, nonconsequentialists could argue that the therapists unjustifiably violated the patient's autonomy when they deceptively used a placebo. Clearly, debates in ethical theory have considerable significance for resolving this case.

The conceptual point concerns the definition of paternalism. Some philosophers insist that paternalism has both strong (or extended) and weak (or limited) forms. Strong paternalism overrides an *autonomous* person's wishes, choices, or actions; weak paternalism overrides a *nonautonomous* person's wishes, choices, or actions (or temporarily intervenes to determine whether a person is acting autonomously). Strong paternalism clearly raises the most serious moral questions, and some philosophers insist that weak paternalism is not even paternalism, at least in any morally interesting sense, because it does not involve a conflict between beneficence and autonomy (because the target of beneficence is not autonomous).

In this case, there could be debate about whether Mr. X's autonomy had been sufficiently compromised both by his pain and by his use of pentazocine, a potentially addictive drug, so as to justify overriding his choices as nonautonomous—whether or not this intervention can be called weak paternalism. In any event, despite their differences about whether a person's diminished autonomy is a necessary condition to justify paternalism, both weak and strong paternalists have to meet some consequentialist conditions that focus on the probability of harm or loss of benefit without intervention and the probability of a net balance of benefit over harm with the intervention. In addition, some ethicists argue, even if the principle of respect for persons is overridden, it still requires that the least insulting, humiliating, disrespectful, and restrictive intervention be chosen (Childress 1982).

Another possible response to this case also focuses on the meaning of the principle of respect for autonomy. Perhaps the therapists did not violate Mr. X's autonomous choices but acted in accord with them. It could be claimed that Mr. X implicitly consented to the modification in medication, even though he continued explicitly to refuse it, because he voluntarily admitted himself to a psychiatric ward where adjustment in medication was a clear expectation and because he accepted the goals of therapy, "to get more out of life in spite of . . . pain." Or it might be argued that Mr. X's current refusal to further modify his use of pentazocine should be put in the context of his *past consent* and his *probable future consent*.

The issue of past consent usually surfaces when a person has previously accepted a course of action that he or she now repudiates. As in the case of implicit consent, the question is exactly what Mr. X consented to when he voluntarily entered the psychiatric ward. Although the appeal to implicit or past consent might succeed if we had no other information about Mr. X's wishes, we do have other information: He expressly refused to allow further reduction in the pentazocine dose. Thus, many would argue, we cannot appeal to implied consent or to past consent to override current express refusals unless we can show that the patient now has diminished autonomy, that is, some defect, encumbrance, or limitation in decision making.

Is it possible for the therapists to appeal to Mr. X's probable future consent and thus invoke the principle of respect for autonomy to justify their actions? The therapists apparently believed that Mr. X retrospectively ratified their decision to use the placebo when he decided to continue the self-control techniques. However, it is difficult to hold that either predicted or actual future consent satisfies respect for personal autonomy. The intervention itself may create the consent, but, even when this danger is not present, the prediction of future consent can only provide some evidence that the criteria for justifying paternalism have been met. That prediction does not itself convert the intervention into respect for autonomy.

The therapists noted that they saw "no option without ethical problems." To be justified, deception must be necessary to meet the goal that is sought. If the goal can be obtained by some other morally appropriate means, deception is unjustified. This claim reflects the conviction that the principle of veracity has at least prima facie moral weight so that any infringement requires justification.

The therapists believed that they had a duty to "use a treatment that had a high probability of success" even if they had to violate "some standard of openness." They thought they had to choose between "openness" and "effectiveness" in seeking a goal that the patient also desired. It is not clear, however, that they had exhausted all moral options. It might have been possible, for instance, to obtain the patient's consent to several medications, including placebos. Such consent might have been obtained at the outset. Indeed, when the placebo was given, Mr. X was informed that a modification of his medication regime would be undertaken, but he did not receive any details. However, because he still insisted on maintaining the same dose of pentazocine (though not the same frequency), he could not be said to have consented to the placebo.

Yet another possibility may not have been adequately explored because of the staff's therapeutic perspective. The staff defined the patient's problem in terms of specific behaviors, and perhaps they paid inadequate attention to the "person responsible for those behaviors" (Kelman 1975). If the therapists had viewed the problem in a different way, they might have considered alternative procedures with high probabilities of success and without serious ethical difficulties.

These cases and problem areas illuminate some complexities in the appeal to principles in the context of actual cases. Not only are there difficult questions about which principles are relevant, there are also difficult questions about their meaning and their weight. Even the appeal to shared principles does not ensure agreement about particular cases because there may be disagreements about the meaning and weight of the relevant moral principles and rules as well as about the facts of the case. The common metaphor of "application" may distort the process of reasoning, especially if it suggests a mechanical or legalistic use of principles and rules. The metaphor of "discernment" may be more helpful as long as it is not combined with efforts to replace principles and rules altogether.

The relation between principles and particular judgments about cases is best viewed as circular or dialectical. Agents move back and forth between them, using principles in their judgments about particular cases but sometimes modifying their interpretation of the meaning and stringency of principles in the light of particular cases. Sometimes it is unclear whether the principles or the particular judgments require modification.

CRITICISMS OF PRINCIPLES

In recent years, several criticisms have been leveled against the prominent role of principles and rules in biomedical ethics (see, for example, DuBose et al. 1994). Some criticisms of particular principles-oriented approaches to bioethics have already been introduced in passing—for example, charges that some such approaches lack adequate theoretical foundations or involve mechanical application. Here I will examine and assess some of the significant criticisms.

Priority of General Moral Norms over Particular Case Judgments

Several critics of principlist approaches contend that priority should be given to particular judgments about concrete cases rather than to general moral norms, such as principles and rules. One version of this criticism emerged in my earlier discussion of situation ethics. Representing the major contemporary form of consequentialism, utilitarians may, as we have seen, appeal to utility to assess particular acts directly (act utilitarianism), or to derive other principles and rules that then determine the rightness or wrongness of particular acts (rule utilitarianism). Act utilitarians hold that principles and rules other than utility can function only as maxims or rules of thumb without prescriptive, binding power. From the standpoint of act utilitarians, both rule utilitarians and rule deontologists are more alike than different; both make too much of principles and rules and too little of the consequences of particular acts. Principles and rules create victims of morality—people suffer bad consequences because of others' adherence to principles and rules.

This criticism, which applies mainly to absolutist versions of principles and rules, fails to note the necessity of principles and rules to solve or to reduce problems of coordination, cooperation, and trust in human interaction. For example, G. J. Warnock (1971) considers the expectations that would be appropriate in an encounter between an act-utilitarian physician and an act-utilitarian patient. Warnock notes that the patient could only expect the physician to try to cure him of his afflictions, "*unless* his [the physician's] assessment of the 'general happiness' leads him to do otherwise" (33). Asking the act-utilitarian physician to declare his intentions truthfully or to promise to consider only the patient's welfare, in accord with the Hippocratic tradition, would not help, because all the physician's promises and declarations would themselves be subject to utilitarian calculation. Trust that the physician would act for the patient's own advantage evaporates because of the physician's lack of commitment to moral principles and rules other than utility. (Similar and more serious problems arise in act deontology. At least act utilitarianism requires that agents attempt to calculate the greatest good for the greatest number; by contrast, act deontologists appeal to intuition, conscience, divine commands, and the like, in the situation, and their predictability becomes even less secure than that of the act utilitarians.)

Revivers of casuistry, which rejects any overarching principle such as utility, hold that moral agents can make discerning judgments about particular cases even though they disagree about principles or rules (Jonsen and Toulmin 1988). For example, in reflecting on the work of the National Commission for the Protection of Human Subjects, Stephen Toulmin (1981), who was a staff philosopher for the commission, argues that the appeal to principles by the commissioners was unnecessary and misleading. For, he insists, the commissioners "were, quite evidently, surer about these shared particular judgments [e.g., about the kind of consent procedures required in biomedical research using 5-year-old children] than they were about the discordant general principles on which, in theory, their practical judgments were based" (32). So, Toulmin contends, appeals to principles do not provide "a more solid foundation" for particular ethical judgments, but rather connect ethical conclusions with nonethical commitments. "Such principles serve less as foundations, adding intellectual strength or force to particular moral opinions, than they do as corridors or curtain walls linking the moral perceptions of all reflective human beings, with other, more general positions—theological, philosophical, ideological, or Weltan-schaulich" (32).

Toulmin's target is not clear, for he shoots indiscriminately at "the tyranny of principles," the "absoluteness of moral principles," "tyrannical absolutism," "the cult of absolute principles," "unchallengeable principles," "a single principle held as absolute," "a morality based entirely on general rules and principles," and so forth. It may be possible and desirable to escape the tyranny of absolute, single, unchallengeable principles, but it may not be possible or desirable to escape all principles.

In addition to arguing for the significance of principles and rules for human interaction, rule utilitarians and rule deontologists contend that particular case judgments imply rules because of the principle of universalizability: To hold that act X is wrong is to imply that all relevantly similar Xs are wrong. Hence, to make a judgment about a particular case is to move toward a principle or rule.

Critics of principlist approaches frequently employ principles and rules, even when they fail to acknowledge them. For example, Joseph Fletcher, who expressly recognized only the ultimate principle of utility and reduced other principles and rules to the status of suggestive maxims, appeared to affirm at least one other strong rule when he held that no "unwanted and unintended baby should ever be born" (Fletcher 1966, 39).

Finally, the factors identified for case analysis by Albert Jonsen, Mark Siegler, and William Winslade in *Clinical Ethics* (1986) are close to moral principles. These four factors—medical indications, patient preferences, quality of life, and external factors—correlate closely with what others call moral principles. For example, medical indications and quality of life both involve principles of beneficence and nonmaleficence; patient preferences involve respect for persons and their autonomy; and the external factors, which focus on the impact of actions on others, including family and society, involve considerations of utility and justice. In fact, these ethical factors or considerations function in their argument about clinical ethics in roughly the way that similar principles and rules function for some other theories of biomedical ethics. They are prima facie or presumptive rather than absolute, but they are more than maxims. Fear of the tyranny of principles that are absolute or simplistic does not warrant avoidance of the language of principles altogether, especially when the moral factors or considerations that are invoked function as principles.

Interactions Among Strangers or Among Friends and Intimates?

Some critics of principlism concede that principles and rules are appropriate in interactions among strangers but not among friends and intimates (Toulmin 1981). Hence, a fundamental question is whether in our society patients and physicians or other health-care professionals interact as friends or as strangers. Dramatic changes in health care have rendered problematic a conception of medicine in terms of friendship—pluralism in values, the decline of close, intimate contact over time between professionals and patients, the rise of specialists who treat only part of the whole person, and the growth of large, impersonal, and bureaucratic institutions of health care have all contributed to the loss of intimacy and community. Trust among strangers cannot presuppose knowledge of their traits of character or their values. Principles, rules, and procedures become increasingly important in the absence of community. As reconceived to fit modern health care, trust may be confidence in and reliance upon health-care professionals to adhere to principles such as autonomy and truthfulness, which do not presuppose knowledge of the professionals' interpretation of benefits and burdens or harms.

In short, principles and rules may provide the basis for interaction among "friendly strangers." Most physicians and patients are not friends, but they are rarely estranged and hostile. Even though they may not have (or at least do not know whether they have) shared conceptions of the good life, including balances of benefits and harms, they can trust each other to respect common principles and rules. As Alasdair MacIntyre (1977) notes,

> When a community of moral and metaphysical beliefs is lacking, trust between strangers becomes much more questionable than when we can safely assume such a community. Nobody can rely on anyone else's judgments on his or her behalf until he or she knows what the other person believes. It follows that nobody can accept the moral authority of another in virtue simply of his professional position. We are thrust back into a form of moral autonomy (210).

Our social situation thus supports claims not only about the importance of moral principles and rules for interaction among strangers but also about the importance of some moral principles and rules over others. Expounding a theory of bioethics for secular, pluralistic societies, Engelhardt (1986) has argued that physicians "must come to terms with the moral commitments and views of individuals from various moral communities while preserving the moral fabric of a peaceable, secular, pluralist society."

Regulatory Bioethics

According to some critics, principlism has become regulatory bioethics and has eschewed a prophetic role for bioethics. Principlists have often attempted to shape public policy in a liberal, pluralistic, democratic society, and these efforts can be construed as regulatory bioethics. And yet, principlists have also prophetically denounced various aspects of health care and its social setting—examples include the criticism of professional paternalism and the unequal distribution of health care.

Some principlists (as well as some casuists and others) have sought to work out acceptable policies in controversial areas such as the use of aborted fetal tissue transplantation research. But which position is prophetic—one that supports a ban on federal funds for human fetal tissue transplantation research because the tissue comes from deliberately aborted fetuses and is alleged to create the risk of additional abortions, or one that opposes a ban because of the possible benefits of the research over the improbable increase in abortions?

Furthermore, principlism has resources for prophetic judgments. Whether principles are discerned in social practices or established by a unified theory, they can serve a critical function, perhaps more readily than a pure casuistry that attempts to operate without principles. General principles provide ways to criticize practices that are not available in case-to-case analysis. As John Arras (1991) has suggested, the casuist in moving from actual case to actual case may be limited to problems or dilemmas as *felt* or *experienced* by practitioners. By contrast, general principles may help identify other cases that should be on the moral agenda, and they may direct our attention to *real* problems and dilemmas that have not yet been experienced as such.

Obsession with Quandaries

Some critics charge that principlism reduces bioethics to quandary ethics by focusing so much on moral dilemmas and problems that have to be resolved. However, even if principlists concentrate on the quandaries that face various parties, they do not suppose that the moral life simply consists of various disconnected moral problems, which are in part created and resolved by appeals to principles. Much of the moral life is a matter of doing what one recognizes to be right, obligatory, and good without any direct appeal to principles and without any perplexity about what one ought to do. Moral agents can recognize that they ought to act as Good Samaritans because of a neighbor's need, without principles-based deliberation. Only when novel situations and conflicts arise, as they sometimes do, must principles be invoked. However common or uncommon, quandaries do have to be faced when they arise. Preventing them is desirable, but preventive ethics, just like preventive health care, is not always successful, and then critical cases have to be faced and resolved. Thus, to concentrate on dilemmas because of their importance and difficulty is not to suppose that they exhaust biomedical ethics.

Neglect of Character and Virtue

A closely related criticism of principles and rules comes from proponents of the primacy of character and virtues. In a framework of character and virtues, as noted above in the discussion of aspects of human action, actions are assessed according to what they express about the agent and his or her motives and traits or character. According to character or virtue ethics, many putatively different frameworks (e.g., principlists and casuists, and deontologists and utilitarians) actually are closer than is usually recognized, for they focus on "What ought I *do*?" in the context of moral dilemmas, quandaries, and problems.

By contrast, proponents of the primacy of character and virtue, by no means a uniform group, first address the question "What ought I to *be*?" They then address the question about what the agent ought to do in light of their conception of good or virtuous character. Virtue theorists usually hold (1) that a virtuous professional can *discern* the right course of action in the situation without reliance on principles and rules, and/or (2) that a virtuous person will *desire* to do what is right and avoid what is wrong.

The first approach is often combined with situation ethics, and it downplays rules and principles in moral decision making. Leon Kass (1980) has articulated this viewpoint: "I increasingly believe that the attempt to replace the often inarticulate yet prudent judgments of discerning physicians with explicit rules or procedures will not lead to better decisions" (1811). Principlists respond that if we try to determine which approach will lead to "better decisions," it is necessary to appeal to principles and rules to identify courses of action that are right, obligatory, wrong, or permitted. And when agents have to justify their conduct, it is not sufficient for them to appeal to their "discernment" or "prudence" or "conscience" without reference to principles and rules. There is simply no assurance that good people will discern what is right.

The second approach to virtues concentrates on the agent's motivation to do what is right, assuming that what is right is clear in most situations and that the major problem is the lack of motivation to do what is right. When there is a conflict between moral requirements and self-interest, the problem may not be one of knowledge but of motivation, and virtues dispose people to act in morally appropriate ways from morally appropriate motives. For example, according to Gregory Pence (1980), "the ultimate argument" why biomedical ethics should be discussed "in the framework of the virtues" is that researchers, physicians, and other professionals can subvert such rules as informed consent if they desire. Thus, it is important to create a climate in which professionals have the right kind of desires. Pence is certainly correct to emphasize the role of virtues in disposing people to right actions, but it is necessary to have an independent assessment of acts in light of moral principles. Virtues include certain motivations to perform right actions, but are not themselves sufficient to determine which actions are right. In many cases, it is simply not clear what a virtuous physician would do—breach confidentiality to warn a person that his or her lover has AIDS? involuntarily hospitalize a patient who is contemplating suicide?

In much (but by no means all) of the moral life, principles of action help to determine which virtues should be developed. Many virtues are correlated with principles and rules, such as benevolence with beneficence, truthfulness with veracity. And many other virtues, such as conscientiousness and courage, are important for morality as a whole.

Neglect of Care in Relationships

A final criticism of principles and rules in biomedical ethics builds on the arguments offered by Carol Gilligan (1982) about male and female moralities. Noting that Piaget and Kohlberg both omitted girls and women from their studies of moral development, Gilligan contends that women are not morally retarded, as some of Kohlberg's tests seem to suggest, but rather speak in a different moral voice, and their voice is not adequately recorded by the tests developed on male models.

In particular, Gilligan notes that women tend to concentrate on narrative, context, and relationships, in which they express care/caring, rather than on tiers of moral principles and rules with their logic of hierarchical justification, as in male perspectives on morality. Gilligan argues that women see and resolve moral problems differently. She emphasizes that what is involved is not gender but socialization and insists that what is needed is a recognition of the complementarity of the two moralities of care and justice, including rights.

Although complementarity is possible within an individual's life over time, it is not yet clear what complementarity implies for some social roles, such as medicine. Consider again the case of the father who did not want to donate a kidney to his dying daughter and asked the physician to lie. Would a physician with a care perspective come to a different conclusion than a physician with a principlist perspective, which could itself lead to several different conclusions? It is hard to predict with confidence that the practical differences between these perspectives would be significant in this case, not only because the socialization process in medicine may inculcate "male" morality, but because the major question is the *moral significance* of the nephrologist's relationships with the father and with the other members of the family. Hence, the physician in that case would have to determine, at least in part through principles and rules, how much weight each relationship should have.

Some moral principles and rules as well as modes of moral reasoning may be more important in some settings than in others, regardless of whether females or males occupy the social roles. If research, medicine, and health care often involve relations among strangers, the appeal to principles and rules may be important and even indispensable, whether the strangers are male or female. Furthermore, principles of respect for autonomy and justice, particularly in the form of equality, strongly support women's rights. Some feminists, who take seriously the social context of oppression of women under patriarchy, wonder whether female caring is to a great extent a product of the oppressive social system (and thus lacks independent standing) and may even help to perpetuate it (Sherwin 1992).

Nevertheless, the moral perspective of care in relationships identifies a major limitation of some principlist approaches and offers an important corrective to such approaches. As Alisa Carse (1991) stresses, "'care' reasoning is concrete and contextual rather than abstract; it is sometimes principle-guided, rather than always principle-driven, and it involves sympathy and compassion rather than dispassion" (17). Although it has similarities to casuistry, the care perspective properly stresses emotional qualities and character traits sometimes neglected by both casuists and principlists. At any rate, principlism must be carefully reformulated in light of the whole range of human moral experience (one test of ethical theories), and this includes women's experiences both as carers and as oppressed persons.

In conclusion, despite the important criticisms of various principlist approaches, principles and rules appear to remain central in biomedical ethics. Whatever revisions are required in principlist approaches, the difficult questions do not concern whether to employ principles and rules, but rather which principles and rules should be adopted, how they should be interpreted, how much weight and strength they should have, which should have priority in cases of conflict, how they are connected to concrete cases, and in what relations and situations they apply. Answering these questions is not easy, but seeking the answers in the context of science, medicine, and health care is the fundamental task of biomedical ethics.

DISCUSSION QUESTIONS

1. Are beneficence and nonmaleficence merely the positive and negative aspects of the same moral principle, or is the moral duty to avoid evil more stringent? Does the ethical slogan in medicine, "first of all do no harm" imply that avoiding harm is a more rigorous or necessary duty for physicians? Would this imply that when a physician must choose between a conservative course (one that can do little harm but also little good) and a more aggressive course (one that can do much harm but also much good), the physician ought to choose the one that does little harm?

2. Do the consequences of actions—the benefits and harms expected—always tell us what is morally required, or are there other characteristics that can determine whether an action is right or wrong (such as whether the action involves violating another's autonomy, lying, breaking a promise, or taking a life)?

3. What should happen when two principles come into conflict? For example, if a physician believes that respecting the patient's autonomy by getting consent from the patient for giving a toxic cancer treatment will do more harm than good for the patient, should the physician be guided by beneficence and omit the request for consent, or should the physician be guided by autonomy and try to obtain consent nevertheless?

4. What is the relationship between the principle of justice and producing the greatest amount of good possible? What should a health planner do when a scarce resource could be allocated in different ways—one of which would produce the greatest amount of good and another of which would distribute the resources more evenly or fairly?

5. Are moral rules (such as the rule to always obtain consent before surgery) always morally binding, or are they only guidelines to be assessed in each case by ascertaining whether the outcome of following the rule is in accord with basic moral principles?

REFERENCES

Arras, John. "Getting Down to Cases: The Revival of Casuistry in Bioethics." *J Med Philos* 16 (1991): 29–51.

Beauchamp, Tom L., Childress, James F. *Principles of Biomedical Ethics*, 4th ed. New York: Oxford University Press, 1994.

Carse, Alisa L. "The 'Voice of Care': Implications for Bioethical Education." *J Med Philos* 16 (1991): 5–28.

Childress, James F. *Priorities in Biomedical Ethics.* Philadelphia: The Westminster Press, 1981.

Childress, James F. *Who Should Decide? Paternalism in Health Care.* New York: Oxford University Press, 1982.

Clouser, K. Danner, Gert, Bernard. "A Critique of Principlism." *J Med Philos* 15 (1990): 219–236.

DeGrazia, David. "Moving Forward in Bioethical Theory: Theories, Cases, and Specified Principlism." *J Med Philos* 17 (1992): 511–539.

DuBose, Edwin R., Hamel, Ron, O'Connell, Laurence J., Eds. *A Matter of Principles? Ferment in U.S. Bioethics.* Valley Forge, PA: Trinity Press International, 1994.

Engelhardt, H. Tristram, Jr., *The Foundations of Bioethics.* New York: Oxford University Press, 1986.

Fletcher, Joseph. *Situation Ethics: The New Morality.* Philadelphia: The Westminster Press, 1966.

Gilligan, Carol. *In A Different Voice.* Cambridge: Harvard University Press, 1982.

Guttmacher, Sally, et al. "Ethics and Preventive Medicine: The Case of Borderline Hypertension." *Hastings Cent Rep* 11 (February 1981): 12–20.

Jonsen, Albert R., Siegler, Mark, Winslade, William J. *Clinical Ethics: A Practical Approach to Ethical Decisions in Clinical Medicine,* 2nd ed. New York: Macmillan, 1986.

Jonsen, Albert R., Toulmin, Stephen. *The Abuse of Casuistry: A History of Moral Reasoning.* Berkeley: University of California Press, 1988.

Kass, Leon. "Ethical Dilemmas in the Care of the Ill." *JAMA* 244 (1980): 1811–1816.

Kelman, Herbert C. "Was Deception Justified—and Was It Necessary? Comments on Self-Control Techniques as an Alternative to Pain Medication." *J Abnorm Psychol* 84 (1975): 172–174.

Levendusky, Philip, Pankratz, Loren. "Self-Control Techniques as an Alternative to Pain Medication." *J Abnorm Psychol* 84 (1975): 165–168.

Levine, Melvin D., Scott, Lee, Curran, William J. "Ethics Rounds in a Children's Medical Center: Evaluation of a Hospital Based Program for Continuing Education in Medical Ethics." *Pediatrics* 60 (August 1977).

Macintyre, Alasdair. "Patients as Agents." In Stuart F. Spicker, H. Tristram Engelhardt, Jr., Eds., *Philosophical Medical Ethics: Its Nature and Significance.* Boston: D. Reidel Publishing Co., 1977: 197–212.

National Commission for the Protection of Human Subjects of Biomedical and Behavioral Research. *The Belmont Report: Ethical Guidelines for the Protection of Human Subjects of Research,* DHEW Publication No. (OS) 78–0012 (1978).

Novack, Dennis H., Detering, Barbara J., Arnold, Robert, et al. "Physicians' Attitudes Toward Using Deception to Resolve Difficult Ethical Questions." *JAMA* 263 (May 26, 1989): 2980–2985.

Pence, Gregory. *Ethical Options in Medicine.* Oradell, NJ: Medical Economics Co., Book Division, 1980.

Ramsey, Paul. *The Patient as Person.* New Haven: Yale University Press, 1970.

Richardson, Henry S. "Specifying Norms as a Way to Resolve Concrete Ethical Problems." *Philos Public Affairs* 19 (1990): 279–320.

Sherwin, Susan. *No Longer Patient: Feminist Ethics and Health Care*. Philadelphia: Temple University Press, 1992.

Singer, Marcus O. "The Golden Rule." *Philosophy* 38 (October 1963): 293–314.

Solomon, William David. "Rules and Principles." In Warren T. Reich, Ed., *Encyclopedia of Bioethics*, Vol. I. New York: Macmillan and Free Press, 1978: 407–413.

Stoppard, Tom. *Every Good Boy Deserves Favor and Professional Foul*. New York: Grove Press, 1978.

Toulmin, Stephen. "The Tyranny of Principles." *Hastings Cent Rep* 11 (December 1981): 31–39.

Veatch, Robert M. *A Theory of Medical Ethics*. New York: Basic Books, 1981.

Walters, LeRoy. "Some Ethical Issues in Research Involving Human Subjects." *Perspect Biol Med* 20 (Winter 1977): 193–211.

Warnock, G. J. *The Object of Morality*. London: Methuen and Co., 1971.

Weinstein, Milton, and Stason, William B. "Allocating Resources for Hypertension." *Hastings Cent Rep* 7 (October 1977): 24–29.

3

The Concepts of Health, Illness, and Disease

ARTHUR L. CAPLAN

SUMMARY

The concepts of health, illness, and disease play a pivotal role in defining the boundaries of medical concern, professional control, and social obligation. Defining what does or does not constitute a disease determines both the authority and power of those charged with alleviating its consequences as well as the scope of the social obligations of those beset by medical problems. Thus, to delineate the proper scope and domain of medicine and the related healing arts, it is necessary to develop a clear and concise understanding of these concepts.

First, the nature of the relationship between health and disease must be established. This relationship, when looked at uncritically, seems to be that health is nothing more than the absence of disease and disease is any impairment in a person's sense of well-being or fitness. However, some philosophers and health-care professionals have pointed out that matters are not so simple as this.

In understanding health or disease, two facts are important. First, disease does not always impair or threaten health. Consider the case of persons who carry the sickle-cell trait. Those with sickle-cell disease are prone to certain blood disorders. Sickle-cell carriers are better protected against malaria than someone lacking this genetic endowment.

Second, some health-care professionals see their jobs as being more than just the alleviation of pain or eradication of disease. They see their role as improving or optimizing functions. While the view that health and disease are conceptual opposites may be valid, establishing this requires a sustained argument.

This chapter considers three major views concerning the analysis of health and disease. The first view suggests that because all organisms are the product of a long course of biological evolution, *health* is the functioning of any organism in conformity with its natural design. Another view holds that *disease* is anything that is statistically abnormal. Health is what has been most commonly detected by statistical measurement as normal (i.e., blood pressure, cholesterol level, IQ, and so on).

A third view suggests that health and disease are concepts that cannot be defined without reference to values. Holders of this position are sometimes referred to as normativists. In this view, health, illness, and disease are inherently value-laden, and to fully understand these concepts, one must realize that decisions about states of the mind or body involve considerations of what is good, bad, desirable, or undesirable.

WHY ARE HEALTH AND DISEASE SO IMPORTANT IN CONTEMPORARY SOCIETY?

Health and disease are concepts that play vitally important roles in our daily lives. This is especially true if we happen to live in one of the nations of the industrialized world. Enormous sums of money are spent on health care. The United States, which is easily the world leader in expenditures for health care, spends nearly 14 percent of its gross national product, more than $1 trillion in 1994, on health care and health-related services. The nations of Western Europe, Scandinavia, Canada, Australia, New Zealand, Korea, Singapore, and Japan spend thousands of dollars per person annually for medical care.

Health affects more than our pocketbooks. Many persons devote a large portion of their time to the pursuit of behaviors and lifestyles that they believe will enhance their health and stave off disease. Many industries and jobs are focused on the provision of services to those who are diseased or to maintaining and improving health. And the legal and welfare programs of many societies rely on definitions of health and disease in deciding how to respond to a wide variety of behaviors and claims by individuals.

Decisions about the meaning of health and disease have direct and important consequences for daily life and the allocation of vast amounts of social resources. Thus, the analysis of the concepts of health, illness, and disease is not a mere exercise in intellectual inquiry or philosophical reflection. How we define these terms has very real legal, social, and economic consequences.

The concepts of health and disease, and the persons and institutions concerned with them, did not always play such central roles in human affairs. As recently as the mid-nineteenth century, physicians and hospitals occupied minor, peripheral roles in nearly every society. Few persons actively pursued health by means of lifestyle, diet, or daily regimens of one sort or another. It is not clear that they could. The prevailing notions of health and wellness in Western societies, that good health and freedom from disease were products of divine grace and social class, were not especially amenable to conscious manipulation by individuals.

During this same time, disease was feared and stigmatized but rarely the object of ministration by organized medicine, health care, or health care institutions. Laymen and family, as well as clerics, were often where the sick and the ill turned. The situation has changed radically. Why is this so and why do these concepts play such a central role in daily contemporary life?

The emergent concern with health and disease in this century is a function of many forces. Conquering the pain associated with medical treatment by means of anesthesia and anesthetics, especially during surgery, opened the door in the late nineteenth century to more aggressive interventions on the part of doctors. The success of twentieth-century medicine and public health services in preventing or reversing many forms of infection, dysfunction, and nutritional deficiency was a key reason for the emergence of popular concern about health and disease. The utility of various modes of conceiving disease, such as the germ theory, from the point of view of prophylaxis and cure compelled changes in the understanding of what disease and health mean. But it was not simply the success enjoyed by medicine and its attendant conceptual models of health and disease that brought the concepts of health and disease center stage over the past 100 years.

The historic connection in many theological writings, particularly Protestant, between health and moral character has played a key role in establishing the cultural importance of health and disease in Western societies. Disease and disability have been seen by many religious traditions as reflections of God's displeasure with sin and with the impure, both in mind and in actual conduct. The current interest in the prevention and avoidance of disease, especially among the wealthy and socially advantaged, reflects this legacy of viewing disease and illness as instruments of divine displeasure.

In a Western world grown far more secular in this century, at least in its public culture, disease, disability, and health have become transformed. Disease is no longer seen as a sign of divine displeasure or a mark of sin. Disease is not seen as having instrumental value; it has taken on intrinsic importance. Often, health, in itself, is interpreted as a sign of good moral character whereas disease is often equated with moral failure.

When those with cancer are told to use their mental powers to visualize dying cancerous cells as a way to dampen the cells' growth, when female workers are told they cannot hold jobs in a particular factory because the chemicals present pose risks to their reproductive well-being; when individuals are told they can use laughter to reverse the course of disease, when experts urge the control of diet, exercise, stress, or sexuality as the key to good health, then disease and health assume a highly individualistic focus. We feel more power to take charge of our disease. But seeing disease and health as subject to human self-determination also means that one's health or the failure to recover from a serious illness can be used as a means of assessing the moral worth and value of human beings.

Technology also has had a role in the emergence of health and disease as central cultural concerns in the Western world. As nineteenth-century science, especially under the influence of Darwinism, began to diminish the boundaries that had made human beings seem special, unique or distinctive, medicine became more willing to treat human beings as possible objects for scientific scrutiny and technologically based interventions.

Throughout this century, particularly in the era since the end of World War II, technology has come to play an increasingly important role in health care. This is reflected in the emphasis of many modern health-care delivery systems on the treatment of acute medical problems in hospital settings. The proliferation of neonatal units, computed tomography (CT) scanners, ultrasound, laproscopy, and organ and tissue transplants is a re- flection of our collective faith in the power of technology and the belief that it can be used to identify and control the evils of disease and disabil- ity. Technology has reified health and disease; it has made it seem as if diseases are real entities in the world that can be observed, identified, manipulated, and eliminated.

Before World War I, there was relatively little that physicians or any- one else could do to combat the effects of acute disease and severe disability. The introduction of antibiotics, vaccines, and transfusions in the decades after the war transformed medicine from a profession focused on diagnosis and caring to one with a serious interest in curing. The expectations of physi- cians and patients have grown considerably in the ensuing decades and, as a result, the desire to be returned to a state of health after the onset of dis- ease or injury now seems more a matter of finding a competent professional than it does a matter for hopes, wishes, and prayers.

Particular political and social values place a special premium on health and the avoidance of disease. Health and the alleviation of disease and dis- ability have key roles to play in highly competitive, capitalist societies. Soci- eties committed to free-market economics can tolerate significant differences in the resources and status held by individual citizens. Such differences can be accepted, however, only if there is general acceptance of the means by which resources are acquired and held. A concern for equality of opportu- nity in economic life in many countries leads inevitably to the assignment of great weight to the preservation of health and the prevention of disease and disability.

The moral assessment of inequalities of power, possessions, and prop- erty is contingent on the view that prevails of the opportunities that have preceded the creation of inequities in the distribution of social goods. If some people are rich because they work hard and others are poor because they are lazy, then so be it. As long as a relative equality of opportunity exists, as long as the initial conditions for competing economically are seen as fair, any differences that result are easier to accept on moral grounds.

If equality of opportunity is a critical moral component of the legal, political, and societal norms of free-market societies, health and disease will be accorded special status. Those who are born with congenital defor- mities and those who suffer from disabling or chronic diseases, especially if they are infants or children, cannot be said to have an equal opportu- nity to compete with their peers for the goods and benefits that a com- petitive society makes available. The alleviation of disease and disability and the promotion of health are important political and cultural goals for the same reasons special priority is given to the provision of basic education, shelter, and food. All these factors influence the extent to which equality can legitimately be said to exist with respect to opportunities and, therefore, to the extent to which the inequalities that result from a free-market approach to the distribution of social resources can be viewed as morally palatable.

Disease and disability have become objects of concern in Western society because they are seen as a threats to equal opportunity and, in turn, to the moral foundation of economic life. The reductions in abilities and capacities that usually accompany diseases are threatening not only because they cause intrinsic harms to those beset by them but also because they undermine the social commitment to the equity of competition and the fairness of the market as efficient methods for distributing social resources. Despite the fact that it may be expensive to redress the effects of disease or to prevent its occurrence, if fundamental inequities exist among people because of serious but remediable differences in their health and well-being, this is a state of affairs that is incompatible with a socioeconomic orientation that seeks to reward striving, performance, and individual achievement. Economics plays a major role in thrusting the concepts of health and disease center stage in developed nations that are organized around competitive markets.

HEALTH, DISEASE, AND THE SCOPE OF MEDICINE

If it is true that health and disease play powerful roles in filling important gaps left by the secularization of public culture and in legitimizing key presuppositions of prevailing socioeconomic arrangements in Western societies, it is obvious why so much attention has centered in recent decades on their meaning and definition. The definitions accorded these concepts play pivotal roles in establishing the boundaries of access to the health-care system, the limits of medical concern and professional control, and also social obligation to share in the burden of alleviating disease, disability, and dysfunction.

Prima facie obligations exist for government to correct the inequalities wrought by disease and illness. Thus, the definition of these terms is more than a philosophical exercise. The answer to the question of what does or does not constitute a disease determines not only how much authority and power are available to those responsible for alleviating the consequences of disease—physicians, nurses, public health officials, social workers, and other health-care professionals—but what government must do to shift resources toward those with special needs resulting from ill health to make economic and social life fair.

There has been much concern on the part of a variety of social commentators and ethicists from both ends of the political spectrum about the

growing power and influence of medicine and other health-care professions in our society. Conservatives worry, for example, that physicians,
nurses, and psychologists will introduce adolescent students to permissive
attitudes toward sexual conduct in the guise of promoting "health" education. Liberals fear that the classification of homosexuality as a disease
rather than a matter of personal behavioral preference or biological
necessity will result in discriminatory treatment of homosexuals and the
promotion of negative stereotypes. The definitions of health, disease, and
illness are seen by many as political issues that require input from both
professionals and laypersons.

Physicians are able to control access to a wide variety of social and economic resources by the use of their authority as gatekeepers of eligibility for
a wide spectrum of public and private programs. Getting a job, receiving life
insurance, receiving permission to immigrate, gaining admission to school,
entering and exiting the armed services, having access to legal compensation, being exculpated from punishment, being able to marry, have children,
and raise a family are all controlled to some extent by physicians and other
health-care professionals. Similarly, decisions about who will or will not be
forced to receive medical care in hospital or institutional settings, who is or
is not free to refuse medication or confinement, and what is or is not an acceptable form of medical treatment are controlled by physicians and other
health-care personnel.

Physicians and other health-care providers not only have the authority to enfranchise some members of society with social benefits or privileges,
they also have the authority to excuse behavior that, without medical ex-
culpation, might be the object of police, judicial, or penal attention. Many
groups have fought long and hard to have particular behavioral dispositions
labeled as diseases. Alcoholics, gamblers, and persons with attention deficits
or chronic fatigue are but a few who have lobbied persistently to have their
conditions labeled diseases. The label of disease excuses certain behavior that
might otherwise be viewed as criminal, sinful, or lazy and thus be subject to
various forms of sanction.

Conversely, many groups, such as homosexuals, the obese, and the deaf,
have struggled to free themselves from being categorized as ill or diseased.
Disease labels, while often exculpatory in terms of liability or responsibility,
carry other burdens, such as the stigma attached to illness and the assumption that persons who are ill or diseased require treatment and cure from
legitimate experts.

If the scope and domain of medicine and the related healing arts are
to be accurately delineated, a clear understanding of the concepts of
health and disease is a necessity. The definitions that are given to these
concepts are critical for understanding the possibilities and limits of health
care and for understanding the moral obligations, rights, and responsibilities that ought to prevail between patients and providers in health-care
contexts.

THE RELATIONSHIP BETWEEN THE CONCEPTS
OF HEALTH, ILLNESS, AND DISEASE

What is the nature of the logical relationship between health, illness, and disease? Many health-care professionals and much of the general public appear to view health and disease as logical opposites; illness and disease are often used as synonyms. When asked if they are healthy or feel well, most people answer affirmatively if they are not suffering from any particular disease or disorder at the time the question is asked. Looked at uncritically, health would seem to be no more than the absence of disease and illness. Disease and illness appear to connote any impairment in a person's sense of well-being or fitness.

But there are powerful reasons for questioning the appropriateness of viewing health and disease merely as conceptual opposites and disease and illness as synonyms. Even if no particular disease is present, it is still possible to say that a person seems healthier or is healthier in certain ways than in others. The average marathon runner or professional athlete is probably healthier, with respect to overall physical well-being, than the average philosophy professor, even if neither happens to be afflicted with a specific disease at the time the comparison is made. Health seems to require the absence of disease or illness as a necessary condition. But it is not clear that this absence is, by itself, sufficient to define the nature of health.

The possibility that health is not simply the absence of disease or illness but refers to something more is reinforced by the activities of some contemporary health-care practitioners. Some see their job as more than simply the alleviation of disease. Psychoanalysts, plastic surgeons, nutritionists, and sports physiologists are interested not only in the prevention or alleviation of disease, but also, and perhaps sometimes only, the promotion of health. If health and disease were logically related to one another as contradictory concepts, it would be impossible to make any sense of the ideas expressed by such terms as "maximize health" or "positive mental health." These ideas, as well as the notion that relative degrees of health can exist even in the absence of disease or illness, appear to be meaningful and coherent.

Not only is the absence of disease not sufficient to establish the existence of health, diseases do not always impair or threaten health. Some diseases are unpleasant and disabling but do not compromise the health of the individual who has them. For example, enduring a short bout of measles or mumps during childhood, either through infection or inoculation, may actually be conducive to health. A person can be riddled with cancer, be delusional, or suffer from hypertension but remain entirely unaware of any symptoms or dysfunction. A person who is the carrier of the sickle-cell trait, although prone to certain problems under certain rare circumstances, is better protected against malaria than someone lacking this genetic endowment.

The fact that one can be functioning well and feel healthy while suffering from a disease also hints that the concepts of illness and disease may actually refer to different states or conditions. Feeling sick is not the same as having a disease; a person can be ill but not diseased and diseased but not feel ill.

Some behaviors that are viewed as diseases—gambling, homosexuality, hyperactivity, or drug addiction—have tenuous logical connections to the concept of health. Certainly it is much less difficult to obtain agreement across social classes and different cultures about the states of the mind and body that constitute diseases than it is to secure agreement about which states are to be viewed as healthy. The use of addictive narcotic drugs and their relationship to health is viewed quite differently in Jamaica, Holland, Bolivia, and Peru than it is in the United States, Singapore, or Saudi Arabia.

Although the view of health and disease as conceptual opposites may be widely accepted, there are reasons for calling this presumption into question. A strong case can be made for the view that the logical relationship between health and disease is not one of contradiction. The conceptual opposite of health might more reasonably be seen as unhealthy and the logical contradictory of diseased as nondiseased. Health and disease may exist as parallel concepts rather than as concepts defined only in terms of one another. Disease may be among the criteria used to define health, but other measures or states may be necessary to attribute this state to an individual.

NORMATIVISM VERSUS NONNORMATIVISM IN THE DEFINITION OF DISEASE

Perhaps the major point of contention among philosophers, physicians, and other health-care experts who have examined the meaning of health and disease is the extent to which value judgments are requisite for or are implicit in the definitions of these concepts. Many physicians and philosophers believe that there is no need to resort to considerations of value in general or morality in particular to identify, understand, or analyze the concepts of health, illness, and disease. Those who subscribe to nonnormativism believe that determinations of health and disease are matters of empirical fact and nothing more.

One of the ways in which the case for assigning a key role to values in the definition of health and disease is made by those who espouse the contrary view, normativism, is to observe that categories of disease vary from culture to culture and historical period to historical period. Moreover, what is supposed to be the same disease or the same state of health can produce very different experiences in different people.

Granted, not everyone has the same experience with disease. One common way of responding is to use the term illness to refer to the subjective perception or the phenomenological experience of disease. If anxiety causes some individuals to hyperventilate but causes a tightening sensation in the chest of others and a headache in still other persons, the wide range of symptoms, responses, and experiences can be captured by the term illness.

Illness is by definition subjective and thus specific to time, place, and culture. Variations in illness are to be expected. It seems beyond dispute that illness, defined only as the experience of health or disease, is heavily influenced by the prevailing values and norms of a given society. Indeed, those who wish to defend the view that health and disease can be defined in purely objective terms without reference to values are more than willing to concede the historical and sociological findings of those such as Foucault, Szasz, Sedgwick, and Canguilhem that disease is irremediably a product of culture, economics, and ideology. But, by segregating the perception of disease and the response a disease elicits in a particular individual living in a particular society under the rubric of illness, those who seek a nonnormative definition hope to be able to find univocal meanings for disease (and sometimes for health) that transcend the specifics of time, place, and person.

What is at stake in the battle over the role played by values is the objectivity of claims about disease and health. If values play crucial roles in shaping the meanings of illness and of health and disease, it appears as if the prospects for objectivity in medicine and health care, which depend on these concepts, are imperiled. If values infuse the analysis of disease, diseases seem to be a product of human invention. Diseases seem to be categories imposed by human beings on human beings, not states that humans possess and that can be discovered by anyone who has learned the criteria and evidence requisite to make a diagnosis. The greater the role of values in the definition of health and disease, the worse the prognosis appears to be for both their objectivity and reality. Ideology and politics loom especially large in the classification of human behaviors and states as indicative of health or disease to the extent to which values appear because values, unlike empirical facts, are seen as very much a product of social forces. If disease and health are matters of ideology and politics, the prospects for an objective, verifiable, science of medicine seem diminished, if not hopeless.

The clearest contemporary expression of the view that health and disease can be defined without explicit reference to moral values or ethical norms has been offered by the American philosopher Christopher Boorse. He argues that although it is true that different social, ethnic, and economic groups do not agree on the reference class of the terms health and disease, and that it is also true that professionals often disagree about the disease status of a particular condition or behavior, it would be wrong to conclude from such facts that an objective definition of health or disease that does not rely on values is impossible to attain.

Boorse contends that although different people or groups disagree about the specific application of a disease definition to particular cases, nothing in their disagreement disproves the possibility of locating an objective, value-free definition of disease. Illness is often subjective and variable. Disease need not be.

All organisms, including humans, are the product of a long course of biological evolution. Human evolution has been driven by a wide variety of environmental demands that have conferred advantages on creatures possessing certain phenotypic and genotypic traits. Because our minds and bodies have evolved in response to our evolutionary past, health consists in our functioning in conformity with our natural design as determined by natural selection.

If kidneys exist as a result of evolving in response to the contingent forces of natural selection, so that their function is to remove impurities from the body, if hearts evolved to pump blood to organs and tissues, if external ears evolved to allow the localization of sound, then in any human (or in any other organism) who has kidneys, heart, or ears, health consists, in part, in having a kidney that removes impurities from the blood, a heart that pumps blood to organs and tissues, and ears that can localize sounds. These organs were designed by evolution to perform such functions, and when they do so, the organism that possesses them can be said to be healthy. If the organs perform especially well, regardless of why that is so, the person who has the organs can be said to have a very healthy heart or an especially sound pair of kidneys.

If there is some failure in an organ system, if it loses the capacity to perform the function for which it was designed by evolution to perform, the condition is indicative of disease, regardless of whether it is perceived as illness. Natural design permits an analysis of health or disease independent of the experience of the person. Illness, but not disease, is in the mind of the beholder. Values need not enter into the definition of the concepts of health and disease because the goals that drive evolution have nothing to do with ethics, morals, ideology, sociology, or values.

Evolution places a premium on survival and reproduction. Survival and reproduction are the only goals that matter for evolution. To attain these goals, all organisms, including humans, have evolved traits that increase their probability of survival and the transmission of genes to the next generation. Organisms that lacked the genotypes and phenotypes requisite for survival and reproduction became extinct; only organisms with traits adequate for survival and reproduction exist today.

Disease can be defined as any impairment of the functions typical of a particular biological species—functions required to achieve the natural goals set, not by politics or culture, but by the twin demands of survival and reproduction. Are concepts such as survival and reproduction themselves value-laden? Neither of these terms is used in any moralistic or evaluative sense—survival and reproduction are merely the contingent by-products of a Darwinian system responding to a specific set of historical circumstances. There is nothing intrinsically good or bad about them—they merely exist.

If one accepts the view that the goals of survival and reproduction have guided the evolution of every living organism on this planet, health and disease can be understood solely in terms of the causal contributions various states, conditions, and behaviors make to the achievement of these ends. No resort to ethics or any other sort of value judgment is necessary. All that must be done is to determine whether the causal contribution of a particular trait or behavior is positive or negative in terms of the overall capacity of a particular organism to achieve its biologically designed ends. The extent to which this is so determines whether the trait or behavior is classified as healthy or diseased.

An especially persuasive argument that values need play no role in the definitions of health and disease is that a nonnormative analysis works as well for assessing the health status of plants and animals as it does for humans. Veterinarians know what it means for a cat or a pig to be sick. Few would want to argue that, before they could say that an animal was sick or dying, they must resort to an examination of the animal's mores or understand the animal's values!

HEALTH AS NORMALITY, DISEASE AS ABNORMALITY

Nonnormativism, the position that disease can be defined without reference to anything other than the empirical assessment of functions based solely on the understanding of the purposes the functions were designed to serve, is closely related to the definitions of health and disease used in contemporary medical texts. Many physicians, if pressed to define health and disease, respond that disease is anything that is abnormal, and health is what is normal.

Normal and abnormal refer to statistical normalcy, not any sort of value judgment about a particular state or behavior. The unusual, the uncommon, and the extreme become candidates for classification as disease. States and behaviors that cluster around the mean or for which there is relatively small variance become the reference class of health.

The statistical concept of health and disease has prevailed in Western medicine for many, many decades. It is a legacy of the ancient theory of "humours" and the more modern concepts of balance or homeostasis that have grounded thinking about health and disease for many centuries. Health for thinkers as diverse as Galen of Pergamum, William Cullen, and Walter B. Cannon consisted of the attainment of a balance or harmony in the workings of the body. Deviations or abnormalities in the composition of bodily fluids or, in later times, of organ systems, connoted disease.

Physicians often equate abnormal measures of blood pressure, blood chemistry, or body weight with disease, regardless of whether dysfunction or pain are present. The primary problem with the attempt to establish a value-free definition of both health and disease, however, is that anything unusual is considered a disease state even when it is not at all clear why it is unhealthy to be abnormal. It seems conceptually bizarre to say that the unusually tall, intelligent, strong, fast, or agile are diseased simply because of their abnormality or deviance from the norm. Those at the extremes of the distribution of any state, trait, or behavior would by definition, therefore, be diseased—an analysis that seems too inclusive and at the same time indifferent to historical attempts to connect difference with dysfunction.

The problem raised by the advantages conferred by some forms of statistical deviancy for the statistical approach to the definition of health and disease is serious. Abnormality is an indication that something may be wrong, but it does not seem, by itself, to constitute disease. If a value-free view of these concepts is to be found, it would seem that the attempt to root disease and health in a functional analysis, perhaps on the basis of the recognition that human beings are biological organisms that have evolved to meet the challenges of a shifting set of environmental demands, has the best chance of succeeding.

PROPONENTS OF NORMATIVISM

Normativists believe that health and disease are concepts that are inherently value-laden. They believe that to understand exactly what these concepts mean or refer to requires one to realize that decisions have to be made about states of the body or mind, and that the decisions must involve considerations of what is desirable or undesirable, useful or useless, good or bad. Normativists argue that no matter how many descriptive facts are known about the body or about the functions of a particular cell or organ system, it is impossible to decide whether a particular state of affairs represents health or disease without some reference to values.

Historically, the primary focus of philosophical attention on the part of physicians and others interested in health care has been the concept of disease. If disease could be adequately defined and interpreted, it was believed that all other questions about the aims, goals, and purposes of health care would be resolved.

Normativism is sometimes confused with alternative forms of healing. Although there are some exponents of normativism in the ranks of those who espouse holistic health or alternative forms of medical intervention such as spiritual or psychic healing, most normativists are only concerned to defend the position that values form an irreducible element in the definition of disease.

Perhaps the clearest illustrations of the ways in which values influence the definition of health and disease emerge from the realm of mental health and mental illness. A cursory glance at nineteenth-century U.S. medical texts reveals that some physicians asserted with all of the authority at their disposal that women who enjoyed sexual intercourse or engaged in masturbation were certainly afflicted with various forms of mental illness and often a variety of corresponding physical ailments as well. Textbooks of the era were replete with diseases of the mind that seemed to afflict only black men and women in astounding numbers. One of the most omnipresent disorders of the day was a condition labeled drapetomania, a horrible plague that denoted an obsessive desire on the part of a slave to run away from his or her owner.

Normativists are much impressed with illustrations of the ways in which values and cultural prejudices tacitly or overtly influence medical determinations of health and disease. They point to contemporary disputes about the disease status of such conditions as homosexuality, premenstrual syndrome, and infertility and ask how anyone could possibly conclude that labeling some particular physical or mental state as diseased or healthy involves nothing more than an empirical assessment of biological functioning.

Both historical and contemporary cases of shifts in beliefs or uncertainties as to the proper classification of various conditions make it clear that values play an inextricable but entirely appropriate role in defining health and disease. Moreover, as normativists point out, a key element of the definition of disease is that the states of the body and mind viewed as diseases in various cultures are so viewed only as a result of the fact that people disvalue them. For example, in a society burdened with overpopulation, infertility might be viewed as a healthy state. In a society wealthy enough to provide financial support for all newborns and biases toward large families, infertility might be seen as a disease state meriting serious attempts at amelioration through surgical or pharmacological intervention.

One of the boldest attempts to formulate a normative definition of disease, which highlights the valuational dimension of this concept, is that of the psychiatrist Charles Culver and the philosopher Bernard Gert. Culver and Gert assert that the core meaning of disease involves the recognition that something is wrong with a person. They claim that diseases are actually a subcategory of a more general category, which they call "maladies." The members of this category include diseases and also injuries, disabilities, and death itself. Culver and Gert believe that what is common to all these conditions is that humans universally view the conditions as evils—people disvalue these states and try to avoid them if they can.

Unlike most nonnormative analyses of health and disease, which view disease and health in terms of deviations from statistical normalcy or from various norms of species–typical functioning, Culver and Gert's position is that it is not dysfunction but the perceived evil associated with dysfunction that is at the heart of understanding the meaning of disease. For instance, in the case of a myocardial infarction, it is not the deviation from normal functioning that makes us classify this event as a disease. Rather, it is the loss of capacities, the onset of pain, and the risk to life itself (the evils associated with this dysfunction) that lead to the disvaluation of this particular deviation from functional normality.

Although the members of different cultural groups or societies may not always agree on what constitutes an evil, every society recognizes certain states of mind or body as evils to be avoided. People may not always agree on the identities of the mental or physical states that represent evils, but they all recognize that a loss of abilities, a loss of freedom, a loss of pleasure, or pain and death are evils. Malady thus has the apparent advantage of unifying what may initially appear to be disparate states such as pain, injury, and death by allowing them to be grouped under the common criterion of states of the body or mind that people disvalue as evils.

A weakness in the normative approach to the analysis of disease is that it makes the status of disease depend on the willingness of the members of society to recognize a particular state of affairs as evil. Those with hypertension may not feel any loss of capacity, but the physician operating with a nonnormative sense of proper physiological functioning can say that disease is present, even if the patient does not. Similarly, a culture that has no written traditions may be unaware and unconcerned about the presence of dyslexia in some of its members. But a psychologist studying the group may be aware that a nondisvalued abnormal condition is present and may wish to intervene to modify the problem so that such a person could learn to read should the person move into another society.

NORMATIVISM VERSUS NONNORMATIVISM— WHAT IS REALLY AT ISSUE?

The debate about the role played by values in the definition of health and disease may appear to be nothing more than an abstract philosophical controversy having few if any consequences for either the clinical practice of health care or the formulation of health policy. However, once the underlying concerns motivating the debate are made clear, it can readily be seen that what is at issue are understandings about the aims of medicine and the scientific status of its practices.

Normativists and nonnormativists are equally concerned with supplying a definition of health and disease that is capable of roughly capturing our intuitions about what ought be classified as disease and who ought to be viewed as healthy. But those offering definitions are also concerned with providing a definition that can help classify ambiguous states of the body or mind or resolve uncertainty where disagreements exist as to the proper classification of a condition as a matter of health or disease.

Aside from the aesthetic appeal of living in a world in which conceptual matters admit of neat and tidy resolutions, there are important reasons for undertaking these definitional efforts. Unless medicine and other health-care professions use definitions of disease and health that are clear and univocal, there is a grave danger that uncertainties will exist on the part of both health-care providers and patients as to the aims, goals, expectations, and hopes they bring to medical encounters. If health and disease are nothing more than socially determined, culturally mediated, and individually subjective concepts, there is some fear that there will be little possibility of placing medicine on a firm scientific footing or of finding consensus among experts and patients about the proper limits of medical concern.

If one doubts that judgments of value are in any way objective, the presence of values in the definition of health and disease make it impossible for health care and medical science to rest on an objective and universal foundation. If, on the other hand, value judgments are seen as amenable to objective, reasoned argument, their presence in the definitions of health and disease do nothing to undermine the objectivity or scientific prospects of medicine and health care.

Why should values and objectivity or even consensus be presumed to be incompatible? If it is possible to obtain agreement among rational human beings that some states of the body or mind are valuable and desirable, but others are not, it ought to be possible to accord an explicit role to values in the definition of disease and health without sacrificing objectivity, precision, or universality. Because among both patients and health-care providers there would seem to be no lack of agreement that, under ordinary circumstances, life is preferable to death, ability is preferable to disability, and pleasure is more desirable than pain, those committed to normativism would appear to have some grounds for optimism that an objective foundation can be found on which to rest value-laden definitions of both health and disease. The foundation may be more difficult to establish for some conditions or states than for others (is it better to be born with the capacity to develop large or small breasts?), but the goods and evils that bring people into the health-care system and motivate others to want to practice the art and science of health care, seem to be a rough area within which consensus can be reached about what is good and what is bad and, therefore, about what is health and what is disease.

The controversy over normativism and nonnormativism, which has occupied center stage in recent thinking about health, illness, and disease, may be more illusory than real. If the motivation for the controversy is fear of the subjective nature of values, it may be possible to defuse the debate by noting that it is possible to achieve agreement and consensus about values as well as about facts. If this position is acceptable, it may be possible to define disease as disvalued dysfunction defined in terms of both human goals and the design of the human body (and the human mind, to the extent to which this can be known). Health would become a valued form of functioning, optimal or maximal, in certain systems or tissues. The extent to which values are seen as a source of difficulty for objectivity in the definition of health and disease will determine the degree to which one's sympathies lie in the normativist or nonnormativist camps.

DISCUSSION QUESTIONS

1. The World Health Organization defines health as total physical, mental, and social well-being. Does that make health the absence of disease? If so, what are the implications for deciding who has authority to make decisions affecting people's health?

2. Is health appropriately limited to physical well-being, or does it also include other dimensions? Are economic, educational, social, and spiritual well-being part of what is meant by health? If so, are professional counselors in these areas health professionals? Do physicians have responsibility for these dimensions of well-being or only for organic well-being? Is mental well-being part of the health professional's responsibility, or is it the task of a separate, caring profession?

3. Is it more important for medicine to focus on curing disease, or is it equally important to promote and preserve health? If a drug were available that would improve intelligence, would it be more ethical to use that drug to improve the intelligence of a severely retarded person rather than someone who was already mentally normal? If so, why?

4. To what extent is one making an ethical or other evaluative choice when one calls a condition a disease? Are there some conditions that are diseases simply because they are statistically unusual?

5. Is it possible to determine what constitutes health by analyzing what constitutes the normal functioning of members of the species? If so, would different assessments have to be made for persons of different ages? Of different genders? If not, is there any scientific way of determining that a person is sick or well?

FOR FURTHER READING

Useful discussions of the way in which values have shaped the understanding of disease can be found in Ronald Bayer's *Homosexuality and American Psychology: The Politics of Diagnosis*, New York: Basic Books, 1981. Two other especially illuminating sources as to the interaction of values and the concepts of health and disease are Thomas Szasz, *The Myth of Mental Illness*, New York: Harper-Hoeber, 1961; and Michel Foucault, *Madness and Civilization*, Tavistock, 1965. The topic is also examined in many of the chapters of Arthur L. Caplan's *Moral Matters: Ethical Issues in Medicine and the Life Sciences*, New York: John Wiley & Sons, 1995.

A historical overview of debates about the definition of health and disease is presented in the anthology, *The Concepts of Health and Disease*, edited by Arthur Caplan, H. Tristram Engelhardt, and James McCartney, San Francisco: Benjamin Cummings, 1981. The clearest exposition of the view that values play no role in the definition of disease can be found in two papers by Christopher Boorse, "On the Distinction Between Disease and Illness," *Philosophy and Public Affairs* 5:49–68, 1975; and "What a Theory of Mental Health Should Be," *Philosophy of Science* 44:542–573, 1976. Arguments for the value-laden character of these concepts are presented in Henry E. Sigerist's classic work, *Civilization and Disease*, Chicago: University of Chicago Press, 1943; Peter Sedgwick, *Psychopolitics*, New York: Harper & Row, 1982; and in Edmund D. Pellegrino and David C. Thomasma, *For the Patient's Good*, New York: Oxford, 1988.

Useful analyses of the role played by the concepts of health and disease in explanations in medicine can be found in *Philosophy in Medicine* by Charles M. Culver and Bernard Gert, New York: Oxford, 1982; and Henrik R. Wulff, Stig Andur Pedersen, and Raben Rosenberg, *Philosophy of Medicine*, 2nd. ed., Boston: Blackwell, 1990. Lawrie Resnek gives an especially insightful analysis of the ontological status of disease in *The Nature of Disease*, New York: Routledge and Kegan Paul, 1987.

4

The Physician–Patient Relationship

HOWARD BRODY

SUMMARY

The physician–patient relationship prompts many basic questions in medical ethics. Under the medical ethic popular before the 1960s, physicians usually placed the moral principle of benefiting the patient (according to the physicians' own view of benefit) on a higher plane than the moral principle of respect for the patient's autonomy. This led to many medical practices now felt to be improperly paternalistic. Medicine today is dominated by a new ethic in which respect for autonomy occupies a central place, and a new model of the physician–patient relationship, a contractual model, moves in the direction of recognizing the greater emphasis placed on autonomy as a moral principle.

The contractual model, in turn, has come under criticism as a flawed or incomplete description of the ethically ideal relationship. To replace or to expand the contractual model, some have proposed contractarian approaches or more explicit discussions of power. Others have tried to elaborate more carefully what respect for autonomy actually requires of the physician. And others have turned to an ethic of virtues, instead of principles or rules, as a guide.

Three additional problems in medical ethics relate directly to the physician–patient relationship—the physician's duty to disclose truthful information; the physician's duty to maintain confidentiality; and the challenges to the physician–patient relationship posed by new economic arrangements in medical practice.

Acknowledgment: Tom Tomlinson, Kenneth Howe, Leonard Fleck, and Robert Veatch made helpful suggestions for revising an earlier draft of this chapter. Tom Tomlinson provided Case 4.2.

What is a chapter about the physician–patient relationship supposed to accomplish? To answer this question, we need to understand a change that took place in the subject of medical ethics roughly between 1965 and 1970. At the risk of greatly oversimplifying a complex history, I will characterize an "old" medical ethics and a "new" medical ethics. The "old" medical ethics had the following features:

1. Ethics was generally thought of as a list of do's and don'ts for the physician.
2. Ethics was based on professional authority. Physicians would determine their own ethics. Nonphysicians did not know medicine and therefore could have nothing useful to say about medical ethics (Veatch 1979).
3. The primary ethical principle was benefit to the patient. So long as he was serving the patient's welfare, the physician could be justified in deceiving, coercing, and doing other things to the patient that would be impermissible in other human relationships.

This account is, again, historically oversimplified; but it highlights the features of the "new" medical ethics below:

1. Ethics is thought of not merely as a list of rights and duties, but also as the study of the underlying reasons for those rights and duties.
2. People trained in moral reasoning, such as philosophers and theologians, can contribute to the subject. Physicians must be ready to give reasons for their ethical views that nonphysicians would find rational and reasonable. Medical ethics is no longer a privileged, in-house medical matter.
3. Patient benefit is only one moral principle among many. Of special importance is the principle of autonomy, often thought of as the right of self-determination.

Old ethics would have addressed the physician–patient relationship by compiling a list of how doctors should treat patients and vice versa (Benjamin 1985). This was, in fact, the form of the first code of ethics adopted by the American Medical Association in 1848. New medical ethics approaches the physician–patient relationship with a more ambitious aim. We want, for practical guidance, to have some handy lists of rights and duties. But we do not want to accept these simply on the basis of habit or custom. We want an underlying theory of the ethical nature of the relationship, so that the specific rights and duties can be seen as flowing logically from the more basic theory (Veatch 1981). And, in addition, we want that theory to fit well with two different considerations: general ethical theory that is pertinent to other human relationships, and the factual reality of medical practice. We want our underlying view of the physician–patient relationship to be both ethically valid and realistic.

One of the appeals of using the physician–patient relationship as a way to start looking at medical ethics is that a cluster of important ethical issues is linked closely to our understanding of that relationship. Three such issues are taken up later in this chapter—truthful disclosure, confidentiality, and the role of financial gatekeeper. A fourth, informed consent, is the subject of Chapter 7.

The focus on the physician–patient relationship suggests that our ethical inquiry is directed at the therapeutic practice of medicine. Physicians do many other things that do not involve relationships with patients—public health and medical research are two examples. The other activities raise different sorts of ethical issues. Ethical issues arising in a health-team setting, where many professionals work together, are not part of our focus, even though the ethically sound team–patient relationship may closely resemble the physician–patient relationship described here. Although studies of the physician–patient relationship by medical psychologists and medical sociologists (Bloom 1963; Parsons 1978) may be useful and informative, their purpose is descriptive; our approach here is normative. The use of the term *physician*–patient relationship suggests that although nurses and other health professionals may consider the same moral principles when determining how they ought to relate to their patients or clients, their exact role responsibilities may differ from that of the physicians.

PATERNALISM AND CONTRACTUAL MODELS

Old medical ethics had a *paternalistic* view of the physician–patient relationship. The nature of paternalism has been discussed in great detail (Buchanan 1978; Gert and Culver 1976, 1979). We use a definition by James Childress (1982): Paternalism is refusing to acquiesce in the wishes or desires of another person for that person's own benefit. When we acquiesce in somebody else's wishes or desires, we recognize the moral principle of autonomy— that a person is entitled to make free choices. When we act paternalistically, we place the moral principle of benefiting that person (according to our view of benefit) on a higher plane than the moral principle of autonomy (Beauchamp and McCullough 1984).

Even before the era of new medical ethics, paternalism in medicine was sometimes viewed with skepticism. Szasz and Hollender (1956) proposed early models for physician–patient relationships. They suggested a range of possible relationships from an extreme of total paternalism on one end to equal and mutual participation on the other and argued that each model had utility for specific medical circumstances. (Obviously a mutual participation model does not work for a patient in a coma, for instance.) But, to the critics who launched the new medical ethics, the old physician–patient relationship was too dependent on a paternalistic stance and offered too few opportunities for alternatives. These critics sought to base an alternative to paternalism on a sound underlying theory, not just on an unreflective distaste for paternalistic behavior. A possible way of establishing an underlying theory led to a label for this approach to the physician–patient relationship—the *contractual model*.

This label was fruitful for philosophers because of an analogy with a similar concept in the history of Western political philosophy, social contract theory (Masters 1975). The "old" political theory stressed the divine right of kings; subjects were supposed to accept the established order and not object to the authority of their "betters"; the free consent or participation of citizens in political affairs played no part in establishing the legitimacy of the ruling system. By the time of the Enlightenment, such a theory seemed intolerably demeaning to the emerging idea of the dignity of the individual. Thus, philosophers began to explore an alternative theory of government, which relied explicitly on the idea of the free consent of the governed. People were viewed as having a choice to either remain outside of government altogether or else agree freely among themselves on ground rules for a just and decent state. By the social contract approach, to argue that a particular form of government is just is to argue that, hypothetically, people would have been willing to choose freely that form of government rather than remain without any form of government at all. And presumably they would choose to do so only if that government respected their most basic and important human rights.

Similarly, old medical ethics might be seen as a system in which the patient's free consent counted for nothing. By the old theory, doctors could appropriately dictate to patients for a variety of reasons—the traditions of the medical profession, the individual physician's commitment to protect the well-being of patients, and the helplessness and dependency that sickness can produce in the sick individual. If this theory and its paternalistic implications are insufficiently respectful to the patient's rights and dignity, an obvious alternative is to ask what sort of relationship parties might freely and rationally consent to, assuming that they were placed in a position of equal power at the beginning. We can first look at the outlines of a contractual model of the physician–patient relationship and then the list of rights and duties implied by a contractual model.

An influential early description of a contractual model was provided by Veatch (1972), who reviewed four possible models to govern the physician–patient relationship in evolving contemporary society. He rejected three of them. The Priestly Model was basically the old model of physician paternalism. The Engineering Model gave full decision-making power to the patient and reduced the physician to the role of technician. The Collegial Model assumed shared decision making in which the physician and patient were regarded as equals on all counts.

The remaining model, the Contractual Model, admitted differential decision-making capacity but respected both parties, physician and patient, as free moral agents with their own goals and interests. By this model, the physician would take responsibility for all purely technical decisions of the sort for which one is specifically prepared by medical training. The patient would retain control over decisions that involved personal moral values or lifestyle preferences. For example, in deciding the treatment of a newly discovered breast cancer that has not yet spread, the physician would decide the relative risks and benefits of a modified radical mastectomy as opposed to mere removal of the lump followed by radiation therapy. But the patient would ultimately decide which surgery to have on the basis of the impact of those risks and benefits on her own life preferences and goals. The physician might be competent to say, for instance, that the 5-year survival rate for mastectomy would be 15 percent better than that for lumpectomy in this particular sort of tumor; but only the patient could decide whether it was *worth it to her* to give up a breast to gain that extra 15-percent chance.

The Contractual Model envisions a process of information exchange and negotiation between the two parties as various decisions are encountered. It also includes the possibility that the patient may freely delegate some decision-making power back to the physician ("I'm confused by all these facts, Doctor. What do *you* think I ought to do?").

The Contractual Model can be fleshed out by listing some of the patient rights (and corresponding physician duties) that someone negotiating this sort of "contract" would be likely to include. Fried (1974), in trying to explain what might be meant by "personal care," stated that a patient in this sort of ethical relationship should be regarded as having four "rights in personal care." Fried listed them as *lucidity* (the right to a full disclosure of pertinent information); *autonomy* (the right to be regarded as a self-determining agent, to be consulted in one's own care); *fidelity* (the right to continuing service aimed toward one's own interests and the rejection of possible conflicting interests); and *humanity* (the right to be treated with compassion and to have one's individual uniqueness taken into account). We could view this list as combining key elements of the new medical ethics (lucidity and autonomy) with preservation of the most desirable, nonpaternalistic strengths of the old professional ethics (fidelity and humanity). It is therefore reasonable to argue that a doctor and a patient, viewed as equally powerful contractors, could freely and mutually agree to this list of four rights as defining an ethically acceptable relationship.

In this way, contractual models can provide a nonpaternalistic alternative to old ethics and, in the process, appeal to acceptable moral theory and include respect for the patient as being of equal moral worth despite the physician's superior technical knowledge. But contractual models have been criticized for intrinsic faults.

CRITICISMS OF CONTRACTUAL MODELS

Although few critics of contractual models have attempted to resuscitate the old paternalistic ethic, many have claimed that contractual models have serious deficiencies as a positive account of what the physician–patient relationship should be. Compared with these flaws, the purely negative accomplishment of contractual models—undermining physician paternalism—may be insufficient justification for adopting such models.

One line of criticism is to reconsider the factual and moral assumptions that were thought to support the old ethic, to see whether they yield useful ethical guidance without necessarily forcing one into a paternalistic stance. Perhaps Pellegrino has been most articulate in defending these assumptions by arguing that an ethic of medicine must be based on two features—the act of profession and the fact of illness. The former refers to the historical tradition of the physician's commitment to the welfare of the patient; the latter refers to the patient's dependency and vulnerability in the face of serious illness. From this basis in the historical tradition of medicine (as opposed to a more superficial grounding in present-day consumerism), a more satisfactory and yet still nonpaternalistic medical ethic might emerge (Pellegrino 1979; Pellegrino and Thomasma 1981, 1988).

Contractual models have also been faulted for mistaking certain important but limited features of an ideal physician–patient relationship for the core or essence of the relationship (Siegler 1981). For example, Twiss (1977) argued that a satisfactory ethical account of the physician–patient relationship ought to explain two special features: the needs of the patient as constituting the major criteria for correct decisions and actions; and the importance of the ongoing integrity of the relationship and the fact that a good physician–patient relationship grows over time in such a way that both physician and patient have a greater stake in it and a deeper commitment to it. Contractual models, it could be charged, fail to explain either of these two aspects satisfactorily.

Contractual models have been charged with these specific shortcomings:

1. Contractual models are based on a factually incorrect assumption, as it is generally not the case that a physician and a patient begin their relationship by explicitly negotiating a contract of any sort.
2. Contractual models focus attention on explicitly stated and shared expectations of the patient and the physician and ignore that much of the relationship is based on implicit expectations.
3. Contractual models focus attention on financial aspects of the physician–patient encounter rather than on its deeper ethical content (Masters 1975).
4. Contractual models focus narrowly on rights and neglect equally important moral concepts such as duties and goals (Masters 1975; Siegler 1980).
5. Contractual models envision the physician–patient relationship as a socially isolated dyad, when in fact both physicians and patients are embedded in social systems and reflect this in their behavior (Masters 1975).
6. Contractual models are legalistic. Since contract is more of a legal than an ethical notion, such models would have us replace medical ethics with medical law (Ladd 1979; May 1975).

7. Contractual models focus narrowly on one moral principle, that of respect for patient autonomy, and ignore other important moral principles such as patient benefit and avoidance of harm (Beauchamp and McCullough 1984).

8. Contractual models encourage "minimalist" thinking. Instead of asking, "How may I cultivate and nourish this relationship over the long term for better service to the patient's welfare?" the models encourage the physician to ask, "What's the least I can get away with in the short run without violating any explicit rights of the patient?" (Callahan 1981; May 1975; Siegler 1980).

Some of these criticisms can be quickly brushed aside by referring to the models of Veatch and Fried. It is, for example, readily apparent on sympathetic reading that these models do not assume explicit contracting as the primary mode of interaction, that they allow for implicit as well as explicit expectations, and that they are in no way limited to the fiscal aspects of the relationship. Further, Fried's four rights in personal care make clear that autonomy is only one important principle and that beneficence is specifically encouraged rather than excluded. The minimalist criticisms, however, seem to strike closer to the mark. So long as one's view of oneself as a free, self-interested negotiator is the *primary* moral conception that one brings into a relationship, one is unlikely to "go the extra mile" for the other party in ways likely to make the relationship grow and flourish over time. Thus, May (1975, 1983) suggested that the religious ideal of "covenant" captured the core notion of the physician–patient relationship better than the word "contract."

Another way to respond to these criticisms is to remember what the idea of contracting means in the original philosophical theories from which our current understanding of individual liberty has emerged. Social contract theory, which philosophers have used to test out possible theories of what constitutes a just society, never supposes that people actually negotiate contracts and thereby form a new society from a more primitive state of existence. Rather, the contracting is a purely hypothetical exercise. A social arrangement is argued to be fair if we can imagine a suitable thought experiment, designed so as to guarantee conditions of fairness, and explain how persons in that set of hypothetical circumstances would freely choose to be governed by that social arrangement (Rawls 1971).

It seems possible to apply that model of contract-by-thought-experiment to the physician–patient relationship; if the conditions are specified carefully, one can argue that something very much like Fried's four rights in personal care are precisely the rules that, hypothetically, contractors would freely choose—whether they were looking at the situation as if they were potential patients or potential physicians (Brody 1987). One could call this a contractarian approach to distinguish it from a contractual model in the more limited sense. Even so, this method assumes that the same general approach that can be used to devise *fair* social and political institutions could be used to describe a *fair* relationship between physician and patient. Those who have attacked the contractual model as overly minimalist would insist that we simply miss the whole point if we think that *fairness* is the ultimate test of a good physician–patient relationship.

Possibly a more promising approach is to go back to what was presumed in the development of the contractual model in the first place—to see the problem of the ethical physician–patient relationship as a problem in the responsible use of power when two parties possess power to a very unequal extent. In general, physicians possess power and are supposed to use that power to benefit the patient, but that same power could readily be misdirected so as to cause harm to the patient. Instead of alluding to the responsible use of power elliptically by speaking of autonomy and benefit, one might insist that we should talk directly about the balance of power between physician and patient, what counts as appropriate uses and as abuses of the physician's power, and how to design relationships that allow free rein for appropriate uses while trying to prevent or discourage abuses (Brody 1992).

Yet another modification of a contractual approach is to question what it means to respect patient autonomy. In a very thoughtful study, Emanuel and Emanuel (1992) examined a paternalistic model of the physician–patient relationship and contrasted it with three other models, which they call informative, interpretive, and deliberative. They note that it is not quite correct to say that the paternalistic model dispenses with patient autonomy; instead, it understands patient autonomy in a very limited sense—the patient is expected to assent to what the physician, in the role of guardian, asserts to be best for the patient. They then argue that the other three models involve a gradually expanding and deepening sense of patient autonomy. The informative model (closest to the way many have interpreted the contractual model) understands autonomy as controlling choices over medical care, when a person's values and preferences are simply taken for granted as given. The physician's role is that of competent technical expert and dispassionate educator. The interpretive model envisions the physician as a counselor or adviser. Autonomous behavior, by this model, is not merely to choose medical care according to one's values; it is to understand those values better and to reflect more seriously on them. Going even farther, the deliberative model understands autonomy as moral self-development in relation to medical choices. The physician acts more as a friend or teacher, trying to get the patient to consider alternative values and preferences and perhaps to modify the initial values that would lead to the choice of a different type of medical care. (The ethical physician, in this model, freely uses moral persuasion, but is careful not to cross the line to manipulation or coercion.)

The Emanuels argue that for most physician–patient relationships, the deliberative model represents the ideal. They would therefore criticize the older contractual model (at least, as it often has been understood) as including much too narrow or too limited a sense of what it means for a physician to respect and to promote patient autonomy.

The Emanuels' approach fits nicely with the need to address power explicitly as an ethical variable in the relationship. As the physician moves from the position of technician and information source to that of counselor, advisor, and friend, the physician acquires relatively more power over the relationship, and that power could be abused. But if we respond to the threat of abuse simply by saying, "Physicians should not be counselors, advisors, or friends," we deprive patients of relationships that they find supportive and helpful in most circumstances and that in many cases actually enhance the patients' autonomy. It seems we must look carefully at the various ways in which physicians, while occupying those roles, might abuse power, and we must work to prevent the abuses while retaining the positive aspects of the roles.

CONTRACT VERSUS VIRTUE

Although many criticisms might be turned aside by going from a contractual to a contractarian model, the latter still arises from a particular philosophical tradition in ethics (the social contract approach). If one rejects that entire tradition as being a good system of ethics, one must also reject the contractarian model. Lately, among those interested in ethical theory, this is exactly what some authors have proposed. MacIntyre (1981) has been especially interested in replacing that philosophical tradition with one more like Aristotle's system of ethics, which stressed the idea of virtue.

MacIntyre's arguments are very complex. We can view MacIntyre as contrasting a bottom-line method of applying ethics with an ethics of virtue, which is based much more on ongoing human activity. In *bottom-line ethics*, all that matters is what comes out at the end—how one behaves or what the consequences are. In virtue ethics, the way one does things along the way also matters. To be quite simplistic, bottom-line ethics is only concerned with winning or losing the game, but virtue ethics is also concerned with how one plays the game.

Virtues, as Aristotle saw them, are sorts of excellences in human activity. If we use playing a game as a metaphor, virtue requires learning the rules of the game carefully, developing one's skills and talents over time by careful practice, and using whatever creativity one has eventually to put the stamp of one's individuality on the way the game is played. To really understand virtues, our observation point has to be the way one's life unfolds over an extended period, not how one carries out one specific action.

Smith and Newton (1984) endorse a virtue ethic when they point out that our philosophical tradition has encouraged us to think about the physician–patient relationship only in terms of rules and rights—purely bottom-line thinking. By reducing everything to rules, it is almost as if we thought we could make the relationship "doctor-proof." It is as if we thought one could ignore whether the doctor is a saint, a sinner, a sophisticate, a nerd, a humanitarian, a technician—just get him to follow the rules, and a good doctor–patient relationship will exist. But Smith and Newton feel this is unrealistic; any deep description of the relationship must include some picture of what sort of person the doctor ought to be. And this picture will reveal certain excellences, or virtues, that we ought to expect and promote among physicians. For example, in an ethics of virtue, the quality of sympathy would probably be singled out as a central excellence of the physician's role. But in bottom-line ethics we do not know what to do with sympathy, as it is hard to reduce it to a right or a rule. Bottom-line thinking reduces qualities like sympathy to frosting on the cake instead of seeing them as central excellences.

A virtue-based ethics contributes to our understanding of the physician–patient relationship by focusing attention on integrity and character, which tend to get left out of bottom-line or contractual discussions. In bottom-line ethics, what I do this week is assessed as right or wrong by whether it fits with the rules, rights, duties, or whatever method my ethical theory stipulates to determine the rightness or wrongness of individual actions. What I do next week is assessed the same way, but there is no necessary connection between the two actions. However, according to virtue theory, this is a peculiar and perverted way of looking at human existence and human morality. It is not enough to say that we desire, as moral people, to follow the rules. This may be fully sufficient if somebody is going to have very limited contact with us and simply expects predictable and appropriate behavior in that one instance. But it is insufficient if we are going to look at our lives as a whole. "He followed the rules" is not what most of us would want our friends to say about us after we die. Instead, we would like our friends to see a life that was connected, that made sense as a whole. We would like to think that the ideals and values we felt most strongly about would be revealed to anyone who took the time to look at how we lived our lives over time. We feel most proud of ourselves when our actions, over time, steadfastly adhere to our values, and we feel least proud when we deviate from those values simply because some individual act is the easy thing to do at the time. Looked at this way, "living a life" can be seen as something quite different and more basic to our human identity than "following the rules" or "exercising our rights" (Drane 1988).

A virtue model of the physician–patient relationship would ask what sort of character an ideal physician ought to have, and what virtues or excellences go to make up that character (Shelp 1985). It would also view the relationship as growing and evolving in such a way that no set of rules set out at the beginning could fully determine its future (an idea similar to "covenant," as argued by May in 1975 and Twiss in 1977). If the relationship is to grow, both physician and patient must find rewards in seeking a common goal, which must be centered on the patient's welfare. And, as the patient grows older and perhaps moves into different social settings, what that welfare consists of may change and the relationship will have to be altered to take this into account. For the relationship to grow and be nurtured in this way, Smith and Newton (1984) suggest that "dialogue" is one critical feature it must include. To keep the relationship going and to keep it focused on the common goal, the physician and patient will have to exchange information in a regular and explicit way. It will not do for each person to assume that he or she can read the other's mind. And it will not do to reduce communication to a cold and legalistic catalogue of medical facts, options, risks, and benefits. Real dialogue lies between these two extremes, but exactly where, for each relationship, is a tricky question. There are no rules of dialogue that guarantee the physician and patient will always get it right. In a somewhat similar vein, Katz (1984) discussed the problem of informed consent under the rubric of "conversation," by which he meant a conversation that includes at least the possibility that the patient will become involved in making decisions.

TRUTHFUL DISCLOSURE

The models of the physician–patient relationship discussed above have important implications for what physicians are obligated to tell patients about their illnesses and treatment. According to the contractarian model, the choosers would pick as a right of the patient what Fried called lucidity, which involves the right to know the truth about one's medical condition. The issue of truth telling in medicine is both closely linked to, but is also distinguishable from, the issue of informed consent. Informed consent involves two of Fried's rights, lucidity and autonomy—the patient has the opportunity both to know the truth and to use that information in deciding on a strategy of care. The concept of autonomy is important in understanding both why truthful disclosure is important for patients and what legitimate exceptions may exist to the physician's duty to disclose (Sheldon 1982). But patients themselves readily distinguish between receiving truthful information and involving themselves in their own medical decisions. An intensive study of hospitalized patients revealed that nearly all wanted information, for a variety of reasons ranging from simple courtesy to a desire to better follow the doctor's advice, but only about 10 percent wanted to participate in the choosing of medical treatment along with the physicians (Lidz et al. 1983).

The right of lucidity runs into some of the same problems that contractual models encounter when contrasted with the long, historical tradition of medical practice. It is difficult to find anyone in the American medical literature of the last decade or so who argues that routine deception of patients is ethical. But any right of lucidity has generally been rejected in Russian medical practice (Veatch 1981). In Italy, although physicians understand the new-found value of promoting patient autonomy, they also realize that frank disclosures to terminal patients may lead to a loss of emotional and social support, which is hardly a good outcome from the patient's point of view (Surbone 1992). Moreover, the entire history of Western medicine before about 1960 is the history of routine deception and withholding of information for fear that frank truth would frighten or harm the patient; voices calling for more disclosure were distinctly in the minority (Reiser 1980). There were some good reasons for the shift, such as new research suggesting that the truth is not as harmful to patients as physicians had previously feared (Kübler-Ross 1969). But the very radical nature of the shift is at least puzzling—about 90 percent of cancer physicians favored nondisclosure of the diagnosis in 1960 (Oken 1961) but in a similar survey 20 years later, 90 percent favored full disclosure (Novack et al. 1979). We might naturally wonder whether this represents new ethical insight or a temporary fad.

One of the deepest analyses of information disclosure by physicians appears in a book by Jay Katz, a psychiatrist interested in medical law (1984). Katz is interested primarily in informed consent, but his observations apply equally to the disclosure issue. He suggests that the long history of nondisclosure can be explained by powerful psychological forces in the physician–patient relationship. These forces feed into each other so that blame cannot be assigned to either doctor or patient alone. A great deal of the problem is the natural human fear of uncertainty, especially when one is facing serious illness and really wants a magical cure rather than a scientific analysis of probabilities and statistics. In most cases of serious illness, a frank conversation would quickly reveal that important facts are unknown or are understood only as statistical probabilities. A cancer patient may naturally wonder, "How long have I got, Doc?" But the physician knows that any information beyond something like, "There is a 34-percent chance that you will survive for 5 years," would require a crystal ball. Medical science cannot tell this patient whether he is in the 34-percent group or the 66-percent group.

Thus, both physician and patient have a psychological interest in maintaining a mutual charade that medicine is much more certain and powerful than it is—for the patient as a way to retain hope in miracles, and for the physician as a way to merit the faith and trust that the patient has. Further, a more severely ill patient may regress psychologically so that the relationship becomes more like a child–parent situation than an adult–adult relationship; the parent usually does not feel that full disclosure of information to the child is needed or helpful. As a result of these and similar forces, both physician and patient may find strategies to dodge real lucidity, and these strategies, over time, become embedded in customary medical practice and the usual expectations that patients have of physicians.

Katz personally favors recognizing the right of lucidity and promoting increased patient autonomy. He argues, however, that this can be achieved in medicine only if we study and take very seriously the strong psychological forces that drive us in the other direction. He also argues that medicine, scientifically, is in a much better position to do this now than at any previous time in its history. To Katz, medicine always was and still is characterized by a great deal of uncertainty and ignorance; but what is different today is our ability to describe and demarcate our uncertainty in scientific terms such as probability, statistics, and quantitative decision analysis (Weinstein et al. 1980). Because we can talk more accurately and more meaningfully with our patients about medical uncertainty, we have much less reason to waver on the right of lucidity.

Thus, there are strong ethical arguments favoring truthful disclosure, and there are important psychological barriers that may influence both physicians and patients. This suggests that it is not enough to teach in an ethics course that the physician *ought* to tell the truth, for instance, to a patient recently diagnosed with a possibly terminal cancer. It is also necessary to teach aspiring physicians *how* to tell the patient this information. The physician, ideally, wants to respect the patient's right to the information necessary to make autonomous choices, to be compassionate toward the patient and offer effective emotional support to help cope with serious illness, and to transmit information necessary for the patient to get on with the agreed-on tasks of medical care, whether that includes performing surgery, administering chemotherapy, or referring a dying patient to the local hospice program. To do all these things at once, and do them well, requires both a careful plan of action and some practice.

Buckman (1992) has provided a very useful practical manual to assist these tasks. He suggests a five-step strategy for approaching the patient with a disclosure of "bad news." He describes the various emotional reactions patients may have to the disclosure (anger, denial, despair, and numerous others) and suggests ways the physician could respond therapeutically to each. In brief summary, Buckman's approach has two important aspects—first, the physician does more listening than telling; second, the physician respects the patient's autonomy much more than would be the case if the physician saw the job as merely telling the truth. The process starts with a careful assessment of what the patient already knows and then an offer to tell the patient more. In most cases, the patient simply asks for the new information, and the physician goes on to the next task of assessing the patient's emotional reaction to the news and deciding which is the most helpful and supportive way to respond to that reaction.

But in some cases, the patient refuses the offer, either temporarily ("I wish you'd wait to tell me later today when my daughter will be here") or indefinitely ("I think I'd feel much better not knowing"). If the reasons for refusing to hear the news aren't clear, the physician can explore them with the patient. But respect for autonomy requires that the physician honor a refusal to hear some information if the patient makes a considered and reasoned refusal, just as much as it requires that the physician disclose information that is crucial to the patient in most other cases. Buckman describes many cases in which the refusal is only temporary—in a day or two the patient feels better able to face the bad news and asks for full details. But he also describes a rare, occasional case in which patients died after some months of treatment, never having received full information about their diagnoses, and who insisted to the end that that was how they wanted it. He even describes a case in which a patient refused to hear that he had been diagnosed with cancer but freely consented to cancer chemotherapy. He told his doctors, in effect, that he wished them to treat him for his disease, and wanted to be informed of the risks and side effects of treatment, but did not want to know what his disease was. It is hard to escape the conclusion that this patient, at some level, "knew" that he had cancer. And yet, if he knew himself well enough to know that he would respond better emotionally so long as that word were not said in his presence, then the physicians very appropriately felt duty-bound to honor his choice. Their willingness to negotiate carefully about what to say and what not to say not only showed respect for autonomy, it also avoided an unnecessarily adversarial stance between physicians and patient—a stance that could have markedly interfered with appropriate, humane treatment.

Before leaving the issue of lucidity, we might note one interesting way that a physician may deceive a patient or practice incomplete disclosure. The physician may administer a placebo pill or treatment that is intended for symbolic purposes only, with the patient allowed to think that the treatment has a pharmacologic or physiologic potency. Although experiments and experience have shown that occasionally placebos can be powerful healing tools, the right of lucidity and respect for the principle of autonomy suggests that their use in medicine should be strictly limited (Brody 1982). Indeed, a proper analysis of lucidity and its implications shows that the physician who is tempted to use a placebo to help the patient is almost always guilty of a limited imagination. For one thing, there are a great many ways in which the powerful symbolism of the physician–patient relationship can be used to promote healing without using a sugar pill or a similar deceptive device (Benson and Epstein 1975). For another, in some situations in which a placebo may actually be beneficial, the patient may be able to give explicit permission for its use. Suppose, for example, that a patient is sure that a pill with possible serious side effects is necessary to relieve his symptoms; the physician thinks the pill works by suggestion only. They may jointly agree on a trial in which the patient will take unmarked pills, some active drug and some placebo, and keep a diary of his symptoms over time to see if the active drug has any advantage. In this example, a placebo is used, but the patient is not deceived and gives free consent (Vogel et al. 1980).

Although the history of medicine reveals a record of deception and nondisclosure, there are sound reasons, referring to the features of the physician–patient relationship discussed above, to favor a policy of truthful disclosure unless the autonomous patient requests a different approach. The rare exceptional case, when telling the truth may produce great harm, must be dealt with under the question of when paternalism may be justified (Childress 1982).

CONFIDENTIALITY

Traditionally, the patient's right to fidelity (as Fried [1974] uses the term) has included a right to have privacy respected and not to have any information disclosed to other parties without permission. One version of the Hippocratic oath states, "What I see or hear in the course of the treatment . . . , which on no account one must spread abroad, I will keep to myself . . ." (Beauchamp and Childress 1983, 330). This sentence suggests two things. One is that, historically, physicians have been expected to maintain confidentiality and patients have been encouraged to take this for granted. The other is that, on occasion, the physician must use individual judgment to decide "what ought to be spoken of abroad" and what should not. That is, occasionally other important moral considerations may override a duty of confidentiality.

The historical basis of confidentiality can, however, be misleading. The old model for confidentiality, which is the picture that many patients still carry in their minds (Weiss 1982), assumes there is one physician, one patient, and information that is largely kept in the physician's memory and that is solely the physician's—to disclose or not. The current health-care situation is radically different, with dozens of physicians and health-care professionals commonly involved in care, the unquestioned need for written records to which many people must have access, the need to transmit information to insurance companies and others with a financial interest to ensure payment for services, and the increasing computerization of this information. If, under these pressures, confidentiality is not to become a "decrepit concept" (Siegler 1982), we need a careful analysis of what confidentiality is and why it is basic to the physician–patient relationship, as well as a sense of its limits.

Privacy and confidentiality should be seen as closely linked with basic human dignity and respect for persons, as are lucidity and autonomy. It will clearly not do, for example, to tie the duty of confidentiality to the solely material harms that could befall the patient if confidentiality were breached. Suppose I know that a patient engages in some unusual sexual practices, I tell his employer, and he is fired as a result. Being fired is a material harm, and I could be blamed for having caused it. But suppose, in another similar case, I know that the employer is very liberal and tolerant so that no material harm will result for the patient. My moral duty to keep what I know to myself is not lessened by this change in circumstances.

A more subtle and satisfactory reason is that patients are routinely called on to disclose private and embarrassing information to physicians, and yet patients are also routinely helped by their physicians' care. If they could not trust physicians to keep the embarrassing information private, many patients might be discouraged from seeking medical help, and this could, over time, lead to both individual and social harm.

This second reason gives a better account of why confidentiality is basic to the physician–patient relationship. Yet it is also unsatisfactory in ways analogous to the discussion above of why the benefit principle ultimately fails to do justice to truth telling. By appealing to patient benefit, the argument undermines itself. In cases in which physicians think that violating confidentiality would benefit the patient in some way, they would be encouraged to seek that benefit at the expense of patient privacy. But that would encourage precisely the state of affairs—patient mistrust in physicians—that the argument seeks to avoid. Thus, even though patients benefit in a variety of ways from having their privacy honored, we may conclude that benefit is not the most basic moral value that explains the importance of confidentiality.

There is a deeper explanation of why confidentiality is central to respecting the patient's human dignity. We assume that who we are as individual persons is centrally bound up with a series of human relationships, roughly depicted by a set of concentric circles with the individual in the middle. The smallest circles represent the few, most intimate relationships and the largest circles depict chance acquaintances and those with whom we have no personal stake or commitment. To a large degree, we define and control this system of relationships by choosing what information about ourselves to reveal to various people. We reveal very minimal information to those on the outermost circles, usually just enough to get some specific task done, like using a credit card to purchase clothing. We reveal a great deal more (though still not everything) to those on the smallest inner circles. Controlling these relationships constitutes a large part of what it means for us to have control over our lives and our identities (Beauchamp and Childress 1983).

If someone proceeds to violate our confidentiality by revealing private information about us without our consent, that person has effectively taken control of our lives and has taken our identities away from us in one important sense. If that person chooses to reveal that information to others, that person, not us, is determining who shall be (to some extent) in a relationship of intimacy with us. If that person uses that information toward some goal that is his, not ours, we and our very identities are being made use of in an undignified and disrespectful way. This account, better than any benefit analysis, shows why fundamental human dignity hinges on confidentiality. As the term "fidelity" implies, violating confidentiality is a particularly gross example of breaking faith with someone who has trusted you.

Thus, confidentiality is central to preserving the human dignity of patients. Occasionally, however, other important moral considerations can cause physicians to disclose information without the patient's consent. Which sorts of moral considerations and what circumstances might be sufficiently strong to override the duty of fidelity? Some cases that appear at first glance to be potential violations of confidentiality do not, on analysis, call for careful weighing of competing moral claims. For instance, health professionals are required by law to report to appropriate authorities certain information—communicable diseases (including sexually transmitted diseases), gunshot wounds, and suspicions of child abuse or neglect. These are all examples of information that a patient may have strong reasons for keeping private and of conditions in which harm can come to the patient if the information is revealed. But it is possible to see these cases as instances in which the physician can report the information, even without the patient's consent, without major moral qualms. The reason is that the laws requiring disclosure of such information are (theoretically) in the public domain, passed by the representatives of the people, and thus fully in the public knowledge. Patients (theoretically) have already consented to disclosure of this sort of information, if they choose to go to a physician, because of their presumed awareness of the law (Marsh 1979). Obviously, the patient may not see it this way. And the physician may certainly desire, as a matter of courtesy, not to reveal the information without warning the patient that the disclosure is about to occur. But the argument suggests that the disclosure of this sort of information, covered by law, need not engender a major moral controversy.

Tough decisions balance confidentiality against other major moral principles. These decisions might be of two general types. First, the other moral principle might be the well-being of the same patient who demands privacy. Imagine a patient who suffers from an alcohol or other dependence problem, which so far he has succeeded in hiding from his family and work associates. If the physician reveals the seriousness of the problem to the patient's friends or family, they might exert pressure for definitive treatment; the patient refuses to consent to this disclosure. The desire to respect confidentiality (the right of fidelity) is in conflict with the physician's desire to save the patient from harm (the right of humanity). This is a good example of a paternalistic interference with a patient's liberty. Thus, the basic arguments about when, if ever, paternalism is justified apply to this case (Beauchamp and McCullough 1984; Childress 1982).

Another general type of dilemma around confidentiality involves conflicting fidelities. The harm threatened by not disclosing some information may not strike the patient, but someone else. If the someone else is someone to whom the physician feels a justified duty of fidelity, aside from and in addition to the fidelity owed the patient within the physician–patient relationship, a moral dilemma will arise.

The easiest competing duty of fidelity to imagine is one's faithfulness as a member of society, which engenders a duty to save the public, or specific individuals, from serious and immediate harm. This duty arose in one of the most widely discussed recent court cases on confidentiality, the Tarasoff case (Beauchamp and Childress 1983). A psychologist learned from a patient of the patient's intent to murder a former girlfriend who had jilted him. The legal dispute, which obscured the ethical issue, was whether it was enough to tell the police (which the psychologist did) or whether there was also an obligation to tell the girl or her family (which was not done). But the central moral conclusion, which was not really in dispute, was that the serious harm threatened to a specific individual was sufficient to override the moral duty to protect confidences.

Deciding when confidentiality may be overridden is one of the most difficult problems in medical ethics (Jonsen et al. 1982). We can distinguish three sorts of situations in which the justification for overriding confidentiality becomes progressively stronger:

1. Revealing the information would produce some considerable public good.
2. Revealing the information would prevent some possible risk of harm to someone, but who that would be is not known for certain.
3. Revealing the information would prevent some very likely harm to specific and identifiable individuals.

A duty to the public at large is not, however, the only duty of fidelity that a physician may feel. As medical practice becomes more complex, and as health-care institutions become more multifaceted and pervasive, several competing loyalties may be encountered. The family physician, for example, may owe a duty to respect the privacy of a patient, but also feel a duty to family members of that patient, who are also members of that physician's practice, and who may have a strong interest in knowing the information. An adolescent who does not want her parents to know she is asking for birth control pills is a common example (Eaddy and Graber 1982). The physician employed by an industrial firm may feel loyalty both to the company and to the employee who seeks help. The physician may wish to reveal to the employer any patient information that would prevent financial losses to the company—for example, an employee's alcohol problem, or the fact that an employee's disability may not be due to a work-related injury but to some previously existing medical problem. Other situations that may create similarly divided loyalties are physicians employed by the military, by prisons (Thorburn 1981), or by athletic teams (McKeag et al. 1984).

These divided-loyalty settings may cause a physician to become too attentive to who signs the paycheck and too unconcerned about the rights of patients. On the other hand, some moral problems may be sidestepped by a frank disclosure of possible competing loyalties. If the company physician is forthright with the employee about the circumstances in which he will feel obligated to report information to the firm, the employee can freely choose what to reveal and what to keep secret. But the "patient's free choice" argument also has its limits—for example, an increasingly common practice of requiring employees to undergo blood tests, such as screens for drug use, which threaten to reveal private information. The company may claim that anyone working for them has given their free consent; after all, if they do not want to participate, they can always find another job. But most of us would find threatened loss of employment so serious a risk that our consent could not be said to be truly voluntary under these circumstances (Graebner 1984).

Control over personal information is becoming increasingly problematic in medicine and in modern life overall. The increasing use of computer systems and sharing of information among computer networks offer many social advantages (such as catching criminals and catching parents avoiding child support payments) but just as obviously present a threat to individual privacy. The changes and reforms likely to occur in U.S. health care over the next several decades will probably produce increased computerization of medical records and increase the possibilities for sharing and distributing medical information over great distances. Physicians will have to attend to their personal practices and to matters of public policy to ensure that they carry out the duty to protect patients' privacy as much as possible.

THE PHYSICIAN AS GATEKEEPER

To this point, we have discussed the physician–patient relationship as if it were uninfluenced by economic considerations. Recently, the health-care marketplace in the United States has become increasingly dominated by managed-care arrangements, in which the physician is expected to make decisions about when patients ought to have access to certain expensive resources (such as hospitalization, laboratory and x-ray tests, and referral to specialists). The term *gatekeeper* has come to designate this relatively new physician role.

The gatekeeper faces a potential conflict of interest. On one hand, the physician might wish to provide everything for patients that might benefit them, even if the cost is high. On the other hand, the physician is expected by the health-care plan (which either pays the physician's salary or controls a substantial portion of the physician's income) to try to cut costs. This conflict has led some to argue that the increase in managed-care arrangements in the United States is a serious threat to the ethical physician–patient relationship (Emanuel and Brett 1993) or that the gatekeeper role is unethical under any circumstances (Levinsky 1984).

Simply to dismiss gatekeeping as unethical seems, however, to ignore several important moral considerations. It assumes, for one thing, that every potential conflict of interest is an actual and serious conflict of interest; in fact, most of us face numerous conflicts of interest in our daily lives and yet manage to navigate them in an ethically responsible manner. Moreover, it assumes that the moral duty of the physician is exhausted once the physician has done whatever is possible to benefit the patient who happens to be there at that moment in time. But it seems reasonable, especially in a world where it has been calculated that physicians could easily spend the wealth of the nation if they actually tried to purchase "everything possibly beneficial" for each patient, to say that the physician has at least *some* moral obligation to act as a wise steward over the pool of scarce and expensive resources that society has placed at the physician's disposal.

If resources are truly limited, whenever a physician uses an expensive resource to benefit one patient (X), there must, somewhere else within the system, be patient Y who has to do without a potential benefit. If X receives a substantial benefit and Y manages without a benefit, there is no problem. But suppose (as happens often in today's health care) the benefit to X is questionable or negligible, but nontreatment or delayed treatment for Y will seriously threaten Y's health or life. Can the physician make the excuse that X was the patient who happened to be there at the moment and Y is some other physician's patient? (How does the physician *know* that Y is not, in actuality, going to turn out to be another patient in his own practice?) If we say that the physician is not morally off the hook *just because* one patient is "his" patient at this particular moment, we have established the principle that the duty to benefit one patient must somehow be balanced against a more general duty to ensure a fair and equitable distribution of scarce or expensive resources—even if *most of the time* the physician's predominant duty is to provide benefits for the present patient, and *only rarely and to a limited extent* is the physician asked to serve as social steward.

Considerations like these have led some to conclude that the physician can act ethically in the gatekeeper role under some circumstances (Brody 1992). That means, in turn, that physicians will have to specify what sorts of gatekeeping arrangements are ethically defensible and what sorts violate key principles of an ethical physician–patient relationship.

To analyze specific gatekeeping arrangements, we need to avoid some common sources of confusion. One source of confusion is the different sorts of relationships that are called "gatekeeper." Some managed-care systems employ health professionals (commonly nurses) to review patients' charts and to decide which patients should be approved to receive a benefit and which should not on the basis of clinical criteria. These professionals never provide care for the patients and never see a patient. In other health-care plans, a physician or nurse practitioner may be asked to make decisions about entitlement to expensive care and to provide the ongoing primary care for the patient. This professional not only faces the patient regularly, but also, in some sense, has to help pick up the pieces if the patient suffers a health setback because a laboratory test was not ordered in time or because the patient was sent home from the hospital too early. The implications of the two different roles for the professional–patient relationship may be vastly different, but both sorts of professionals have been called "gatekeepers."

Another confusion is to assume (often implicitly) that the ideal model of ethical medicine was the old physician–patient relationship before managed-care plans came into existence. Because the managed-care physician has a financial incentive to do less for the patient, presumably we have gone downhill from the ethical high ground into an ethical swamp. This way of looking at the issue ignores that under the customary fee-for-service system, every physician faced a potential conflict of interest with every patient—

the physician could always make extra money by ordering unnecessary tests or performing unnecessary surgery. In the United States, many people tend to assume that doing more is always good for the patient and doing less is always bad, but the facts do not support that simplistic view; it often turns out, for instance, that primary-care physicians who take care of patients at lower cost than do specialists produce just as good or even better health outcomes (Franks et al. 1992).

To avoid these confusions and determine which gatekeeping arrangements might be ethically most defensible, we might be guided by three general rules. First, the resource allocation system as a whole, within which the physician–gatekeeper functions, must be fair. It hardly seems defensible for one physician to be saying "no" to a patient who might benefit from care, while elsewhere in the system patients with much lower levels of medical need have easy access to expensive resources. ("System" refers both to the local system, such as a single managed-care plan, and to the national system within which that plan operates) (Cassel 1985; Daniels 1986).

Second, full disclosure to patients of the financial arrangements within the health-care plan and any financial pressures placed on the personal physician seems mandatory. Respect for patient autonomy requires that patients be given an opportunity to question any medical decision that could conflict with their interests because of financial inducements or constraints. There are occasional reports of managed-care plans that explicitly forbid their physician–gatekeepers from disclosing such financial arrangements to patients, apparently lest such knowledge prompt patients to join a rival plan. Ethical physicians ought not to work for a health-care corporation of this sort.

Financial incentives should also be reasonably nonintrusive into the decisions for individual patients. For example, consider two plans that use financial inducements to remind their physicians of the need to contain costs. One plan extracts a penalty from each physician every time he keeps a patient in the hospital for what the plan managers consider to be too many days. The other plan looks at overall practice patterns and at the end of the year pays a small bonus to physicians who seem to use hospital resources most prudently. The first plan seems more likely to induce a physician to cause a patient harm by early discharge than does the second plan.

CONCLUSION

The old medical ethic evolved over many centuries and was largely an internal product—physicians talked with other physicians and eventually came to agreement about how they should treat patients. The new medical ethics has, by contrast, been shaped by a constructive give-and-take among physicians, philosophers, and other scholars and practitioners. This give-and-take helps to ensure that physicians meet two tests—that our model of the physician–patient relationship has a solid foundation in ethical theory and that it fits with the reality of clinical practice as that practice is situated in the modern world.

This discussion has emphasized the importance of respect for patient autonomy as a fundamental reflection of the dignity of the individual person. At the same time, the discussion has shown that other moral principles besides autonomy must be taken into account to arrive at ethical guidance. We have noted, for instance, how a duty to avoid pressing harm to others might lead to disclosing information that would ordinarily be kept confidential; we have seen that a duty to allocate scarce resources wisely must balance the more traditional physician's duty to benefit the patient who is presently being cared for. We have also seen that ethical wisdom requires that attention be paid to questions of virtue, character, and integrity—how to live one's life—and not merely what rules one ought to follow in making this decision today.

Physicians have traditionally been rather powerful figures in our culture. Today's health-care environment has in some ways reduced their power because physicians must increasingly practice as members of corporations or organizations, which restricts choices and judgments in many ways. The environment has, in other ways, increased physicians' power, as explored in the discussion of problems associated with the gatekeeper role. How to use power wisely and responsibly remains a central ethical question. When the physician builds a relationship with the patient in which the power can be shared over time, the ground is prepared for ensuring that the patient gets the most benefit out of medical care and also exercises autonomy to the optimal degree (Brody 1992).

DISCUSSION QUESTIONS

CASE 4.1

A 38-year-old paraplegic white male is admitted to the community hospital for treatment of a urinary tract infection that causes high fever and prostration. The presumed source of infection is an indwelling suprapubic catheter. The patient had suffered a spinal cord injury in an accident approximately 4 years previously. Since his rehabilitation he has worked as a public relations manager for a radio station. The week before hospitalization, he was informed abruptly that he would be laid off in just a few weeks. He has been extremely upset about how he will support his family, which consists of his wife and two young adopted children, and what he will do when his medical benefits lapse when he loses his job.

In the hospital, the patient appears as an extremely anxious man who is insecure and fearful. Additional history reveals that he is being bothered by flashbacks to his previous hospitalization for the spinal cord injury, and that many unresolved emotional problems relating to that injury and the resulting life crises are haunting him. As part of his anxiety, he indicates an insistence that he be kept fully informed of all developments and that no significant information about his illness be withheld from him. The family physician gives him this assurance because this is routine procedure for this physician regarding all patients. However, the physician is worried about the patient's emotional response to illness and the multitude of emotional risk factors that may complicate the patient's response to treatment.

A rare gram-negative organism is identified as the source of the urinary tract infection and an intravenous antibiotic, amikacin, is ordered. The next morning on rounds, the family physician notes that the patient has begun to respond to the antibiotic, feels a little better, and has a lower temperature. However, there is also an incident report in the chart. Because of a pharmacy error that was not discovered by the nurses in the unit, the patient initially received 500 mg of aminocaproic acid, a drug used to treat a disorder of blood coagulation. Because the usual dose of aminocaproic acid is 4 to 5 grams, the 500-mg dose given erroneously to this patient represents an almost insignificant amount. No side effects were noted from the medication, and in fact nothing of consequence occurred to the patient other than a brief delay in receiving the correct medication, amikacin. The amikacin appears to be working and the delay does not seem to have hindered the patient's response.

The family physician wonders whether he should inform the patient, who is feeling a little better but still acts very anxious and ill at ease, about the medication error. The physician reasons that the information is totally unrelated to the course of management of the patient's illness because the patient does not appear to have been jeopardized and nothing about the patient's treatment need be changed in response to the error. Furthermore, the likely result of imparting this knowledge will be to increase the suspicion and vigilance with which the patient watches nursing staff in administration of all his medication; this is unlikely to provide the kind of relationship with staff that is needed for the patient's care and is also very likely to worsen all the patient's emotional risk factors, which may hinder a good response to treatment. Nevertheless, the physician feels that he would be breaking a promise if he withheld the information.

---

1. Should the family physician tell the patient about the medication error?

2. If the family physician is entitled to withhold this information, would it have made a difference if the patient had actually suffered harm from the medication error or if the patient's treatment was significantly changed as a result of the error?

3. If the family physician decides that it is justifiable to withhold this information now, is the physician required at a future time when the patient might be in a better emotional state to inform the patient of what he has done?

4. Because the error was made by other health-team members, must the physician get their consent before disclosing the information?

CASE 4.2

When the hospital nurse reports for duty at 7:00 A.M., she discovers that one new patient admitted the previous evening is Mr. Turner, a 46-year-old male. The nurse is uncertain of the details and will be responsible for Mr. Turner's care during her shift, so she reviews Mr. Turner's chart. She notices that Mr. Turner is currently under the care of Dr. Brown, who came to the emergency room to see him, admitted him, and wrote the orders.

As she is reading the chart, Dr. Green walks up. "I see Bill Turner's name is on the board under Dr. Brown's case list. I've been Turner's family doctor for 10 years now. I wonder why he didn't call me for this illness, and how he came in under Dr. Brown's care. Let me see his chart, will you?"

The nurse knows that the hospital recently had a staff conference on confidentiality. One point emphasized was that access to charts should be restricted to staff members who have a "need to know" because they are actually involved in caring for the patient during that hospital stay. Curiosity or personal acquaintance with the patient were cited as common but indefensible reasons for looking at the chart. By this stated policy, Dr. Green has no right to see Mr. Turner's chart. But it would be highly unusual for a nurse to refuse to give a doctor a chart, especially when the doctor has provided care for the patient in the past. Dr. Green could easily complain to the nurse's supervisor and get the nurse into trouble.

---

1. Assess the "need to know" policy. Does Dr. Green's long-established relationship with the patient provide such a "need to know"? Do you agree with the nurse's assessment that the chart should be withheld?

2. The case description gives us no clue *why* Mr. Turner might not want Dr. Green to see his chart. Can you imagine some circumstances in which Mr. Turner *would* want Dr. Green to see his chart? Can you imagine circumstances in which Mr. Turner *would not* want Dr. Green to see his chart? How could you determine which set of circumstances actually existed?

3. What should the nurse say to Dr. Green?

REFERENCES

Beauchamp, T. L., Childress, J. F. *Principles of Biomedical Ethics*, 2nd ed. New York: Oxford University Press, 1983.

Beauchamp, T. L., McCullough, L. B. *Medical Ethics: The Moral Responsibilities of Physicians*. Englewood Cliffs, NJ: Prentice-Hall, 1984.

Benjamin, M. "Lay Obligations in Professional Relations." *J Med Philos* 10 (1985): 85–103.

Benson, H., Epstein, M. D. "The Placebo Effect: A Neglected Asset in the Care of Patients." *JAMA* 232 (1975): 1225–1227.

Bloom, S. W. *The Doctor and His Patient*. New York: Russell Sage Foundation, 1963.

Brody, H. "The Lie that Heals: The Ethics of Giving Placebos." *Ann Intern Med* 97 (1982): 112–118.

———. "The Physician–Patient Relationship: Models and Criticisms." *Theor Med* 8 (1987): 205–220.

———. *The Healer's Power*. New Haven: Yale University Press, 1992.

Buchanan, A. "Medical Paternalism." *Philos Public Affairs* 7 (1978): 370–390.

Buckman, R. F. *How to Break Bad News: A Guide for Health Care Professionals*. Baltimore: Johns Hopkins University Press, 1992.

Callahan, D. "Minimalist Ethics." *Hastings Cent Rep* 11(5) (1981): 19–25.

Cassel, C. K. "Doctors and Allocation Decisions: A New Role in the New Medicare." *J Health Politics Policy Law* 10 (1985): 549–564.

Childress, J. F. *Who Shall Decide? Paternalism in Health Care*. New York: Oxford University Press, 1982.

Daniels, N. "Why Saying No to Patients in the United States Is So Hard." *N Engl J Med* 314 (1986): 1380–1383.

Drane, J. F. *Becoming a Good Doctor: The Place of Virtue and Character in Medical Ethics*. Kansas City, MO: Sheed and Ward/The Catholic Health Association, 1988.

Eaddy, J. A., Graber, G. C. "Confidentiality and the Family Physician." *Am Fam Physician* 25 (1982): 141–145.

Emanuel, E. J., Brett, A. S. "Managed Competition and the Physician-Patient Relationship. *N Engl J Med* 329 (1993): 879–882.

Emanuel, E. J., Emanuel, L. L. "Four Models of the Physician–Patient Relationship." *JAMA* 267 (1992): 2221–2226.

Franks, P., Clancy, C. M., Nutting, P. A. "Gatekeeping Revisited—Protecting Patients from Overtreatment." *N Engl J Med* 327 (1992): 424–429.

Fried, C. *Medical Experimentation: Personal Integrity and Social Policy*. New York: American Elsevier, 1974.

Gert, B., Culver, C. M. "Paternalistic Behavior." *Philos Public Affairs* 6 (1976): 45–57.

———. "The Justification of Paternalism." In W. L. Robison and M. S. Pritchard, Eds., *Medical Responsibility*. Clifton, NJ: Humana Press, 1979.

Graebner, W. "Doing the World's Unhealthy Work: The Fiction of Free Choice." *Hastings Cent Rep* 14(1) (1984): 28–37.

Jonsen, A. R., Siegler, M., Winslade, W. J. *Clinical Ethics*. New York: Macmillan, 1982.

Katz, J. *The Silent World of Doctor and Patient*. New York: Free Press, 1984.

Kübler-Ross, E. *On Death and Dying*. New York: Macmillan, 1969.

Ladd, J. "Legalism and Medical Ethics." *J Med Philos* 4 (1979): 70–80.

Levinsky, N. G. "The Doctor's Master." *N Engl J Med* 311 (1984): 1573–1575.

Lidz, C W., Meisel, A., Osterweis, M., et al. "Barriers to Informed Consent." *Ann Intern Med* 99 (1983): 534–543.

MacIntyre, A. *After Virtue*. Notre Dame, IN: University of Notre Dame Press, 1981.

Marsh, F. H. "The 'Deeper Meaning' of Confidentiality Within the Physician-Patient Relationship." *Ethics Sci Med* 6 (1979): 131–136.

Masters, R. D. "Is Contract an Adequate Basis for Medical Ethics?" *Hastings Cent Rep* 5(6) (1975): 24–28.

May, W. F. "Code, Covenant, Contract, or Philanthropy?" *Hastings Cent Rep* 5(6) (1975): 29–38.

———. *The Physician's Covenant: Images of the Healer in Medical Ethics*. Philadelphia: Westminster Press, 1983.

McKeag, D., Hough, D., Brody, H. "Medical Ethics in Sport." *The Physician and Sports Medicine* 12 (1984): 145–150.

Novack, D. H., Detering, B. J., Arnold, R., et al. "Changes in Physicians' Attitudes Toward Telling the Cancer Patient." *JAMA* 241 (1979): 897–900.

Oken, D. "What to Tell Cancer Patients." *JAMA* 175 (1961): 1120–1128.

Parsons, T. "Health and Disease: A Sociological and Action Perspective." In W. T. Reich, Ed., *Encylopedia of Bioethics*. New York: The Free Press, 1978.

Pellegrino, E. D. "Toward a Reconstruction of Medical Morality: The Primacy of the Act of Profession and the Fact of Illness." *J Med Philos* 4 (1979): 32–56.

Pellegrino, E. D., Thomasma, D. C. *A Philosophical Basis of Medical Practice*. New York: Oxford University Press, 1981.

———. *For the Patient's Good: The Restoration of Beneficence in Health Care*. New York: Oxford University Press, 1988.

Rawls, J. A. *A Theory of Justice*. Cambridge: Harvard University Press, 1971.

Reiser, S. J. "Words as Scalpels: Transmitting Evidence in the Clinical Dialogue." *Ann Intern Med* 92 (1980): 837–842.

Sheldon, M. "Truth Telling in Medicine." *JAMA* 247 (1982): 651–654.

Shelp, E. E., Ed. *Virtue and Medicine*. Boston: D. Reidel, 1985.

Siegler, M. "A Physician's Perspective on the Right to Health Care." *JAMA* 244 (1980): 1591–1596.

———. "Searching for Moral Certainty in Medicine: A Proposal for a New Model of the Doctor-Patient Encounter." *Bull NY Acad Med* 57 (1981): 56–69.

———. "Confidentiality in Medicine—A Decrepit Concept." *N Engl J Med* 307 (1982): 1518–1521.

Smith. D. G., Newton, L. "Physician and Patient: Respect for Mutuality." *Theor Med* 5 (1984): 43–60.

Surbone, A. "Truth Telling to the Patient." *JAMA* 268 (1992): 1661–1662.

Szasz, T. S., Hollender, M. H. "The Basic Models of the Doctor-Patient Relationship." *Arch Intern Med* 97 (1956): 585–592.

Thorburn, K. M. "Croaker's Dilemma: Should Prison Physicians Serve Prisons or Prisoners?" *West J Med* 134 (1981): 457–461.

Twiss, S. B. "The Problem of Moral Responsibility in Medicine." *J Med Philos* 2 (1977): 330–375.

Veatch, R. M. "Models for Ethical Medicine in a Revolutionary Age." *Hastings Cent Rep* 2(3) (1972): 5–7.

———. "Professional Medical Ethics: The Grounding of Its Principles." *J Med Philos* 4 (1979): 1–19.

———. *A Theory of Medical Ethics*. New York: Basic Books, 1981.

Vogel, A. V., Goodwin, J. S., Goodwin, J. M. "The Therapeutics of Placebo." *Am Fam Physician* 22 (1980): 105–109.

Weinstein, M. C., Fineberg, H. V., Elstein, A. S., et al. *Clinical Decision Analysis*. Philadelphia: Saunders, 1980.

Weiss, B. D. "Confidentiality Expectations of Patients, Physicians and Medical Students." *JAMA* 247 (1982): 2695–2697.

5

Limiting Procreation

JUDITH AREEN

SUMMARY

This chapter examines the development of controls on contraception, sterilization, and abortion. In the first stage, limitations on procreation in marriage were prohibited by religious authorities. Sexuality was also discouraged, not only outside marriage but also to a great extent within marriage. With the rise of the modern secular state, civil law was increasingly employed to regulate marriage and procreation. In the United States, the first national law restricting access to contraception, the Comstock Act, was passed in 1873. Increasingly, however, the right of secular authorities to regulate private behavior came under attack. Debate increased about whether the law should regulate the use of contraception, sterilization, or abortion.

In the second stage, the use of sterilization to limit procreation was not only permitted but also mandated at least for certain mental patients and criminals. Mandatory sterilization laws were passed in a number of states by the early twentieth century, only a few decades after medical science first developed safe procedures for sterilizing men and women. The U.S. Supreme Court upheld the constitutionality of such statutes in 1927 in *Buck v. Bell*. That decision has never been overruled.

In the third stage, some governmental restrictions on limiting procreation have been struck down as unconstitutional. The modern era began in 1965 when the U.S. Supreme Court announced in *Griswold v. Connecticut* that there is a right of privacy protected by the Constitution of the United States and that the right empowers a married couple to decide whether to use contraception. A later decision of the Court extended the right to use contraceptives to single individuals. In 1973 in *Roe v. Wade*, the Court held that the right of privacy includes the right of a pregnant woman to seek an abortion at least during some stages of pregnancy. The Court has extended the right to seek an abortion to some pregnant minors but has not yet addressed the issue of whether a state may intervene in a pregnancy for the benefit of the fetus over the objection of the pregnant woman.

Abortion remains the most controversial method of limiting procreation because the interests of another living being—the fetus—are at stake. The intensity of disagreement about the morality of abortion as well as the complex interrelationship in this country between morality and constitutional rights are underscored by the fact that the Supreme Court is more closely divided than in 1973 as to whether *Roe v. Wade* was correctly decided.

Knowledge of ways to limit procreation has existed for millennia. Egyptian papyri between 1900 and 1100 B.C. contain recipes for contraceptive preparations (Noonan 1966). Religious prohibitions on the use of contraception, sterilization, or abortion to limit procreation are also very old. Consider the biblical account of Onan. Er, Onan's older brother, had been killed:

> Then Juda [Onan's father] said to Onan, "Go to your brother's wife, perform your duty as brother-in-law, and raise up seed for your brother." Onan knew that the descendants would not be his own, so whenever he had relations with his brother's wife, he let the seed be lost on the ground, in order not to raise up seed for his brother. What he did displeased Yahweh, who killed him also (Genesis 38:8–10).[1]

With the rise of the modern secular state, restrictions on marriage and procreation were incorporated into the civil and criminal law. But the right of secular authorities to regulate the private behavior of individuals later came under challenge. John Stuart Mill, for example, argued that "[t]he only purpose for which power can rightfully be exercised over any member of a civilized community, against his will, is to prevent harm to others. His own good, either physical or moral, is not a sufficient warrant" (1859, 9). In turn, the argument has gained force that contraception, abortion, and sterilization are a form of private conduct that should not be regulated by the law.

Mill might well have objected to this extension of his position. He made clear that his conception of liberty did not extend to giving parents unlimited power over children. He criticized the fact that parents were not required to sacrifice or to secure an education for their children. He also supported population control measures such as laws forbidding marriage unless the parties could show that they had the means of supporting a family. Thus, if the birth rate had fallen low enough to threaten the economic viability of a society, Mill himself might have supported restrictions on contraception, sterilization, or abortion.

The extent to which contraception, sterilization, and abortion should be regulated by public authorities continues to be the subject of much debate. Of the three, abortion is the most controversial method of limiting procreation because the interests of another living being—the fetus—are at

---

[1]The passage has sometimes been interpreted to condemn masturbation. The text provides no support for this position. Indeed, the text arguably does not support the widespread interpretation that the passage condemns contraception as opposed to Onan's failure to carry out a levirate marriage, that is, marriage with the wife of a deceased brother. The objective was to maintain the family line in a society that set great store by blood ties and, consequently, had little use for adoption. [The Anchor Bible: Genesis, p. 300 (E. A. Speiser intro., trans. and notes, 1964).]

stake. The debate about whether abortion is morally wrong is thus complicated by a more basic debate over whether a fetus is entitled to the same moral or legal protection as any citizen.

This chapter is organized into three sections. Each is devoted primarily to a historical stage in the development of controls on contraception, abortion, and sterilization. In the first stage, any limitation of procreation by married couples was prohibited, first by religious and later by secular authorities. Sexuality was also discouraged, not only outside marriage, but to a great extent within marriage as well. The second stage, mandatory sterilization of individuals for eugenic purposes, began in the late nineteenth century when medical science first developed procedures for safely sterilizing men and women. The third stage, constitutional protection of the right of individuals to decide whether or not to limit procreation, began in 1965 with the decision of the Supreme Court in *Griswold v. Connecticut*[2] to protect the use of contraceptives by married couples. In 1973, this right of privacy, as it was denominated, was extended to the decision to seek an abortion, at least during some stages of fetal development.

CONTRACEPTION, VOLUNTARY STERILIZATION, AND THE DUTY TO PROCREATE

The Legacy of the Past

There was little discussion of procreation by secular philosophers before this century. In his treatise *Politics*, Aristotle approved of abortion early in pregnancy when a couple had too many children, but otherwise devoted little attention to the subject (Barnes 1984). By contrast, procreation has always been a central concern of the major Western religious traditions.

The early Christian church opposed any limits on procreation. This position was derived in part from the belief that marriage is a state inferior to celibacy. In St. Paul's language, marriage is for those who "cannot exercise self-control"; therefore, "it is better to marry than to burn" (1 Corinthians 7:9–10). Even within marriage, sexual liberty was discouraged by holding that the only acceptable purpose for sexual relations is procreation. St. Paul accordingly denounced abortifacient and contraceptive drugs (Galatians 5:20) (Noonan 1978).

The early Christian moralists appear to have been strongly influenced in their views on sexuality by the Stoics, who sought to control bodily desires by reason. Epictetus, for example, considered immoderation in bodily activities irrational, for it made a man dependent on his own body (Oates 1940). Seneca, the first-century Stoic and statesman, proclaimed:

---

[2]381 U.S. 479 (1965).

All love of another's wife is shameful; so too, too much love of your own. A wise man ought to love his wife with judgment, not affection. Let him control his impulses and not be borne headlong into copulation. Nothing is fouler than to love a wife like an adulteress (Noonan 1966).

In the fourth century, St. Augustine distinguished between lust and sexual relations for the purpose of procreation. He took the position that in marriage only the former is sinful. He therefore explicitly condemned the use of contraception by married couples (401) (Augustine/Wilcox 1955).

The Protestant reformation brought no change in position on contraception. Because he relied heavily on Augustine for his theology, Martin Luther followed him on marriage. Luther taught that God created man and woman differently "not for lewdness but to be true to each other, be fruitful, beget children, and support and bring them up to the glory of God" (Luther/Fischer 1959, 37).

In the Jewish tradition, the duty of procreation is considered the first "mitzvah" or obligation. Most commentators derive the duty not solely from the admonition to "increase and multiply" (Genesis 1:22), but also from the charge to the sons of Noah (Genesis 9:1, 7) or to Jacob (Genesis 35:11) (Feldman 1968, 46). The duty, however, has been interpreted to apply only to men. Thus although the story of Onan was interpreted to prohibit coitus interruptus, the Talmud prescribed two contraceptive methods—a potion called the Cup of Roots and a vaginal sponge—that women could employ, although only in limited circumstances (Feldman 1968; Gordon 1976).

Secular legal restrictions on interference with procreation date back at least to the first century B.C. Contraception appears to have been lawful in the early Roman Empire, but concern about the falling birth rate of the upper classes led to the passage of legislation in 18 B.C. and 9 A.D. prohibiting the childless from holding certain high offices and restricting their rights of inheritance (Noonan 1966).

Secular regulation of marriage in England was not established until well into the Middle Ages (Helmholz 1974). In Roman law, marriage had been a relatively private matter. No special formula or ceremony was required to contract a valid marriage. There was no requirement of intervention by any sort of public official, and there was no registration of marriages. Divorce was allowed without a decree by any court. It was against this background of freedom in marriage practice that the Christian view of marriage developed. Not surprisingly, the establishment of control over marriage by the Church was a "long and disputed process," which was not accomplished even as late as the thirteenth century (Helmholz 1974, 5). Ultimately, the civil law came to reflect the positions of the Church:

"As the first cause and reason of matrimony," says Ayliffe, "ought to be the design of having an offspring"; so the second ought to be the avoiding of fornication. And the law recognizes these two as the "principal ends of matrimony," namely, "a lawful indulgence of the passions to prevent licentiousness, and the procreation of children according to the evident design of Divine Providence" (Bishop 1852, 175).

In addition to legal restrictions on childlessness and marriage, procreation was controlled indirectly by sanctions imposed on having children outside marriage—both the kind of community sanctions for adultery immortalized in *The Scarlet Letter* and legal disabilities placed on children conceived out of wedlock.

In the nineteenth century, the law began to regulate access to contraceptives directly. In the United States, the first national law restricting access to contraception, the Comstock Act, was passed in 1873. Its passage may have been in part a reaction to an increasing use of contraceptives that was reflected in the sharp decline in the national birth rate. It is estimated, for example, that in the year 1800, white women in the United States had an average of 7.04 children. By 1870, the number was down to 4.55 (by 1940 it had dropped to 2.10) (Gordon 1976).

The Comstock Act bears the name of the young man most responsible for securing its passage, Anthony Comstock, who was secretary of the New York Society for the Suppression of Vice. He has been described as a "deeply religious man with a strong sense of personal sin" (Haney 1960, 19). Born in 1844, he believed that his mission was to improve the morals of other people by ridding the country of obscene literature and photographs (Smith 1964).

The Comstock Act prohibited the use of the mails for the sending of any "obscene . . . book or other publication of an indecent character, or any article or thing designed or intended for the prevention of conception" (Smith 1964, 276). Importation of these items was also forbidden by the Act. The reasons identified by historian Carl Degler for passage of the law are remarkably similar to those advanced by early Christian moralists:

> . . . The reasons . . . fell into two categories. One was a fear that if people practiced contraception they might overindulge in sex, a practice that seemed fraught with unknown consequences. The sexual urge might get out of control. Even an advanced feminist like Charlotte Perkins Gilman had doubts about contraception in the 20th century because she thought it would lead to overindulgence. The second category of argument against contraception was that it represented an interference with nature's as well as God's intentions. According to this line of thought, sexuality presumably had been tied to reproduction for a purpose; to sever that connection was to oppose the natural and religious order as people of the 19th century perceived it (Degler 1980, 191).

The Beginning of the Modern Era

The seeds of change were sown in the nineteenth century when use of contraceptives spread. By midcentury, the women's rights movement in the United States was pressing for "voluntary motherhood." They did not support contraception, however, but favored abstinence as the preferred method for limiting the number of children:

> The Voluntary Motherhood advocates' . . . concern for all the needs of women . . . led them to recognize a number of contradictions. First, they realized that while women needed freedom from excessive childbearing, they also needed the respect and self-respect motherhood brought. . . . Second, they understood that while women needed freedom from pregnancy, they also needed freedom from male sexual tyranny, especially in a society that had almost completely suppressed accurate information about female sexuality and replaced it with information and attitudes so false as to virtually guarantee that women would not enjoy sex. Abstinence as a form of birth control may well have been the solution that made most sense in the particular historical circumstance. Abstinence helped women strengthen their ability to say no to their husbands' sexual demands, for example, while contraception and abortion would have weakened it (Gordon 1982, 45).

Most feminists did not change their minds about contraception until the early twentieth century when Margaret Sanger organized and led the modern movement for birth control. Influenced initially by Emma Goldman, a leading radical, and later by Havelock Ellis and other sexual-liberation theorists, Sanger ultimately drew most of her political support by turning from working-class issues to eugenics (Gordon 1976). In 1919, for example, she announced: "Birth control is nothing more or less than the facilitation of the process of weeding out the unfit, or preventing the birth of defectives or of those who will become defectives" (Kennedy 1970, 115).

During the twentieth century, a number of religious groups altered their position on the subject of contraception. In 1930, the bishops of the Anglican church voted to accept methods other than sexual abstinence to avoid parenthood. By 1959, when the World Council of Churches endorsed contraception, the Protestant consensus in its favor was considered overwhelming (Fagley 1960).

The Catholic Church, by contrast, did not change its position at least with respect to "artificial" contraception, although by the end of the eighteenth century the Catholic theological consensus no longer insisted on procreative purpose in marital intercourse. In the nineteenth century, Jean Gury, a French Jesuit, taught that intercourse might "manifest or promote conjugal affection" (Noonan 1978, 213). His view was very influential. In *Casti Connubi*, an encyclical letter issued in 1930, Pope Pius XI approved marital intercourse at times when the wife would be unlikely to conceive because "there are . . . secondary ends, such as mutual aid, the cultivating of mutual love, and the quieting of concupiscence which husband and wife are not forbidden to consider so long as these are subordinated to the primary aim [of begetting children]." A papal commission appointed just after the Second Vatican Council (1963–1965) recommended the approval of contraceptives in marriage (Noonan 1978). Pope Paul VI nonetheless reaffirmed the traditional condemnation of artificial birth control in 1968:

> [Consider] how wide and easy a road would thus be opened up towards conjugal infidelity and the general lowering of morality. Not much experience is needed in order to know human weakness, and to understand that men—especially the young, who are so vulnerable on this point—have need of encouragement to be faithful to the moral law, so that they must not be offered some easy means of eluding its observance. It is also to be feared that the man, growing used to the employment of anti-conceptive practices, may finally lose respect for the woman, and, no longer caring for her physical and psychological equilibrium, may come to the point of considering her as a mere instrument of selfish enjoyment, and no longer as his respected and beloved companion (Paul VI 1968, 11).

He also reaffirmed approval of recourse to infecund periods:

> If [there] are serious motives to space out births, which derive from the physical or psychological conditions of husband and wife, or from external conditions, the Church teaches that it is then licit to take into account the natural rhythms immanent in the generative functions, for the use of marriage in the infecund periods only, and in this way to regulate birth without offending . . . moral principles (Paul VI 1968, 10).

Significant legal change first occurred in the United States in 1936 when a federal court held that the Comstock Act did not prohibit the distribution of contraceptives prescribed by doctors.[3] By this time, however, a number of states had passed "little Comstock laws" that in some instances were even more restrictive than the original act. These were not successfully challenged until 1965, when the Supreme Court, in *Griswold v. Connecticut*,[4] held unconstitutional as applied to a married couple a Connecticut statute that prohibited the use of contraceptives. The basis for the decision was not that the Constitution provides a right of access to contraceptives, but that it provides married couples with a right of privacy. This privacy right was found to be impermissibly infringed by the Connecticut statute.

[3] *United States v. One Package*, 86 F.2d 737 (2nd Cir. 1936).
[4] 381 U.S. 479 (1965).

It is worth spending some time on *Griswold* and the way it linked procreation and privacy because the opinion laid the foundation for far more controversial Court decisions in the 1970s and 1980s involving abortion and the rights of pregnant minors.

The word privacy does not appear anywhere in the U.S. Constitution. How then did the Court find a right of privacy? Justice Douglas, writing for the Court, explained:

> The association of people is not mentioned in the Constitution nor in the Bill of Rights. The right to educate a child in a school of the parent's choice—whether public or private or parochial—is also not mentioned. Nor is the right to study any particular subject or any foreign language. Yet the First Amendment has been construed to include certain of those rights. . . .
>
> The foregoing cases suggest that specific guarantees in the Bill of Rights have penumbras, formed by emanations from those guarantees that help give them life and substance. Various guarantees create zones of privacy. The right of association contained in the penumbra of the First Amendment is one, as we have seen. The third amendment in its prohibition against the quartering of soldiers "in any house" in time of peace without the consent of the owner is another facet of that privacy. The Fourth Amendment explicitly affirms the "right of the people to be secure in their persons, houses, papers, and effects, against unreasonable searches and seizures." The Fifth Amendment in its Self-Incrimination Clause enables the citizen to create a zone of privacy which government may not force him to surrender to his detriment. The Ninth Amendment provides: "The enumeration in the Constitution, of certain rights, shall not be construed to deny or disparage others retained by the people" (482–484).

Emphasizing that the Connecticut statute before the Court prohibited the *use* of contraceptives, including use by married couples, Justice Douglas linked procreation and privacy by adding, "Would we allow the police to search the sacred precincts of marital bedrooms for telltale signs of the use of contraceptives? The very idea is repulsive to the notions of privacy surrounding the marriage relationship."

Recognition by the Supreme Court of rights not explicitly protected by the Constitution (such as the right of privacy announced in *Griswold*) has been criticized by many legal scholars as placing too much power in the hands of unelected judges. Professor John Ely, for example, notes that "appeal to some notion to be found neither in the Constitution nor . . . in the judgment of the political branches, seems especially vulnerable to a charge of inconsistency with democratic theory" (Ely 1980, 5). By contrast, Professors Heymann and Barzelay (1973) contend:

> [The] family unit [is] an integral part of [our constitutional system.] . . . [The] immensely important power of deciding about

matters of early socialization has been allocated to the family, not to
the government. . . . For the Court to have declined strict review of
state legislation that limits the private right to choose whom to marry
and whether to raise a family, or to decide within wide bounds how
to rear one's children, would have been to leave the most basic sub-
structure of our society and government [to] political whim
(Heymann and Barzelay 1973, 772–773).

Professor Charles Black (1970) has said that *Griswold* is not so much a case
that the law tests as a case that tests the law:

If our constitutional law could permit such a thing to happen then
we might almost as well not have any law of constitutional limitations, partly because the thing is so outrageous in itself, and partly
because a constitutional law inadequate to deal with such an outrage would be too feeble, in method and doctrine, to deal with a very
great amount of equally outrageous material. Virtually all the inti-
macies, privacies and autonomies of life would be regulable by the
legislature . . . (Black 1970, 32).

Whether or not the Court was justified in finding a right of privacy in
the Constitution, it is important for our purposes to notice the way *Griswold*
became a stepping stone to the establishment of a right of *access* to contraceptives. In 1977, in *Carey v. Population Services International*,[5] the Supreme
Court decided a case involving a New York statute that regulated access to
contraceptives. The statute prohibited anyone other than a licensed phar-
macist from distributing contraceptives to persons over 16 years of age, and
prohibited anyone from selling or distributing contraceptives to anyone under
the age of 16. A restriction on sale, of course, would not have to be enforced
by the kind of offensive methods that led the Court in *Griswold* to overturn
a prohibition of use. The Court nevertheless struck down the first restriction:

. . . *Griswold* may no longer be read as holding only that a State may
not prohibit a married couple's use of contraceptives. Read in light
of its progeny,[6] the teaching of *Griswold* is that the Constitution protects individual decision in matters of childbearing from unjustified
intrusion by the State.

By the 1980s, the legal right to limit procreation through the use of
contraceptive measures was so firmly established that private suits began to
reach the courts in which women sued sexual partners for deceiving them
about their infertility.

---

[5]431 U.S. 678 (1977).
[6]The primary case the Court cited was *Roe v. Wade*, discussed in the text at note 17, *infra*.

Consider the facts in one recent California case.[7] Barbara A. hired John G., a lawyer, to represent her in a family law matter. On two occasions they had sexual intercourse with each other. Before they engaged in sexual intercourse the first time, Barbara demanded that John use a condom because she did not want to become pregnant. He assured her, "I can't possibly get anyone pregnant." Relying on this representation, Barbara A. proceeded. She did become pregnant. It was a tubal pregnancy; and, as a consequence, Barbara was forced to undergo surgery to save her life. Her fallopian tube was removed and she was rendered sterile by the surgery. She sued John G. for physical, emotional, and financial injuries resulting from the pregnancy, and won.

The Supreme Court had more difficulty in *Carey v. Population Services* with the issue of whether to uphold the restriction on distribution of contraceptives to minors. A majority of the justices could not agree on a single opinion. A plurality of four[8] argued that because the Court in an earlier case had struck down a blanket requirement of parental consent on the choice of a minor to terminate her pregnancy, a blanket prohibition on the distribution of contraceptives had to be unconstitutional as well. They reasoned: "The State's interests in protection of the mental and physical health of the pregnant minor, and in protection of potential life are clearly more implicated by the abortion decision than by the decision to use a nonhazardous contraceptive." As to the claim that access to contraceptives would lead to increased sexual activity among the young, the four justices replied, "The same argument . . . would support a ban on abortions for minors, or indeed support a prohibition on abortion, or access to contraceptives, for the unmarried. . . . Yet, in each of these areas, the Court has rejected the argument, noting in *Roe v. Wade*, that 'no court or commentator has taken the argument seriously.'"

Justice White agreed that the statute at issue in the case was unconstitutional, but only because the State had failed to prove that the prohibition "measurably contributes" to the deterrent purposes the State advanced as justification for the restriction. He agreed with Justice Stevens who said "I would describe as 'frivolous' the argument that a minor has the constitutional right to put contraceptives to their intended use, notwithstanding the combined objection of both parents and the State." Justice Powell also concurred to make clear that he too would uphold a requirement of prior parental consultation. Chief Justice Burger and Justice Rehnquist dissented. According to Justice Rehnquist:

> Those who valiantly but vainly defended the heights of Bunker Hill
> in 1775 made it possible that men such as James Madison might later
> sit in the first Congress and draft the Bill of Rights to the Constitution.

---

[7]*Barbara A. v. John G.*, 145 Cal. App. 3d 369 (Cal. Ct. App. 1983).

[8]Justices Brennan, Stewart, Marshall, and Blackmun.

The post-Civil War Congresses which drafted the Civil War Amendments to the Constitution could not have accomplished their task
without the blood of brave men on both sides which was shed at
Shiloh, Gettysburg, and Cold Harbor. If those responsible for these
Amendments, by feats of valor or efforts of draftsmanship, could have
lived to know that their efforts had enshrined in the Constitution the
right of commercial vendors of contraceptives to peddle them to
unmarried minors through such means as window displays and vend-
ing machines located in the men's room of truck stops, notwithstanding the considered judgment of the New York Legislature to the contrary, it is not difficult to imagine their reaction (717).

The division on the Court continues a longstanding debate over how
much minors' rights are limited and how to implement the limits. Even John
Stuart Mill, perhaps the leading proponent of the principle of autonomy,
qualified his position with respect to minors:

It is, perhaps, hardly necessary to say that this doctrine is meant to
apply only to human beings in the maturity of their faculties. We are
not speaking of children or of young persons below the age which
the law may fix as that of manhood or womanhood. Those who are
still in a state to require being taken care of by others must be protected against their own actions as well as against external injury (Mill
1859, Chapter 1).

Although there seems to be widespread agreement that minors must be protected from their own imprudence, there is less agreement on when protection is needed and on whether the ultimate power to protect minors
should be vested in their parents or in the state.

Consider the challenge brought in 1981 in federal court in New York[9]
to state restrictions on marriage and illegitimacy. The case was about whether
the state should permit minors to marry to legitimize the birth of their child
despite the opposition of their parents. The plaintiffs, Maria Moe, age 15,
and Raoul Roe, age 18 (the names are fictitious, reflecting the willingness of
the judicial system to protect the privacy of minors who litigate on personal
matters) wanted to marry. The law in New York provided at that time that
all male applicants for a marriage license between ages 16 and 18 and all
female applicants between ages 14 and 18 had to obtain "written consent to
the marriage from both parents of the minor or minors." Maria, who was
pregnant, requested consent from her mother, a widow, to marry Raoul, but
her mother refused, apparently because she wanted to continue receiving
welfare benefits for Maria. Maria then challenged the New York law as a
violation of the constitutional right to marry. The court denied her request

---

[9]*Moe v. Dinkins*, 533 F. Supp. 623 (S.D.N.Y. 1981), affirmed 669 F.2d 67 (2d Cir. 1982).

and upheld the statute on the basis that the right to marry does not protect the rights of minors to the same extent it protects the rights of adults.

CASE 5.1

In 1981, the right of parents to oversee the reproductive activities of their adolescent children was also at issue in the decision of the United States Department of Health and Human Services to issue regulations requiring any family planning program that received federal funds to notify within 10 working days the parents or guardians of any minor who was given contraceptives. The regulations were later invalidated by a federal judge, who found that they were not consistent with the expressed intent of Congress in authorizing funding for family planning programs.[10] Can the result in this case be squared with the holding in the case of Maria Moe and Raoul Roe? Assume you have been asked to advise your Congressman on whether to vote for proposed new legislation that would legalize the notification requirement. What are the strongest arguments for and against such legislation? What would you advise, and why?

There has been almost no litigation over the use of (voluntary) sterilization to limit procreation despite the fact that by 1977, sterilization had become the contraceptive measure used most by married couples in the United States. One partner in each of some 6 million couples, constituting one-third of all couples practicing birth control, has undergone sterilization (Areen 1985).

This relative absence of public controversy does not reflect greater consensus on the ethics of sterilization, as religious objections to contraception generally also apply to sterilization. There are additional religious objections, moreover, that apply only to sterilization. Pope Pius XI's 1930 encyclical on marriage, for example, holds: "[p]rivate individuals have no other power over the members of their bodies than that which pertains to their natural ends; and they are not free to destroy or to mutilate their members, or in any other way render themselves unfit for their natural functions, except where no other provision can be made for the good of the whole body" (Pius XI 1930, 43).

The fact that sterilization is generally irreversible distinguishes it from other contraceptive measures. Its irreversible character also makes it particularly important to ensure that any consent to sterilization is both informed and voluntary. To prevent abuse in the wake of publicized reports of young black girls being sterilized in circumstances that suggested deceit or coercion,

---

[10] *Planned Parenthood Federation of America v. Heckler*, 712 F.2d 650 (1983).

the federal government has taken the position that federal funding may not be used to pay for the sterilization of minors of mentally incompetent adults.[11] Federal money can be used to fund voluntary sterilization for competent adults, but only after they have given informed consent in writing. They must also be informed that their right to future care or treatment or to other federally funded benefits will not be affected if they reject sterilization.

MANDATORY STERILIZATION FOR EUGENIC PURPOSES

No medically safe method of sterilizing men or women was developed until almost the end of the nineteenth century (O'Hara and Sanks 1956). Once the new technology was available, a period of widespread governmental intrusion on reproductive choice began with the passage of eugenic legislation that authorized mandatory sterilization designed to "save" society from the offspring of "defective" citizens. The first such state sterilization law was passed in 1907, in Indiana, where Dr. Sharp of the State Reformatory mounted a campaign for the measure. His purpose was not only eugenic, but "to reduce sexual overexcitation in delinquent boys" (Kevles 1985, 108). Between 1907 and 1917, fifteen more states enacted eugenic sterilization laws. Most of these laws gave the state the power to compel the sterilization of habitual or confirmed criminals, epileptics, and the "insane" (Kevles 1985).

In 1927, the Supreme Court considered the constitutionality of one of these statutes in *Buck v. Bell*.[12] In an opinion by Justice Oliver Wendell Holmes, Jr., the Court upheld a Virginia law that authorized the forcible sterilization of 18-year-old Carrie Buck, who was alleged to be "feeble minded," and who had already given birth to one daughter. Holmes' opinion reflects the social Darwinism that was popular at the time:

> . . . We have seen more than once that the public welfare may call upon the best citizens for their lives. It would be strange if it could not call upon those who already sap the strength of the State for these lesser sacrifices, often not felt to be such by those concerned, in order to prevent our being swamped with incompetence. It is better for all the world, if instead of waiting to execute degenerate offspring for crime, or to let them starve for their imbecility, society can prevent those who are manifestly unfit from continuing their kind. The principle that sustains compulsory vaccination is broad enough to cover cutting the Fallopian tubes. Three generations of imbeciles are enough.

---

[11]42 C.F.R sections 50.201 to 50.210.
[12]274 U.S. 200 (1927).

The Supreme Court has never overruled *Buck*.[13] Seventeen states, moreover, currently authorize the involuntary sterilization of some persons (Areen 1985). It is estimated that some 70,000 people have been subjected to compulsory sterilization in this country since the beginning of the century (Areen 1985).

The rationale provided by the Supreme Court in *Buck* for mandatory sterilization does not stand up well in the light of modern scientific knowledge. First, no hereditary basis has been established for criminal behavior. Science has found no genetic basis for murder or stealing, for example. Second, although there is evidence of a genetic component to intelligence, great debate exists over the relative influence of heredity and environment (Jensen 1972; Layzer 1974). Finally, errors can be made in attempting to measure a person's intelligence. It is striking that mistakes appear to have been made in the very case that went to the Supreme Court. Carrie Buck's daughter Vivian, who died at the age of 7, was considered a "bright child" by her second grade teachers. A physician who examined Carrie Buck in the 1970s reported that she also was not mentally retarded. He judged that she had been sterilized because her infant daughter was considered "slow" and because she was the unwed daughter of an "antisocial" woman some thought was a prostitute (Areen 1985, 835). Thus, there were not "three generations of imbeciles."

In recent years, a growing number of state courts have established standards that must be met before a retarded person may be sterilized:

1. Those advocating sterilization bear the heavy burden of proving by clear and convincing evidence that sterilization is in the best interests of the incompetent.
2. The incompetent must be afforded a full judicial hearing at which medical testimony is presented and the incompetent, through a guardian appointed for the litigation, is allowed to present proof and cross-examine witnesses.
3. The judge must be assured that a comprehensive medical, psychological, and social evaluation is made of the incompetent.
4. The judge must determine that the individual is legally incompetent to make the decision whether to be sterilized, and that this incapacity is in all likelihood permanent.
5. The incompetent must be capable of reproduction and unable to care for offspring.

---

[13]It was arguably narrowed by *Skinner v. Oklahoma*, 316 U.S 535 (1942), in which the Court held unconstitutional a statute that authorized the involuntary sterilization of certain, rather arbitrary, categories of criminals. The Court explained: "We are dealing here with legislation which involves one of the basic civil rights of man. Marriage and procreation are fundamental to the very existence and survival of the race. The power to sterilize, if exercised, may have subtle, farreaching and devastating effects. In evil or reckless hands it can cause races or types which are inimical to the dominant group to wither and disappear. There is no redemption for the individual whom the law touches. Any experiment which the State conducts is to his irreparable injury. He is forever deprived of a basic liberty."

CASE 5.2

Sonya is a severely retarded 13-year-old with an IQ of about 25 to 30 (the equivalent of a mental age of 1–2 years), blind, and with pronounced neurological problems. She was born a normal child. At the age of 5 months, she was severely injured in an automobile accident that caused brain damage and temporary paralysis. Unable to cope with the event, Sonya's mother took her to live with her grandmother, who is 61 years old. Sonya, her two sisters, and her aunt have been living with her grandmother ever since. Sonya regularly attends a special school but has missed many sessions lately because of her physical problems. Sonya has reached puberty and is experiencing pain connected with menstruation. She is unable to care for her most basic hygienic needs and is irritable and disoriented during the menstruation process. Her grandmother, wanting to free Sonya from her pain and disorientation during her periods, as well as to protect her from the consequences of rape, seeks to have a hysterectomy performed, which would both terminate Sonya's menstrual cycle and sterilize her. If you were the judge, would you authorize sterilization? Why or why not? Do you find the reasoning in *Buck v. Bell* helpful? Why or why not?

6. Sterilization must be the only practicable means of contraception.
7. The proposed operation must be the least restrictive alternative available.
8. To the extent possible, the judge must hear testimony from the incompetent concerning his or her understanding and desire, if any, for the proposed operation and its consequences.
9. The judge must examine the motivation for the request for sterilization (Areen et al. 1984, 1283).

Are these safeguards sufficient to protect against possible abuse of the power to sterilize? What justifications, if any, might there be for sterilizing a mentally impaired person? Consider the case of Sonya F (Case 5.2).[14]

ABORTION, FETAL RIGHTS, AND THE RIGHT OF PRIVACY

Once constitutional protection was granted for the use of contraceptives, it was inevitable that the question of the constitutional status of abortion would arise. Abortion and infanticide have often been used to limit procreation

[14]*Wentzel v. Montgomery General Hospital,* 293 Md. 685, 447 A.2d 1244, certiorari denied, 103 S.Ct. 790 (1983).

when contraceptive measures fail. Abortion, from this perspective, is simply another form of birth control, and one that should be entitled to the same constitutional protection.

On the other hand, infanticide is condemned both legally and morally as murder. If a fetus is entitled to the same protection as an infant, abortion should also be considered murder. The resolution of the moral and legal status of abortion, in short, appears to be closely tied to the moral status of the fetus.

The Status of the Fetus

Unfortunately, there is no agreement in our society on the moral status of a fetus. Many hold that from the moment of conception, a fetus should have the same moral status as a born human being. Philip Devine, for example, begins with the rule against infanticide. He argues there are two possible justifications for the rule: (1) the infant is a member of the human species (species principle); and (2) the infant will, in due course, think, talk, love, and have a sense of justice (potentiality principle). Because principles (1) and (2) are also true of fetuses, it follows that, from conception on, fetuses should also be protected and abortion considered murder (Devine 1978).

What if the life of the pregnant woman is at stake? Baruch Brody argues that the principle of self-defense does not permit abortion even in this instance because the fetus is not attempting to take the woman's life. He suggests considering the situation in which A needs a medicine to stay alive. C owns some medicine but will give it to A only if A kills B. Brody concludes that just as it is not permissible for A to kill B in this instance, it is not right for a woman to abort a fetus even when her own life is at stake (Brody 1975).

Nancy Davis has challenged the position taken by Brody and others that a pregnant woman has no right to abort even when her life is at stake. Davis argues that the pregnant woman has a stronger claim to life than the fetus when the two rights are in conflict because there is "a morally relevant asymmetry between the woman and the fetus" (Davis 1984):

> [I]f we ask ourselves what is plausible in the view that [the fetus] does owe a debt to the woman who carries it, [we would note that a] pregnant woman provides life-support to the developing fetus through her body, and the fetus is, in turn, parasitic upon her: a fetus thus survives off a woman (that is, at her expense), not in partnership with her. Since the life and well-being of the fetus are sustained through its physical dependence on the woman's body, the very fact of being pregnant undermines a woman's autonomy. She cannot choose what she shall do without thereby choosing for someone else, and she must therefore take into account the possible risks of even the most mundane sorts of activities: driving a car, lifting a bucket, taking an aspirin. While providing assistance to a postfetal person may involve a significant reduction of a benefactor's freedom of choice

and action, pregnancy involves a physical invasion of the body. . . . The relationship between the pregnant woman and the dependent fetus can thus be seen to be inherently asymmetrical. . . . The supposition that the asymmetry is of moral significance may well underlie the widespread conviction that abortion is defensible whenever the pregnancy poses a threat to the woman's life. . . . It may [also] have considerably more permissive implications. . . . If the woman's claims are strong enough to justify abortion—with the assistance of a third party—when it is undertaken to preserve her life, then they *may* be strong enough to justify it in other cases as well (200–205).

Others take the position that fetuses should not have the same moral status as persons, including pregnant women. H. Tristram Engelhardt, for example, argues:

Even if the fetus is a human organism that will probably be genetically and organically continuous with a human person, it is not yet such a person. Simply put, fetuses are not rational, self-conscious beings—that is, given a strict definition of persons, fetuses do not qualify as persons. One sees this when comparing talk about dead men with talk about fetuses. When speaking of a dead man, one knows of whom one speaks, the one who dies, the person whom one knew before his death. But in speaking of the fetus, one has no such person to whom one can refer. There is not yet a person, a "who" to whom one can refer in the case of the fetus (compare: one can keep promises to dead men but not to men yet unborn). In short, the fetus in no way singles itself out as, or shows itself to be, a person . . . (Engelhardt 1982, 96).

Suppose we had a social practice of naming fetuses once a woman knew she was pregnant. Would that affect how the fetus should be regarded? What significance, if any, should be attached to the fact that no such practice exists? Even if one concludes that fetuses are not entitled to the same respect as born persons, however, it does not follow that we can be indifferent to their well-being. Engelhardt cautions, "It is one thing to say that an entity lacks the dignity of being a person strictly, and another thing to say that it does not have great value" (Engelhardt 1982, 100). A person who believes that abortion is always morally permissible, for example, might nonetheless think punishment appropriate for a person who wantonly kicked a pregnant woman in an effort to injure the fetus.

A third group takes an intermediate position on the moral status of the fetus. Judith Jarvis Thomson states, "We shall probably have to agree that the fetus has already become a human person well before birth. By the tenth week, for example, it already has a face, arms and legs, fingers and toes; it has internal organs, and brain activity is detectable" (Thomson 1971, 3–4). Warren Quinn favors what he terms a "process theory" of the fetus:

[T]he fetus is a being to some extent capable of losing a fully human future life, the very kind of life we now enjoy. [I]t is hard for me to see how the loss of an object of this significance, the loss of the very thing that for ourselves we hold most important in the world, could have no moral weight. In any case, there is surely no precedent for thinking that it could be ignored, for there are simply no other situations in which such losses are at issue where a morally sensitive agent ignores them. The fetus, I feel, must have a right that its future welfare counts for something and thus that there be a sufficiently strong moral case for sacrificing its good. And to the extent that the ties of biological kinship themselves add special weight, it will have an especially strong version of this right against its parents. [A]s the fetus becomes more fully human the seriousness of aborting it will approach that of infanticide. In this way the process theory . . . validates the . . . moral intuition that later abortions are more objectionable than earlier ones (Quinn 1984, 53–54).

Can the Morality of Abortion Be Separated from the Status of the Fetus?

Judith Jarvis Thomson has argued that abortion may be morally acceptable even if a fetus is granted the same moral status as an adult. Imagine that you wake up one morning to find yourself in a hospital bed next to a famous, unconscious violinist found to have a fatal kidney ailment. The Society of Music Lovers canvassed all the available medical records and found that you alone had the right blood type to help. They therefore kidnapped you and plugged the violinist's circulatory system into yours, so that your kidneys could be used to extract poisons from his blood as well as your own. The director of the hospital says "We're sorry the Society did this to you— we would never have permitted it if we had known. But still, they did it, and the violinist is now plugged into you. To unplug you would be to kill him. But never mind. It's only for nine months. By then he will have recovered from his ailment and can be safely unplugged from you"(Thomson 1971, 48–49).

Thomson concludes that to allow the violinist to use your kidneys is a "kindness on your part" but not "something you owe him." She explains, "the right to life consists not in the right not to be killed, but rather in the right not to be killed unjustly. [This is how] to square the fact that the violinist has a right to life with the fact that you do not act unjustly toward him in unplugging yourself, thereby killing him. For if you do not kill him unjustly, you do not violate his right to life. . . . [Now] the gap in the argument against abortion stares us plainly in the face: it is by no means enough to show that the fetus is a person, and to remind us that all persons have a right to life—we need to be shown also that killing the fetus violates its right to life, i.e., that abortion is unjust killing" (1971, 57). Thomson adds that this is not an argument that abortion is always moral. On the contrary, if it would take only one hour to save the life of the violinist, for example, then it would be "indecent" to refuse (Thomson 1971, 61). The point is that a person should not be required to be more of a Good Samaritan when pregnant than at other times.

The analogy used by Thomson has been criticized for overlooking the responsibility that the pregnant woman has for placing the fetus in a vulnerable position. Except in the case of pregnancy due to rape, the woman did indulge in intercourse and thus is "among those who are at least partially responsible [for] the fetus being in need of a life-support system" (Tooley 1983, 45). Thomson replies:

> [Suppose] people-seeds drift about in the air like pollen, and if you open your windows, one may drift in and take root in your carpets or upholstery. You don't want children, so you fix up your windows with fine mesh screens, the very best you can buy. As can happen, however, [one] of the screens is defective, and a seed drifts in and takes root. Does the person-plant who now develops have a right to the use of your house: Surely [not] (Thomson 1971, 59).

Donald Regan has also attempted to expand the Good Samaritan analogy to pregnancies that do not result from rape (Regan 1979). He concedes that except in cases of rape the pregnant woman has done something that provides some reason to compel her to aid the fetus. But she has not done as much as has a parent to establish a relationship with a child, nor a voluntary rescuer to establish a relationship with the object of the rescue. In addition, no other potential Samaritan is required to bear burdens as physically invasive as the burdens of pregnancy and childbirth. He concludes that laws forbidding abortion are at odds with the general principles of Good Samaritan law.

To what extent can moral disagreement about abortion be resolved by appeals to analogies, by appeals to our moral instincts or judgment about other situations and circumstances, or by refining our concept of a "person" or a "human being"? Is our collective concept of a "person" or "human being" a determining influence on our moral view of abortion, or is our moral view of abortion, supported on other grounds, the determining factor, to which our concept of a "person" or "human being" is adapted?

The Constitutional Status of Abortion

In 1973, in *Roe v. Wade*,[15] the Supreme Court invalidated a Texas statute that made it a criminal act to perform most abortions. Justice Blackmun's opinion for the Court contains a long, historic section devoted to proving that most restrictions on abortion are not ancient, but originated in the

---

[15]410 U.S. 113 (1973).

latter half of the nineteenth century. A major obstacle to his thesis was the Hippocratic Oath, which prohibits giving an "abortive remedy" to any woman (Edelstein 1943, 3). Justice Blackmun turned to scholarly sources to demonstrate both that the Oath was the code of a minority medical group and that most Greek thinkers approved of abortion, at least early in the pregnancy. Aristole, according to his *Hist. Anim.*, for example, thought that the fetus, if male, did not become animate until about the fortieth day after conception and, if female, about the ninetieth day after conception (Barnes 1984). His views were later adopted by early Christian writers including St. Augustine.

The Romans shared many of the Greeks' attitudes. The Stoic philosopher Seneca wrote without apology, "We destroy monstrous births, and drown our children if they are born weakly and unnaturally formed" (Noonan 1966). There was, in the code of Justinian, an attempt to limit abortion, but the reason was to protect the right of the father to his children—the child's interests do not seem to have mattered (Rachels 1986).

At common law, abortion was not a crime prior to "quickening," that is, the point when the pregnant woman first feels fetal movement. Even after quickening, abortion was punished less harshly than the murder of a born person.

As late as 1800, there was no legislation in the United States on abortion, yet by 1900 virtually every state made most abortion a crime due in large part to an aggressive campaign against abortion launched by physicians affiliated with the American Medical Association begun at the end of the Civil War (Mohr 1978).

The basis for the decision of the Supreme Court in *Roe* was the right of privacy first announced in *Griswold*. Although the Court in *Roe* held that a right of privacy belongs to the pregnant woman, it also stated that the right does not include an unlimited right to "do with one's body as one pleases." In summarizing its holding, the Court added that during the first trimester of pregnancy the abortion decision "must be left to the *medical judgment of the pregnant woman's attending physician*" (emphasis added). The *Roe* decision thus grants women only a conditional power to decide whether to have an abortion, a power that may be vetoed by the medical profession. The Court never explained what it meant when it invoked a medical judgment standard, moreover. In practice, a physician is likely to decide on the basis of his or her own moral judgment. Is this an appropriate basis on which to make an abortion decision? Will it encourage women to shop for a physician whose moral judgment is compatible with their own? Is that bad?

The Court in *Roe* also made clear that the right of privacy is to be balanced against other rights. Thus the Court held that after the end of the first trimester of pregnancy, states are free to regulate the abortion procedure in ways that are "reasonably related to maternal health." The Court stated that states might, for example, require that late-term abortions be performed in hospitals rather than in out-patient settings.[16]

The Court also held that a fetus is not a "person" as that term is used in the Fourteenth Amendment of the Constitution. States nonetheless are free to legislate to protect the life and health of fetuses, just as they can (and do) legislate to protect other nonpersons, such as animals or personal property. States may not regulate or proscribe abortion, however, in pursuing their interest in "the potentiality of human life" until after the fetus is "viable."

The Court defined a viable fetus as one "potentially able to live outside the mother's womb, albeit with artificial aid." Thus, the Court did not set viability at the end of the second trimester as sometimes reported. Rather, it explicitly drew a technology-dependent line, one that will advance closer to conception as medical science increases its ability to save ever younger fetuses. Is this an appropriate line for protecting fetuses? It could be argued that viability is the modern equivalent of birth in the sense that it is the time when, at least in theory, the fetus could survive being separated from the mother and thus is the point when the fetus should be given the same moral deference as an infant. Would it be preferable to have a line that is linked to brain capacities or other characteristics of the fetus?

The holding in *Roe* permits states to proscribe the abortion of viable fetuses; it does not mandate that result. The Court added that the abortion of even viable fetuses may not be proscribed by state law "where it is necessary, in appropriate medical judgment, for the preservation of the life or health of the mother." Only about half the states have acted to limit late abortions (Areen 1985, 181).

In 1992, the Court in *Planned Parenthood v. Casey*[17] rejected the trimester framework established in *Roe* as not essential to the holding of *Roe* and in its place established an "undue burden" standard to decide which limitations imposed by state law are constitutional. Under the new standard, the Court explained, it is constitutional for states to impose a mandatory 24-hour waiting period before an abortion may be performed, and to require the provision of information about the consequences of abortion to the fetus as part of the process of obtaining informed consent.

Examining the Relationship Between Law and Morality

The existence in our society of profound disagreement on the moral status of the fetus as well as the moral status of abortion makes it extremely difficult to decide how the law should treat abortion. Any law will be in conflict

---

[16]In *Akron v. Akron Center for Reproductive Health*, 462 U.S. 416 (1983), the Court held that such a requirement was not constitutional before well into the second trimester of pregnancy because early abortions have become so safe.

[17]505 U.S. 833 (1992).

with the strongly held moral position of parts of the society. Such a law is likely, therefore, to be strongly resisted. Some contend that in such a situation, the law should tolerate different views by leaving the decision to individuals. Mario Cuomo (1984), the former Governor of New York, believes abortion to be morally wrong, for example, yet argues the law should not forbid abortion:

> I believe that legal interdicting of abortion by either the federal government or the individual states is not a plausible possibility and even if it could be obtained, it wouldn't work. Given present attitudes, it would be "Prohibition" revisited, legislating what couldn't be enforced and in the process creating a disrespect for law in general (Cuomo 1984).

Is the danger of disrespect sufficient reason to eschew prohibiting abortion? Are the arguments of Thomson and Regan more persuasive that legal prohibitions on abortion impose a disproportionate burden on pregnant women to be Good Samaritans?

A third argument against a legal prohibition of abortion rests on the claim that an accurate understanding of our constitutional heritage dictates that abortion as well as other limits on procreation should be left to private rather than public control:

> The Constitution was consecrated to the blessings of liberty for ourselves and our posterity—yet it contains no discussion of the right to be a *human* being; no definition of a person; and, indeed, no express provisions guaranteeing to persons that right to carry on their lives protected from the "vicissitudes of the political process" by a zone of privacy or a right of personhood. . . . But the Constitution is not a totalitarian design, dependent for its success upon the homogenization or depersonalization of humanity. The judiciary has thus reached into the Constitution's spirit and structure, and has elaborated from the spare text an idea of "human" and a conception of "being" not merely contemplated but required. [This conception recognizes] the fundamental personal character of a right to reproductive autonomy (Tribe 1978, 893, 923).

The argument for leaving abortion to private choice is buttressed for some by recognition that pregnancy is a burden imposed only on women. Because women's interests have not often been protected in the political system, according to this view, it was appropriate for the Court to protect their interests by removing the debate from the political arena.

On the other hand, to those who think abortion immoral, the argument that the abortion decision should be a matter of individual choice is equivalent to saying that murder should not be a crime simply because some people think it proper.

Additional Legal Issues Concerning Abortion

Three important legal issues were explicitly not decided in *Roe*, but have been addressed in subsequent Supreme Court cases: the rights, if any, of fathers; the rights of pregnant minors; and public funding of abortion. A fourth issue, the right to intervene for the benefit of a fetus over the objection of the pregnant woman, has not been addressed by any federal court although there are several state court decisions on the point.

THE RIGHTS OF FATHERS

In *Planned Parenthood of Central Missouri v. Danforth*,[18] in 1976, the Supreme Court considered a Missouri statute that required a pregnant woman to have the consent of her spouse before an abortion could be performed. Faced with having to empower one spouse or the other to make the decision in the event of conflict, the Court reasoned, "Since it is the woman who physically bears the child and who is the more directly and immediately affected by the pregnancy, as between the two, the balance weighs in her favor." The right of privacy first announced in *Griswold* as grounded in the marital relationship thus has evolved into an individual right that permits a wife to limit procreation by aborting a fetus even in the face of an objection from the man who is her husband and the father of the fetus.

Although the logic of the Court's decision is clear, its broader implications are more fully illustrated by an example posed by George Harris. Imagine a wife, Michelle, who discovers she is pregnant and who decides to have an abortion because a child would interfere with her career. She has never told her husband Steve of her feelings because she knows that he wants a family, but believes she will eventually talk him out of it. That very day Steve is in an automobile accident that leaves him sterile. He tells Michelle that if she will not have the abortion, he will assume full economic and parental responsibility for the child, who is the only biologically related child he will ever be able to father. *Danforth* means Michelle is legally free to refuse. Is her refusal moral? Harris contends that it is not:

> Due to the fact that both men and women have a morally legitimate interest in procreation, couples have an obligation to be forthright and informative about their desires and reservations about family planning. . . . [It] is understandable, though neither mature nor laudable, for a person who is deeply in love with someone with significantly different life plans, perhaps as a result of self-deception, to think that the other person can be brought around to seeing things

---

[18]428 U.S. 52 (1976).

the other way. But it is not excusable. . . . [It] would be wrong to Steve
for Michelle to have the abortion (Harris 1986, 598–599).

Conversely, consider a woman who deliberately deceives a man with
whom she has a sexual relationship by telling him that she is taking birth
control pills. When she gets pregnant, he again makes clear that he does
not want to be a father and offers to pay for an abortion. She refuses, and
later sues him for child support. In the judgment of all courts that have
ruled on this issue, he must pay.[19] The rationale generally given is that
any other result would harm the child. One lower court suggested that a
better resolution in the face of maternal deceit would be to require the
mother to provide as much child support as she possibly can, and to hold
the father liable only for the difference, if any, between what the mother
can afford and the needs of the child. That court was overruled on appeal,
however.[20]

THE RIGHTS OF MINORS

In 1979, the Supreme Court in *Bellotti v. Baird*,[21] considered the right of a
pregnant minor to obtain an abortion. As a general rule, except in emergencies, parents must consent before any medical procedure can be performed on their child. The issue in *Bellotti* was whether a state statute that
embodied that traditional legal rule with respect to abortions was constitutional. A majority of the Court decided the statute was unconstitutional,
but no rationale for the decision was supported by a majority of the Justices. A plurality of four Justices held that "mature minors" must be able to
decide for themselves whether to have an abortion. Because the term is a
new one in constitutional law, it is very unfortunate that the Justices provided only a sketchy definition. They explained that a "mature minor" is
one who is "mature enough and well enough informed to make her abortion decision." The plurality also stated that the determination of who is a
"mature minor" need not be made by a court, but can be made by an administrative agency or officer. Finally, they cautioned that it is a determination that must be made on a case-by-case basis; thus, a state cannot pass a
law that declares all 17-year-olds to be "mature minors."
 The Justices next held that even a minor who does not qualify as mature must be able to have a court order an abortion, even in the face of parental objections, if the court determines it would be in her best interests.

[19]See, e.g., *People in Interest of S.P.B.*, 651 P.2d 1213 (1982).
[20]*In re Pamela P. v. Frank S.*, 110 Misc.2d 978, 443 N.Y.S.2d 343 (1981), reversed 88 A.D.865, 451
N.Y.S.2d 766 (1982), affirmed 59 N.Y.2d 1, 462 N.Y.S.2d 819, 449 N.E.2d 713 (1983).
[21]443 U.S. 622 (1979).

The principle of carving out an exception for mature minors to age-based legal standards is not only new, but potentially extremely far-reaching. Should Maria Moe, for example, have been able to attempt to convince the court that she was mature enough to decide to marry the father of their son?[22] Should a 17-year-old be able to convince a court that he or she is mature enough to vote in a presidential election? Is abortion different? If so, why?

PUBLIC FUNDING

In a series of cases, the Supreme Court has repeatedly held that public funding of abortions is not required by the Constitution. In *Harris v. McRae*,[23] for example, the Court upheld the Hyde Amendment, a law passed by Congress that prohibits federal funding of even medically necessary abortions:

> [R]egardless of whether the freedom of a woman to choose to terminate her pregnancy for health reasons lies at the core or the periphery of the due process liberty recognized in [*Roe v.*] *Wade*, it simply does not follow that a woman's freedom of choice carries with it a constitutional entitlement to the financial resources to avail herself of the full range of protected choices. [A]lthough government may not place obstacles in the path of a woman's exercise of her freedom of choice, it need not remove those not of its own creation. Indigency falls in the latter category. The financial constraints that restrict an indigent woman's ability to enjoy the full range of constitutionally protected freedom of choice are the product not of governmental restrictions on access to abortions, but rather of her indigency. Although Congress has opted to subsidize medically necessary services generally, but not certain medically necessary abortions, the fact remains that the Hyde Amendment leaves an indigent woman with at least the same range of choice in deciding whether to obtain a medically necessary abortion as she would have had if Congress had chosen to subsidize no health care costs at all.

Compare the rationale of the three dissenting Justices—Brennan, Marshall, and Blackmun:

> *Roe* and its progeny established that the pregnant woman has a right to be free from state interference with her choice to have an abortion—a right which, at least prior to the end of the first trimester, absolutely prohibits any governmental regulation of that highly

---

[22]The problem is presented on pages 113–114 of the text.
[23]448 U.S. 297 (1980).

personal decision. The proposition for which these cases stand thus is not that the State is under an affirmative obligation to ensure access to abortions for all who may desire them; it is that the State must refrain from wielding its enormous power and influence in a manner that might burden the pregnant woman's freedom to choose whether to have an abortion. The Hyde Amendment's denial of public funds for medically necessary abortions plainly intrudes upon this constitutionally protected decision, for both by design and effect it serves to coerce indigent pregnant women to bear children that they would otherwise elect not to have.

Feminist Catherine MacKinnon (1984) has criticized the rationale of *Roe v. Wade* for ignoring the needs of women. In her view, *Harris v. McRae* follows logically from *Roe*, but for reasons quite different from those articulated by the Court:

Most [women who seek abortion] did not mean or wish to conceive. In contrast to this fact of women's experience, the abortion debate has centered on separating control over sexuality from control over reproduction. . . . Liberals have supported the availability of the abortion choice as if the woman just happened on the fetus. The political Right imagines that the intercourse which precedes conception is usually voluntary, only to urge abstinence, as if sex were up to women. . . . Continuing this logic, many opponents of state funding of abortions, such as supporters of the Hyde Amendment, would permit funding of abortions when pregnancy results from rape or incest. Thus they make exceptions for those special occasions during which they presume women did not control sex. From all this I deduce that abortion's proponents and opponents share a tacit assumption that women significantly do control sex.

Feminist investigations suggest otherwise. . . . Under conditions in which women do not control access to our sexuality, [the decision in *Roe v. Wade*] facilitates women's heterosexual availability. The availability of abortion removes the one remaining legitimized reason that women have had for refusing sex besides the headache. . . . It is not inconsistent, then, that framed as a privacy right a woman's decision to abort would have no claim on public support and would genuinely not be seen as burdened by that deprivation. Privacy conceived as a right from public intervention and disclosure is the opposite of the relief that [*Harris* and other abortion funding cases] sought for welfare women. State intervention would have provided a choice women did *not* have in private. [Indigent] women, women whose sexual refusal has counted for particularly little, needed something to make their privacy effective. The logic of the court's response resembles the logic by which women are supposed to consent to sex. Preclude the alternatives, then call the sole remaining option "her choice." The point is that the alternatives are precluded *prior* to the reach of the chosen legal doctrine. They are precluded by conditions of sex, race, and class—the very conditions the privacy frame not only leaves tacit, but which it exists to *guarantee* (MacKinnon 1984, 46–53).

If you were a member of Congress, would you support or oppose use of public funds for abortions for indigent women? How would—or should—the fact that many citizens think that abortion is a serious moral wrong affect your choice?

MEDICAL INTERVENTIONS FOR FETUSES

A final issue that *Roe v. Wade* did not resolve is whether the Constitution limits judicial or legislative action intended to protect fetuses when the action also poses risk to, or restricts the liberty of, the pregnant woman. Consider the facts of a recent Georgia case (Case 5.3).[24]

In reaching your decision it is important to notice that the woman was not seeking an abortion. Thus *Roe v. Wade* arguably has no bearing on the matter. On the other hand, one could argue that because the woman has a constitutional right to have an abortion (because her life is at stake), surely she also has the right to subject the fetus to vaginal delivery, whatever the risks. This argument raises the question of what is an abortion. When the

---

CASE 5.3

A woman came into the hospital in her thirty-ninth week of pregnancy. She was diagnosed as having a complete placenta previa, a condition in which the placenta blocks the opening of the womb. In the judgment of the examining physician, there was a 90 percent certainty that the child could not survive vaginal delivery and a 50 percent chance that the mother would also die if vaginal delivery were attempted. A caesarian section was recommended, as it normally is in such circumstances. The woman, for religious reasons, refused to consent to the recommended procedure. The hospital then sought a court order. The trial court granted temporary custody of the fetus to the state. It also ordered the mother to submit to a caesarian in the event that a sonogram confirmed that her condition made vaginal delivery too dangerous. If you were asked to review the decision of the trial court on appeal, how would you decide the matter?

---

[24]The facts are based on *Jefferson v. Griffin Spalding County Hospital Authority*, 247 Ga. 86, 274 S.E.2d 457 (1981).

Court in *Roe* held that a woman has a right, at least early in the pregnancy, to have an abortion, did that mean a right to have the fetus killed, or only a right to terminate the pregnancy by having the fetus removed from her body, in which case the fetus might survive? If *Roe* is read narrowly as granting only a right to terminate the pregnancy, it does not empower a woman to have the fetus killed except when fetal death is a necessary result of the removal procedure.

But to conclude that *Roe* does not empower the woman to refuse a caesarian does not mean that she does not have other principles to invoke to justify her refusal. She might, for example, invoke the principle of respect for autonomy. In addition to overriding her autonomous refusal, implementing the trial court's decision would involve a physical invasion of her body. Surely the right of privacy protects against coerced surgery—or does it? Recall that the Supreme Court has never overruled *Buck v. Bell*, which upheld forcible sterilization for eugenic purposes. Does it follow that a woman could be forced to undergo surgery for the benefit of her fetus (e.g., implantation of a shunt to offset a blocked ureter) although the surgery posed some risk and no benefit to the woman herself?

CONCLUSION

The first restrictions on contraception, sterilization, and abortion were religious in origin. With the rise of the modern secular state, civil law was increasingly employed to regulate marriage and procreation. As the view gained strength that private behavior, including procreation, should not be subject to secular regulation, debate increased as to whether, and if so, to what extent, the law should govern contraception, sterilization, and abortion.

By the late nineteenth century, there were stringent legal restrictions on access to contraceptives or abortion in most states. By the early twentieth century, a number of states had passed statutes authorizing the involuntary sterilization of certain mental patients and prisoners. The legal pendulum then began to swing toward individual choice. In 1965, a decision of the Supreme Court of the United States established that the right of privacy embodied in the Constitution includes the right to decide whether or not to use contraception. In 1973, the Court held that the right of privacy also encompasses a woman's decision to seek an abortion, although later decisions made clear that poor women have no constitutional right to public funds to pay for an abortion. Although the *Roe* decision has been reaffirmed by the Court on several occasions, the Court is now more closely divided than ever on the issue. A number of difficult related questions remain unresolved, moreover, including the extent to which the law can coerce a pregnant woman to act, or not to act, in order to benefit the fetus.

DISCUSSION QUESTIONS

1. Should minors have the same right of access to contraceptives as adults? Should parents be notified if contraceptives are provided to their minor children?

2. Should government-sponsored limitations on procreation for the purpose of limiting the size of the population ever be permitted? When? Is there a morally relevant difference between direct limitations (such as mandatory sterilization) and indirect limitations (such as limiting the amount of welfare available to poor families who have more than three children)?

3. At what point during fetal development does a fetus achieve the status of a full member of the moral community? What is the moral significance of each of the following: conception, implantation, the development of central nervous system tissue, measurable brain activity, the ability to survive outside the womb albeit with mechanical aid, quickening (perception of fetal movement by the mother), birth, ability to use language, ability to reason?

4. No court has ever ordered a parent to give a kidney to a child, yet more than 20 courts have ordered pregnant women to undergo surgical procedures that pose risks to the life of the woman for the sake of a fetus. Is it appropriate to impose greater obligations on pregnant women than on parents? Should a court order a pregnant women to stop using heroin during the pregnancy for the sake of her fetus? Should a court order a pregnant woman not to drink? Should a court order a pregnant woman not to go skiing? Should physicians be required to report when pregnant women are engaged in activities that may harm the fetus they carry? Should such court orders be enforced by jailing pregnant women who refuse to comply? If the obligations of pregnancy become too onerous, will more women avoid seeking medical care or elect to have abortions?

REFERENCES

Areen, J. *Cases and Materials on Family Law,* 2nd ed. New York: Foundation Press, 1985.

Areen, J., King, P., Goldberg, S., Capron, A. *Law, Science and Medicine.* New York: Foundation Press, 1984.

Augustine, St. *De bono coniugali* (The Good of Marriage) (Wilcox trans.). New York: Fathers of the Church, Inc., 1955.

Barnes, J., Ed. *The Complete Works of Aristotle* (Rev. Oxford trans.). Princeton, NJ: Princeton University Press, 1984.

Bishop, J. P. *Commentaries on the Law of Marriage and Divorce and Evidence in Matrimonial Suits,* Vol. I. London, 1852.

Black, C. "The Unfinished Business of the Warren Court." *Wash L Rev* 46 (1970): 3–45.

Brody, B. *Abortion and the Sanctity of Human Life: A Philosophical View.* Cambridge, MA: MIT Press, 1975.

Callahan, D. *Abortion: Law, Choice and Morality.* New York: Macmillan, 1970.

Cuomo, M. "Religious Belief and Public Morality: A Catholic Governor's Perspective." Paper delivered at the University of Notre Dame, September 13, 1984.

Davis, N. "Abortion and Self-Defense." *Philos Public Affairs* 13 (1984): 175–207.

Degler, C. *At Odds: Women and the Family in America from the Revolution to the Present.* Oxford, England: Oxford University Press, 1980.

Devine, P. *The Ethics of Homicide.* Ithaca, NY: Cornell University Press, 1978.

Edelstein, L. *The Hipppocratic Oath.* Baltimore: Johns Hopkins University Press, 1943.

Ely, J. *Democracy and Distrust: A Theory of Judicial Review.* Cambridge, MA: Harvard University Press, 1980.

Engelhardt, H. T. "Medicine and the Concept of Person." In T. Beauchamp and L. Walters, Eds., *Contemporary Issues in Bioethics,* 2d ed. Belmont, CA: Wadsworth, 1982: 94–101.

Fagley, R. *The Population Explosion and Christian Responsibility.* New York: Oxford University Press, 1980.

Feldman, D. M. *Marital Relations, Birth Control and Abortion in Jewish Law.* New York: Schocken, 1968.

Gordon, L. *Woman's Body, Woman's Right.* New York: Penguin, 1976.

———. "Why Nineteenth-Century Feminists Did Not Support 'Birth Control' and Twentieth-Century Feminists Do: Feminism, Reproduction, and the Family." In B. Thorne and M. Yalom, Eds., *Rethinking the Family: Some Feminist Questions.* New York: Longman, 1982.

Haney, R. *Comstockery in America.* Boston: Beacon Press, 1960.

Harris, G. W. "Fathers and Fetuses." *Ethics* 96 (1986): 594.

Helmholz, R. *Marriage Litigation in Medieval England.* Cambridge, MA: Cambridge University Press, 1974.

Heymann, R., Barzelay, D. "The Forest and the Trees: *Roe v. Wade* and Its Critics." *B.U.L. Rev.* 53 (1973): 675–784.

Jensen, A. *Educability and Group Differences.* London: Methuen, 1972.

Kennedy, D. *Birth Control in America: The Career of Margaret Sanger.* New Haven, CT: Yale University Press, 1970.

Kevles, D. J. *In the Name of Eugenics: Genetics and the Uses of Human Heredity.* New York: Knopf, 1985.

Layzer, D. "Heritability Analysis of IQ Scores: Science or Numerology?" *Science* 183 (1974): 1259–1266.

Luther, M. *The Large Catechism.* (R. E. Fischer, trans.) Philadelphia: Fortress Press, 1959.

MacKinnon, C. "*Roe v. Wade*: A Study in Male Ideology." In J. Garfield and P. Hennessey, Eds., *Abortion: Moral and Legal Perspectives.* Amherst, MA: University of Massachusetts Press, 1984.

Mill, J. S. *On Liberty* (Rapaport, Ed.) Indianapolis: Hackett Publishing, 1978.

Mohr, J. C. *Abortion in America: The Origins and Evolution of National Policy, 1800–1900*. Oxford, England: Oxford University Press, 1979.

Noonan, J. *Contraception: A History of Its Treatment by Catholic Theologians and Canonists.* Cambridge, MA: Harvard University Press, 1966.

———. *The Morality of Abortion: Legal and Historical Perspectives.* Cambridge, MA: Harvard University Press, 1970.

———. "Contraception." In W. Reich, Ed., *Encyclopedia of Bioethics.* New York: Free Press, 1978: 204–216.

Oates, W., Ed. *The Stoic and Epicurean Philosophers: The Complete Writings of Epicurus, Epictetus, Lucretius and Marcus Aurelius.* New York: Random House, 1940.

O'Hara, J., Sanks, T. "Eugenic Sterilization." *Georgetown L J* 45 (1956): 20–24.

Paul VI. "Humanae Vitae." Trans. as "Humanae Vitae (Human Life)." *Catholic Mind* (Sept. 1968): 35–48.

Pius XI. "Casti Connubi." ("On Christian Marriage"). *Catholic Mind* (1930): 21–64.

Quinn, W. "Abortion: Identity and Loss." *Philos Public Affairs* 13 (1984): 24–54.

Rachels, J. *The End of Life.* Oxford, England: Oxford University Press, 1986.

Regan, D. "Rewriting *Roe v. Wade*." *Mich L Rev* 77 (1979): 1569–1646.

Seneca. *Fragments*, F. Haase, Ed. (Quoted in Noonan, 1966.)

Smith, P. "Comment: The History and Future of the Legal Battle over Birth Control." *Cornell L Rev* 49 (1964): 275–303.

Speiser, E. A. *The Anchor Bible: Genesis.* New, York: Doubleday, 1964.

Thomson, J. "A Defense of Abortion." *Philos Public Affairs* (1971): 47–66.

Tooley, M. *Abortion and Infanticide.* Oxford, England: Clarendon, 1983.

Tribe, L. *American Constitutional Law.* Mineola, NY: Foundation Press, 1978.

Veatch, R. *Case Studies in Medical Ethics.* Cambridge, MA: Harvard University Press, 1977.

Warnock, M. *A Question of Life.* London: Blackwell, 1985.

Cases

Akron v. Akron Center for Reproductive Health, 462 U.S. 416 (1983).

Barbara A. v. John G., 145 Cal. App. 3d 369 (Cal. Ct. App. 1983).

Bellotti v. Baird, 443 U.S. 622 (1979).

Buck v. Bell, 274 U.S. 200 (1927).

Carey v. Population Services International, 431 U.S. 678 (1977).

Griswold v. Connecticut, 381 U.S. 479 (1965).

Harris v. McRae, 448 U.S. 297 (1980).

Jefferson v. Griffin Spalding County Hospital Authority, 247 Ga. 86, 274 S.E.2d 457 (1981).

Moe v. Dinkins, 533 F. Supp. 623, affirmed, 669 F.2d 67 (2d Cir. 1982).

In re Pamela P v. Frank S., 110 Misc.2d 978, 443 N.Y.S.2d 343 (1981), reversed 88 A.D. 865, 451 N.Y.S.2d 766 (1982).

People in Interest of S.P.B., 651 P.2d 1213 (1982).

Planned Parenthood of Southeastern Pennsylvania v. Casey, 505 U.S. 833 (1992).

Planned Parenthood Federation of America v. Heckler, 712 F.2d 650 (D.C.Cir. 1983).

Planned Parenthood of Central Missouri v. Danforth, 428 U.S. 52 (1976).

Roe v. Wade, 410 U.S. 113 (1973).

Skinner v. Oklahoma, 316 U.S. 535 (1942).

Thornburgh v. American College of Obstetricians and Gynecologists, 476 U.S. 747 (1986).

United States v. One Package, 86 F.2d 737 (2d Cir. 1936).

Wentzel v. Montgomery General Hospital, 293 Md. 685, 447 A.2d 1244, certiorari denied, 103 S.Ct. 790 (1983).

6

Human
Experimentation

A. M. CAPRON

SUMMARY

We often think of the German concentration camp experimentation as the epitome of unethical research, yet the regulations governing research in Germany at the time were as advanced as any in existence. The German experience is compared with the development of research ethics in the United States beginning with criticism of the ethically questionable American research in the 1960s.

Key terms, such as *research* and *therapy*; *therapeutic* and *nontherapeutic*; and *benefit*, though commonly employed, are characterized by a host of subtle nuances that make their meanings unclear. The very definitions of these terms carry ethical freight.

Research involving human subjects needs to be justified by appealing to ethical principles. Such principles include respect for persons (regardless of competence), beneficence, nonmaleficence, and justice. The emergence of ethical and legal guidelines for human experimentation and the participation of the government in the establishment of such standards mark important developments in bioethics. This chapter outlines the steps involved in the regulatory process and explores such documents as the Nuremberg Code and the Declaration of Helsinki as well as federal and state regulation of research with human subjects.

Next, the discussion turns to current ethical issues such as highly risky research, risky behavior and beneficence, randomization, disclosure of the null hypothesis, double-blind studies, placebos, waiver of consent, research design, and the use of fetuses and abortuses. Each is analyzed within a theoretical framework that emphasizes the interplay of two central factors—risk and consent.

Evaluating research involving human beings is a difficult and puzzling task. Such research is at once both necessary and problematic, both socially laudatory and ethically dangerous. On the good side, it has enabled physicians to exercise the highest form of beneficence by creating tools with which they can truly do good for their patients. On the bad side, some of the darkest

moments in medical annals have involved abuses of human research subjects. Even ignoring such extreme instances of maleficence, the whole practice of exposing human beings to risk for the sake of knowledge collides with
the traditional Hippocratic injunction, "First, do no harm."

Historically, scientific investigation has been central to advances in
modern health care because it is only through such research that medicine—
which for thousands of years relied on magic, superstition, and unproven
remedies—has been transformed into a powerful (albeit imperfect) force for
human betterment. Well within the memory of physicians practicing today,
the stethoscope was the major piece of medical technology, and quinine,
digitalis, and aspirin were the major drugs. Biomedical scientists have totally transformed that picture in the past 45 years—and the transformation
has been so rapid and so total that those who have grown up in this new
world may well take it for granted. Nonetheless, risking the health or even
the life of one person to gain knowledge is potentially very dangerous. It
can destroy the moral position of physicians and, worse yet, the well-being
of those who have entrusted them with their lives.

Despite such risks, American society continues to allow and indeed to
encourage human experimentation, perhaps from the realization that as
amazing as the changes that have occurred in the field of medicine may be,
much remains to be learned. The need for knowledge extends beyond the
discovery and perfection of new diagnostic and therapeutic methods—from
human gene therapy to artificial organs to effective cancer cures—to encompass, perhaps even more important, the development of means to vali-
date and calibrate existing therapies. There is a critical need for data that
would establish the relative safety and effectiveness of perhaps most of what
is now done in medicine, done without proof of efficacy, done out of tradition or habit, done often very differently from town to town or hospital to
hospital, or even physician to physician, without proof of which approach,
if any, is really the best.

Plainly, these moral tensions make the subject of human research pivotal in any study of bioethics. Yet, today, the subject is often naively viewed
as one of settled ethical principles, detailed statutory and regulatory requirements, and multifaceted procedures. History suggests that such claims must
be viewed skeptically: the principles may be less conclusive and the guidelines less protective than they appear.

A HISTORICAL COMPARISON

Consider two historical examples. In each case, a government, abetted by a
physician's revelations of shocking experiments, promulgated general guidelines and then detailed regulations. In the first case, the official rules did
not prevent horrible abuses; the second case is still unfolding.

German Regulations, 1900–1945

The first story began in 1900 when the Prussian government issued a directive to the heads of clinics and similar establishments "absolutely prohibiting" medical interventions "for purposes other than diagnosis, therapy, and immunization" when:

1. The person in question is a minor or is not fully competent on other grounds;
2. The person concerned has not declared unequivocally that he consents to the intervention;
3. The declaration has not been made on the basis of a proper explanation of the adverse consequences that may result from the intervention (Der Minister der geistlichen 1900).

The directive also specified that interventions required the explicit approval of the director of each medical institution and the keeping of records to show that the subject met the three qualifications.

This document is notable for many reasons. First, it did not speak directly of research; instead, it implied its coverage by what it excluded, which blurred the boundary lines around practices that mix diagnosis, therapy, or immunization with investigation. Second, it gave special protection to vulnerable persons who are unable to consent on their own behalf. Third, it required not merely consent but disclosure. Fourth, it placed responsibility on the institution where the research was conducted, not merely on the individual investigator.

Why did the Prussian government attend to this issue at this time? Professor Erwin Deutsch suggests that "unethical, rough and even criminal experiments were taking place and being reported in [biomedical] journals" (1979, 23). This gave rise to a countercurrent in journals and books, of which the best known is the turn-of-the-century pseudonymous memoir of Vikenty Veressayev, a Russian physician who provided a "martyrology of the unhappy patients offered up [by his fellow physicians] as victims to science" (1901, 365). Many studies he described involved venereal diseases because these conditions had to be studied in humans in the absence of an appropriate animal model. For example, one physician, to establish that a specific microorganism was the cause of gonorrhea, inoculated unwitting patients and repeatedly showed that infection (painful and not always curable) occurred. The memoirist also described experiments involving transplanting cancers, exposing people to typhoid and scarlet fever (sometimes through injections), and manipulation of the brain of a woman who then had seizures, lapsed into a coma, and died shortly thereafter. With the exception of this last case, Veressayev wrote, "these bizarre disciples of science proceeded upon their way without encountering any effective opposition, either from their colleagues or the medical press."

The 1900 directive was followed up by more detailed German regulations in 1931; these regulations distinguished between "new therapy" which was "therapeutic experimentation and modes of treatment which serve the process of healing . . . even though the effects and consequences . . . cannot yet be adequately determined," and "human experimentation" which consists of "operations and modes of treatment . . . carried out for research purposes which are nontherapeutic" (Sass 1983, 105).[1] The horrible events of the following fourteen years in the Nazi prison camps demonstrate, however, that neither official endorsement nor high aspirations—embodied here by requirements for consent and risk limitation—are necessarily enough to guarantee that an ethical code will protect subjects from abuse or worse.

American Regulations since 1966

The second story follows a remarkably similar sequence. In September 1965, James A. Shannon, the Director of the U.S. National Institutes of Health (NIH), sought the advice of the National Advisory Health Council (NAHC) concerning the ethical implications of the changes that were occurring in biomedical research, which had moved from mere observation of patients to "manipulation [of] not only the diseased individual but also [of] normal individuals" (Frankel 1972, 30). Dr. Shannon stressed that

> since such investigation departs from the conventional patient-physician relationship, where the patient's good has been substituted for by the need to develop new knowledge, . . . the physician is no longer in the same relationship . . . and indeed may not be in a position to develop a purely or wholly objective assessment of the moral nature or the ethical nature of the act which he proposes to perform (National Advisory Health Council 1965).

---

[1]The guidelines for new therapy required: (a) cost-benefit balancing, (b) previous animal testing, where possible, (c) consent or proxy consent after appropriate information has been provided, (d) use without consent only to save lives or prevent severe harm or because of special circumstances, (e) special consideration in cases involving minors, (f) rejection of the exploitation of the needy, (g) special care in use of live microorganisms, (h) acceptance of full responsibility by the facility's chief physician, (i) written documentation, and (j) publication that respects the patient's dignity.

In addition to these requirements, the guidelines for human experimentation also specified: (a) no human experimentation without consent, (b) no human experimentation until laboratory and animal research has been completed, and therefore no unfounded or random use of humans, (c) no use of minors if they are endangered, and (d) no use of dying persons.

Physicians were charged with the duties of introducing new therapy in suitable cases and conducting human experimentation in order to promote the progress of medicine. They were also charged with the "grave responsibility . . . for the life and health of each individual undergoing New Therapy or Human Experimentation" (Sass 1983, 104–105). The importance of these factors was reiterated in the mandate given to teachers in medical schools to stress these special duties.

At its next meeting, in December 1965, the NAHC resolved that the Public Health Service (PHS) should support clinical research involving human beings "only if the judgment of the investigator is subject to prior review by his institutional associates to ensure an independent determination of the protection of the rights and welfare of the individual or individuals involved, of the appropriateness of the methods used to secure informed consent, and of the risk and potential medical benefits of the investigation." This recommendation became the basis for an order by the Surgeon General on February 8, 1966, mandating prior peer review of federally supported research (U.S. Public Health Service 1966a).[2] In December 1966, the order was further modified, in light of comments from the American Psychological Association and the American Sociological Association; certain behavioral science experiments were to be exempted from the requirement of informed consent or even awareness of the people being studied (U.S. Public Health Service 1966b).

As in Germany, the governmental directive coincided with criticism of existing research practices by a physician who had compiled a list of unethical experiments which likewise included operations performed without consent, exposure of patients to infections, and the transplantations of cancers from one patient to another (Beecher 1966). More than 20 examples published by the physician were drawn from a larger group in excess of 100, all appearing during a single year in a single, prestigious medical journal. Despite the horrifying nature of the revelations, he concluded that the best protection for patients lay in the conscience of the investigator. This article—which the author followed with a book on the same subject (Beecher 1970)—caused quite a stir and probably contributed to Dr. Shannon's goal of creating a more profound sense of research institutions' ethical responsibilities (Frankel 1972).[3] (Only later—with the discovery of other, even larger experiments that had been conducted by American physicians, both before and after World War II, involving lack of knowledge or actual deception of

---

[2]A revision was issued on July 1, 1966, to make clear that the "assurance" of review by a peer panel could be submitted for an entire research institution rather than for each individual project. An assurance had to include (1) agreement with the principles of the policy; (2) a description of the method of review; (3) the competencies represented in the review committee; (4) the administrative mechanism for surveillance and advice; and (5) the manner in which the institution would assure itself that the advice of the committee would be followed. John F. Sherman, NIH Deputy Director, recalls that NIH officials also "hoped that the use of a single but institutionally oriented assurance would, in most, if not in all situations, stimulate consideration also of reviews by a similar process of projects not supported by PHS grants" (Frankel 1972, 35).

[3]This was only reinforced by the publication shortly thereafter of another detailed examination of human experimentation by M. H. Pappworth (1968, 200) who also drew on reputable journals (emphasizing British over American) but who reached a less tolerant conclusion: "the voluntary system of safeguarding patients' rights has failed and new legislative procedures are absolutely necessary."

subjects—would the degree of need for attention to such responsibilities become fully apparent.)

Over the years, the initial PHS policy statement has evolved into detailed regulations based on a statutory requirement (National Research Act 1974) for prior review of research protocols at each institution, no longer just by an investigator's scientific peers but by a multidisciplinary group, at least one of whom must not be affiliated with the institution. The regulations of the Department of Health and Human Services (HHS 1983), the government department with the greatest involvement in research with human subjects, form the basis for oversight by most of the other two dozen departments and agencies that conduct or support such research (President's Commission 1981).

It is the existence of these federal rules, as well as the extensive scrutiny the issues have received (Levine 1986), that gives rise to the sense that the problems in human experimentation have all been neatly cabined if not totally resolved. Ought the horrible abuses perpetrated by distinguished physicians during the Nazi era in Germany, despite that nation's similar (indeed, in some ways even stronger) official rules, disturb the complacent view of the present American situation? Deutsch (1979) suggests that the German guidelines did not arouse public interest and had "ein obskurses Dasein" (an obscure existence), whereas in the United States, the guidelines interact closely with public opinion. There is no question that the requirements for ethically and legally acceptable human studies are widely accepted among researchers and that the rules and procedures are applied even in cases where they are not mandatory (for example, in studies not supported by federal funds). Are such differences between the present situation and that which prevailed when subjects were misused—in the United States as well as abroad—sufficient to conclude that research with human subjects is now no longer ethically problematic? Or, even when professional codes and governmental rules are perfectly applied, do certain difficult issues remain, as inherent features of this enterprise?

DEFINITIONS

Taxonomy seems important to students of many fields, and writers on human experimentation have devoted a great deal of attention to drawing categories. In the end, of course, an ethicist will want to know, What is the moral significance of such differences? Is the matter simply a procedural one? For example, formal review by a committee (such as an Institutional Review Board, or IRB) may be required for research but not for therapy. Or are substantive differences also implied? By labeling something as therapy, does a physician claim to have wider leeway to proceed without as much disclosure of risks or even without consent, on the ground that the intervention is routine? Are physicians less obligated to provide, and patients to accept, experimental interventions? Such questions are raised rather than resolved by the framing of definitions.

Two, Three, or Many Categories?

In medicine, every intervention by a physician could be regarded as an experiment, because each person is different and the exact outcome of medical interventions must therefore remain somewhat uncertain (Blumgart 1969; Ivy 1948). Further compounding the confusion, the practice of medicine does involve a mixture of techniques (the well-proven, the merely historically accepted, and the truly novel) and a mixture of motives (to help the individual, but also to teach the practitioner things of value for future cases). The same is also true in research outside the biomedical arena; for instance, policy analysts and behavioral scientists are interested both in present practices and in developing and testing new ones.

Nonetheless, some rough lines can be drawn. As concluded by a governmental commission that for several years in the mid-1970s examined research with human subjects, "the term *practice* refers to interventions that are designed solely to enhance the well-being of an individual patient or client and that have a reasonable expectation of success" (National Commission 1978a, 2). In the medical sphere, practices usually involve diagnosis, preventive treatment, or therapy; in the social sphere, practices include governmental programs such as transfer payments, education, and the like.

"By contrast, the term *research* designates an activity designed to test a hypothesis, permit conclusions to be drawn, and thereby to develop or contribute to generalizable knowledge (expressed, for example, in theories, principles, and statement of relationships)" (National Commission 1978a, 3). In the polar cases, then, practice uses a proven technique in an attempt to benefit one or more individuals, while research studies a (usually novel) technique in an attempt to increase knowledge.

These definitions have several implications. First, use of an unproven technique is not necessarily research unless the way in which it is used is designed to permit generalizable knowledge to be gained—not just to see what results from using the technique in a particular instance. Conversely, not each intervention carried out with the intent of benefiting the patient (or other subject) automatically qualifies as practice; adequate information must exist to provide a reasonable basis for believing it will achieve the intended result.

Of course, distinctions between research and therapy are not solely matters of intellectual curiosity; the label research carries with it requirements for protocol review. Consequently, a tension arises between an investigator's desire to design a formal research program that will yield scientifically valid results and the desire simply to do some experimentation or innovation that, not being cast in the form of research, seems more like treatment. Jay Katz tells of listening at a national meeting to an interesting paper on the treatment of leukemia in young children. The investigator reported that he had performed more than half a dozen bone marrow biopsies during a two-week interval in order to monitor the efficacy of the anti-leukemic drugs employed. During the discussion period I expressed surprise that he had been able to receive IRB committee approval for a project that exposed infants to considerable discomfort. He responded that committee review had been unnecessary because his was not a research project, but a therapeutic intervention (Katz 1987, 5).

Cases of this sort suggest a need to recognize a region—between pure instances of research and of practice—of "innovative therapy" (National Commission 1978a) or "nonvalidated practices":

> A practice might be nonvalidated because it is new; i.e., it has not been tested sufficiently often or sufficiently well to permit a satisfactory prediction of its safety or efficacy in a patient population. It is equally common for a practice to merit the designation "nonvalidated" because in the course of its use in the practice of medicine there arises some legitimate cause to question previously held assumptions about its safety or efficacy . . . At the time of the first substantial challenge to the validity of an accepted practice, . . . subsequent use of that modality should be considered nonvalidated. . . . (Levine 1986, 4).

Since nonvalidated practices are not carried out according to a research plan ("protocol"), they cannot be justified by their benefit to science; because they lack a valid basis in science, they cannot be defended for the benefit they will provide to those with whom they are used. The more unproven the procedure and the more risk its use creates, the more troublesome is this state of affairs. The solution, of course, is to employ a nonvalidated practice in the context of an appropriate research plan or to substitute a proven treatment.

This will not always be possible, especially when attempting to cure problems (such as life-threatening conditions) for which no satisfactory therapy exists and when the need to intervene is too urgent to allow a formal research plan to be adopted. But the failure to convert situations of nonvalidated practice into either real research or pure practice occurs much more frequently than is justified by the number that are truly on the frontiers of biomedical and behavioral science. Rather, there are other impediments—practical and psychological—that stand in the way.

Testing a new practice requires much more effort than simply trying it out on an individual. The average practitioner's outlook differs from a researcher's; physicians feel justified in using a nonvalidated treatment because the general uncertainty of much of medical practice makes it acceptable to proceed with good intentions rather than face the lack of proof. Moreover, "human experimentation" has strongly negative connotations. The suggestion that physicians enroll their patients in a research project rather than use a nonvalidated practice is resisted because physicians see this as a request to sacrifice patients' well-being for the good of science or they fear that their patients would, at least, perceive the request that way.

Nonetheless, the resistance to experimenting should not be lightly dismissed. Danger can arise when professionals have conflicting loyalties—to the goals of science and to their obligations as caregivers to protect and enhance their clients' well-being. Because of this tension, society has adopted means of overseeing the relationship of practitioner-qua-researcher and patient-(or citizen)-qua-research subject to minimize the harmful effects on the interests of the latter as well as to augment the beneficial effects to subject and to society. The existence of such safeguards has probably done much to legitimize the place of human research in society; by reassuring the public, these safeguards make it more acceptable for practitioners to ask for participation in an experiment. Yet procedures and delays entailed in these safeguards tar experimentation anew with unfavorable connotations for practitioners, who argue that what they are doing is "just practice" (even if unvalidated), and hence they ought not to be subjected to the rigors of formal research review.

Therapeutic versus Nontherapeutic Research

A further example of the ways in which mere definitions can carry ethical freight is found in the terms *therapeutic* and *nontherapeutic* research. These terms are commonly employed to distinguish research that is carried out as a part of patient care from that which involves subjects for whom the procedure being examined is not expected to have any value. In revising its 1964 code for biomedical investigators, The Declaration of Helsinki, in 1975 the World Medical Association proposed the phrase *clinical research* for medical research combined with professional care, and *nonclinical biomedical research* for nontherapeutic research.

Whatever terminology is used, the distinction is certainly clear, but not without danger. Modifying "research" with "therapeutic" may well lull an investigator and any persons called on to review the research into treating the project as inherently more justified than "nontherapeutic" research because of the assumed intention to provide a benefit to the patient–subject. Yet, in order to be justified as research, the project must aim to answer questions about the intervention being tested (such as whether it is safe and provides a net benefit). Thus, there can be no assumption that patient–subjects will derive any benefit (i.e., therapeutic results).

The risk of being led to misevaluate the research because of the benign label therapeutic is at least as great for patients as for practitioners. Although many codes suggest that greater protection is needed for participants in nonclinical research than in research combined with professional care, the reverse may be the case, especially regarding the standards for informed consent because patients are less likely than normal volunteers to be in a good position to consider the physical, psychological, and monetary risks and benefits in consenting to participate. A patient's emotional ties to the physician, his or her need for treatment (especially when conventional methods have proven ineffective), and the human tendency to overrate the benefits and underestimate the risks of a research technique, justify setting higher requirements for consent and imposing additional safeguards when therapy is combined with experimentation, lest investigators even unwittingly expose consenting patient–subjects to unreasonable risks (Capron 1972).

Benefits to Others

Part of the definition of practice as opposed to research is that it involves interventions "designed solely to enhance the well-being of an individual. . . ." (National Commission 1978a, 2). Yet there are some activities (such as vaccination) that are accepted practices because of their expectation of success but are not intended solely to benefit the individual, and there are others (quarantine, organ and tissue donation) that are intended solely to benefit others and not the individual. Although appearing to fall outside the definition of practice, such activities clearly are also not research.

Faced with this definitional problem, the National Commission insisted that the apparent inconsistency not be allowed "to confuse the general distinction between research and practice" (National Commission 1978a, 3). The reason given, however, seems disingenuous:

> Even when a procedure applied in practice may benefit some other person, it remains an intervention designed to enhance the well-being of a particular individual or group of individuals; thus, it is practice and need not be reviewed as research.

This rationale is either tautological (a "procedure applied in practice" is a "practice") or unpersuasive (if only a few people suffer from a disease, an intervention aimed at discovering a cure for that disease would be "designed to enhance the well-being of a particular . . . group of individuals," but it would still be "research," not "practice"). It would be better simply to recognize that sometimes practices of proven value are carried out for the purpose of benefiting someone other than the persons immediately subjected to the intervention.

This recognition yields an important ethical conclusion: Practice sometimes shares an important feature with research, namely, benefiting others. In research, the benefit to others is a benefit to science from an increase in generalizable knowledge, but in the case of certain practices, the benefit flows to other individuals (the recipient of donated blood) or to society at large (protection by a quarantine from an infectious person). The willingness of society to accept the gift of such benefits—and sometimes even to extract them from an unwilling person—in the context of biomedical, as well as behavioral or social, practices and programs is a point worth remembering when evaluating the legal and ethical issues posed by research (Fox 1974).

JUSTIFICATIONS AND PRINCIPLES

In an era dependent on science and technology, it may seem unnecessary to examine the justifications for research with human subjects because such research is an indispensable link between theory or initial observations and the application of scientific findings and technology developments to benefit people and society at large. But in ethical terms, such scrutiny is needed because the question is not whether to have all possible research or none at all but rather how much research to have at what cost, when cost includes possible harm to values other than the advancement of knowledge.

Research: Necessary or Optional?

As philosopher Hans Jonas eloquently argued nearly 2 decades ago, value conflicts do not occur when science employs inanimate objects, but once feeling beings "become the subjects of experiment, as they do in the life sciences and especially in medical research, this innocence of the search for knowledge is lost and questions of conscience arise" (Jonas 1969, 219). The promotion of progress is a valid social goal but not, in his view, one to which individuals must be committed simply as members of society and beneficiaries of the current state of scientific knowledge.

Those who take the contrary view, that there is a social imperative in medical research, do not actually disagree with the view that other values must enter into the evaluation of research projects and the enterprise as a whole. Instead, they point to the enormous harm that is caused by well-meaning but misinformed biomedical (and social) interventionists using methods that have never been adequately tested, and they stress "the necessity for controlled trials to determine whether what is traditional does harm rather than good" (Eisenberg 1977).

Since the risks of medical research are small—comparable to the rates for accidental injury in the general population (Cardon et al. 1976)—there is a strong argument that patients should participate in evaluation studies on the risks and benefits of the practices to which they are routinely subjected, at least as to those practices whose morbidity and mortality exceed those encountered in research. However, this justification is insufficient for treatments on the frontiers of knowledge, especially those that contribute to some far-off goal of eventual understanding (or even cure) and those that involve more than minimal risks. For the latter, support of, and involvement in, research is a noble choice rather than a moral obligation. Progress is, after all, an optional not a mandatory goal, and its pursuit must take place within limits established by other values, including the value of individual autonomy.

Basic Ethical Principles in the History of Human Research

The bioethical principles that get the most attention in the context of human subjects research are respect for persons, beneficence, and justice (National Commission 1978).

Respect for Competent Persons

Respect for persons has two rather different implications for research: The first emphasizes respect for the personhood or personal rights of research subjects, the second their personal well-being. To respect personal rights in either Kantian or utilitarian terms implies that those in charge of a project must provide prospective subjects with information that will enable them to decide whether it is acceptable according to their own values and goals and must then permit the subjects to choose whether or not to participate, rather than manipulating the information or coercing the choice.

This requirement may seem so basic as to require no comment, but it has presented problems both in historical experience and in theory. Deviations from the requirement of consent have sometimes been so shocking that it is well to remember that there have also been fine examples of physicians throughout history who respected the freedom and dignity of the subjects with whom they conducted research, such as the nineteenth-century American pioneer physician William Beaumont, who made a true collaborator of the patient whose internal workings he observed for many years through the opening left created by an injury, and Walter Reed, who sought the consent of subjects for his yellow fever study not merely in English but also in Spanish for the Spanish-speaking.

Such respect was, of course, horribly absent in the work of the Nazi physicians in the concentration camps. The terrors inflicted upon unconsenting subjects in experiments in which numerous inmates died in low-pressure environments (designed to simulate the effects on pilots of flying at, or falling from, high altitudes), from exposure to freezing air or water, from being used as human incubators and vaccine subjects for typhus, and from being given poisons—to name just a few categories of "research"—so blinded the investigators that in many instances they missed important scientific findings. The horror of the civilized world at what was revealed during the trial of 23 Nazi physicians at Nuremberg is embodied not only in the conviction of 16 of them for war crimes and crimes against humanity (with seven condemned to death) but also in the judges' statement of principles, commonly called the Nuremberg Code, which begins: "The voluntary consent of the human subject is absolutely essential."

A similar fate did not await Japanese researchers who had carried out similarly barbarous experiments in Manchuria during World War II. Indeed, the existence of these abuses was not even generally known for more than 35 years because, in exchange for not being publicly tried and punished, the Japanese investigators agreed to cooperate with their American captors and share the information they had gathered about biological warfare through their experiments with Chinese captives (Gomer et al. 1981).

Between 1930 and 1945 Japan conducted human experiments in biological warfare and physical response to infection both through controlled research on prisoners of war and through field trials on mainland China. The main research installation was Unit 731, located near Harkin, which was operated by Lieutenant General Ishii. At least 3000 people were reported killed; some died as a result of the experiments, others were killed to observe the progression of the experiment, and others were killed when they became too weak to continue. At least two other sites were in operation, one near Changchun and one near Nanjing. Complaints from the People's Republic of China have identified at least 11 cities believed to be the targets of "field tests." A reported 700 victims contracted plague as a result of these attacks.

Unit 731 was "a large, self-contained installation with sophisticated germ and insect breeding facilities, a prison for the human experimentees, testing grounds, an arsenal for making germ bombs, an airfield, its own special planes and a crematorium for the human victims" (Gomer et al. 1981, 45). It was capable of producing eight tons of bacteria per month. Experiments were conducted on the human response to anthrax, botulism, brucellosis, cholera, dysentery, hemorrhagic fever, plague, smallpox, syphilis, tick encapalitis, tsutsugamushi, tularemia, typhoid, and typhus. Other experiments included prolonged exposure of the liver to x-rays, freezing body parts to try various methods of thawing, pumping the body full of horse blood, and vivisection.

Although officials of the United States were fully aware of the nature of the experimentation and that American prisoners of war had been used, they concluded that the value of the information obtained far outweighed the value of prosecution because the research greatly augmented scientific knowledge and was believed to be unobtainable anywhere else due to the tight controls on human subject research. The prosecution of the Japanese would have led to admission of this information at trial, which the American officials decided posed a threat to national security because the scientific findings would become available to all countries of the world. The Japanese were offered protection from the Russians in exchange for their full cooperation.

In the period after World War II, American complicity with the abuse of subjects by the Japanese was not known. Instead, leaders of biomedical research proclaimed their adherence to the principle of consent. Yet the behavior of American investigators sometimes was otherwise, such as in chemical and biological testing by American military and intelligence agencies from the 1940s to the 1960s.

The original rationale was that such testing was necessary for defensive purposes, on the belief that World War II enemies had used such techniques in interrogations, brainwashing, and in attacks designed to harass, disable, or kill Allied personnel and that in the future it would be important to understand how these substances worked and how their effects could be detected. As the potential for offensive use of these substances was recognized, the testing emphasis shifted and included a search for information on how unsuspecting people would respond. Therefore, as part of the testing procedures, unwitting subjects were used in real-life settings.

Two deaths have been directly linked to these experiments. In 1953, Harold Blauer was a patient at New York State Psychiatric Institute. As part of the United States Army Chemical Corps experiments, Blauer was injected with a synthetic mescaline derivative without his knowledge. He died of circulatory collapse and heart failure as a result of the drug. In 1975, the Secretary of the Army announced that Blauer had died while serving as an unwitting subject in Army drug testing. His daughter, Elizabeth Barrett, filed suit and charged negligence in the creation and administration of the program and conspiracy to cover up the results (Barrett 1981).[4]

Dr. Frank Olson was an aerobiologist assigned to the Special Operations Division of the United States Army Biological Center at Camp Detrick, Maryland. At a meeting in 1953, five Army and Central Intelligence Agency (CIA) scientists received a dose of LSD in an after-dinner drink. Twenty minutes later they were informed of its presence in the drink. It is unclear whether these scientists ever agreed to be subjects. Olson became seriously depressed and committed suicide 9 days later. The CIA provided no information to Olson's family concerning its involvement in his death; this information only emerged years later as a result of an action for damages brought against the government.

Although other allegations of severe harm and even death have not been proven (*Nevin* 1983), there is no question that many experiments were performed by American investigators from 1946 to 1965 without the knowledge, much less the consent, of the subjects and otherwise in violation of the existing codes (U.S. Senate 1977; *San Francisco Chronicle* 1986).

Respect for Incompetent Persons

The fulcrum on which respect for a person's right to autonomous choice rests is the determination of the person's capacity to make the decision at hand. But how should one apply "respect for persons" when the subject is incapacitated? In the Belmont Report, the National Commission found a second "ethical conviction" embedded in respect for persons: "persons with diminished autonomy are entitled to protection" (1978, 4), in other words, respect for their personal well-being.

One situation in which the reach of this principle might be tested arises when parents of a young child with an illness that is usually fatal, such as cancer, refuse to allow an experimental treatment because they believe that the chances for long-term remission are so slim that it would be better to

---

[4]In May 1987, Mr. Blauer's daughters obtained a $700,000 award against the government in the District Court in Manhattan (Lubasch 1987).

allow the child to die in peace (Holder 1987). Because the child is incapable of making the choice personally, the question is whether the parents' refusal should be binding. On the one hand, the regulations applicable to new drugs make consent a crucial requirement, so that it would not seem reasonable for the physicians simply to treat the child because they are convinced of the wisdom of this course. Moreover, the unproven nature of the treatment makes it unlikely that refusing it would be labeled neglect of the child such as to cause a court to transfer care and custody of the child to someone other than the parents. On the other hand, the extreme nature of the situation—when use of an unapproved treatment offers the child's only chance of surviving—might lead a court to ignore the niceties of the law.

Plainly, this aspect of respect for persons is more difficult to apply than the consent requirement for competent persons. Certain strategies have been developed for minimizing the difficulties, such as relying on the assent of subjects who are capable of understanding some or all of the experiment but who are legally too young to give consent, which must be obtained from the child's legal guardian (usually the parents) (National Commission 1977; HHS 1983, §§46.402b and 46.408a).

When treatment, rather than research, for an incompetent is at issue, the law has generally recognized and ethicists have generally endorsed, a surrogate decision maker (usually the next-of-kin or someone designated before the patient became incompetent) making the decision that the incompetent would have made based on his or her known choices and values. Of course, in many cases such a substituted judgment is impossible because the patient was never competent (for example, a young child) or did not express a preference relevant to the medical choice in question. In such circumstances, the surrogate is supposed to make in the person's best interests a decision that encompasses treatment choices that the average person would find reasonable under the circumstances. How applicable are such standards to human research? Would the surrogate need to know not only the incompetent person's preferences about treatment but also his or her willingness to take risks and to participate in research when part of the benefit is intended to flow to science and to other patients? In one study designed to examine the side effects of long-term use of urinary catheters in the elderly, nearly one-third of family members who thought their mentally incompetent relatives (who resided in two nursing homes) would not want to be used for research nevertheless allowed their doctors to include them in the study (Warren et al. 1986). Alternatively, if a surrogate makes a choice according to the best interests standard, what presumption ought the surrogate apply regarding the reasonableness of taking risks in experiments for the benefit of others?

Beneficence

In effect, the second facet of respect for persons—the obligation to protect the personal well-being of those who are incapable of deciding for themselves—might be seen as an aspect of the principle of beneficence, which was said by the National Commission to give rise to two obligations: "(1) do no harm; and (2) maximize possible benefits and minimize possible harms" (1978, 6). Both aspects of beneficence are thus quite compatible with respecting the well-being of the most vulnerable human subjects, those lacking the capacity for autonomous choices.

But when one turns to the first half of the respect for persons principle, the potential for direct conflict with beneficence in human research is enormous. The no-harming or "nonmaleficence" facet of beneficence poses the least risk of trespassing on respect for the choices of autonomous agents. Indeed, the no-harm principle can be derived not only from Hippocrates' oath and *Epidemics* (Jonsen 1978), but, like respect for persons, also from Kant, because actively to do a person harm is to use him or her as a means to some end (good or perverse) not of his or her own choosing. As the nineteenth-century researcher Claude Bernard held, one should not injure one person regardless of the benefits that might come to others (Bernard 1865).

Yet Dr. Bernard's oft-quoted personal code—among experiments "those that can only do harm are forbidden, those that are harmless are permissible, and those that may do good are obligatory"—illustrates the collision between autonomous choice and the benefit-maximizing aspect of beneficence.[5] After all, this aspect of beneficence goes far beyond the categorical imperative; lacking a common root with respect for persons, it is not surprising that it can easily come into conflict with that principle.

This problem is well illustrated by research conducted between September 1950 and November 1952 among more than 1000 women who received prenatal care at the University of Chicago's Lying-In Hospital. The researchers doubted the then-accepted use of diethylstilbestrol (DES) to prevent miscarriages; with the goal of improving women's health care, but wishing not to upset the pregnant women, they conducted a double-blind study without informing the women of either the study's design or the true nature of the drug they were receiving (*Mink* 1978). Only when the children of these women began, some 20 years later, to manifest unusually high rates of cancer and other reproductive tract abnormalities did the subjects learn of the experiment's existence. In 1982, a suit brought on behalf of the subjects and their offspring was settled by the University of Chicago agreeing to provide free, lifetime care of adenocarcinoma for any daughter of a subject and to provide other health-related redress for potential victims. In evaluating

---

[5]The text analyzes the problems regarding those experiments said by Dr. Bernard to be "obligatory." As Beecher points out, the rest of Bernard's "splendid sentiments" are equally problematic: He forbids harmful experiments (but such harm is often not known in advance), and he holds harmless ones to be permissible, when in fact they are unethical "unless they are properly organized [including provisions for third-party review and subject-consent?] and give promise of value" (1970, 226).

the tension between beneficence and autonomy in this case, is it relevant that at least some of the women would have received DES anyway (as standard treatment), that the study showed DES to be ineffective in preventing miscarriages (thereby benefiting these and many future women), and that the harm that eventually occurred was not anticipated and would not have been included in any statement of risks had the women given informed consent at the time of the study?

Quite plainly, the professional goal to search out and try to achieve what is thought to be best for others will sometimes be at odds with the rights of autonomous individuals. If respect for persons is given primacy, as it typically is in contemporary ethical and legal documents on human subjects research, the principle of beneficence becomes a side constraint on the actions of investigators; that is, at a minimum, a researcher should conduct only experiments that have been designed in a manner that minimizes their possible harms; a person's willingness to be a subject is not an adequate sanction for performing an experiment if the investigator could reasonably have reduced the experiment's risks.

This view of the two principles does not remove the tension between them but does permit practical action to occur without abandoning either principle. There is, however, another irony inherent in the two halves of the beneficence principle itself. The nonmaleficence half of the principle emphasizes the paramountcy usually (perhaps erroneously) given this value in interpreting the Hippocratic tradition primum non nocere. Given the limited understanding and meager therapeutics of medicine in ancient Greece—and, indeed, until the middle of this century—the advice "above all, do no harm" was sound. Today, however, intervening despite risks of further harm is often of extreme benefit to patients.

Furthermore, applying the do-no-harm principle to human research (especially nonclinical research unrelated to subjects' well-being) would preclude all experiments; any intervention risks generating some harm. Yet to take this do-nothing posture contradicts the second half of the beneficence principle because the failure to increase biomedical (as well as behavioral and social) knowledge defaults on the obligation to maximize benefits and minimize harms. Certainly, as already remarked, the justification for research as a societal good, which deserves both collective and individual support, is that it not only improves the lot of mankind but also helps to avoid some of the harm that would otherwise be perpetrated because of our present state of ignorance and misguided attachment to practices that are in fact wasteful of resources or actually harmful to individuals. Thus, both a person wishing to carry out a research project and someone who opposes the project could, based on an agreed set of facts about the risks of the project compared to the risks of the present state of practice, support their positions by reference to opposite halves of the principle of beneficence as articulated by the National Commission and adopted by other commentators (Levine 1986).

Justice

As important as the principle of justice is in the Western tradition, it has traditionally played only a minor role in discussions of human research. Failures to respect this principle are, regrettably, legion. One, of which every American needs to be aware, began in 1932 but was not publicly revealed (and halted) until 1972. During those 40 years, the PHS carried out a "study in nature" of untreated syphilis among rural black men near Tuskegee, Alabama, who were kept in ignorance of the experiment and steered away from receiving effective treatment, lest that interfere with the investigators' data (Brandt 1978; Tuskegee Syphilis Study 1973).

Although it would generally be agreed that certain gross instances of abuse of research subjects—such as the Tuskegee study and the experiments in the Nazi camps—involved unfair treatment of the subjects, this is simply another way of saying that they manifested a total disrespect for the subjects as persons. The more particular sense of justice as an ethical principle— namely, the comparative use of the concept, which holds that it is unfair to treat like cases differently—is not implicated by these examples, since the experiments conducted by the Nazi physicians would not have been fair even had they selected their victims randomly from among all the inmates, or even from among all Germans.

When this sense of the word justice is employed, the resulting questions—Who deserves to bear the burdens of research? Who deserves to enjoy its benefits?—are interesting and complex. There are many ways of measuring fair distribution. In an egalitarian democracy, these ways include "(1) to each person an equal share; (2) to each person according to individual need; (3) to each person according to individual effort; (4) to each person according to societal contribution; and (5) to each person according to merit" (National Commission 1978a, 9).

Converting these possible criteria for fairness into operative principles for human research is both conceptually and practically difficult. In many spheres, society gives justice preeminence over other principles. In the collection of taxes, for example, progressive taxation is premised on the idea that it is fair to extract a larger share of income from a wealthy person than from a poor one. However, in human experimentation, where respect for the choices of autonomous persons is also a guiding principle, a classic conflict emerges: If autonomy is accorded the primary position it usually enjoys in human-subjects research, the selection of subjects dictated by justice is possible if all the fairly selected potential subjects actually agree to participate. Thus, a just distribution of the burdens of research operates primarily as a side constraint in the design of experiments, not as justification for enrolling unwilling subjects in attempting to distribute research risks fairly in society.

The practical problems in implementing the principle of justice in research are great, even if justice plays a limiting rather than an activating role.

Because the connection between many research projects and eventual benefits to people are often remote and difficult to draw even after-the-fact, much less to predict reliably in advance, deciding among research projects with an eye to achieving a fair distribution of their fruits is probably wasted effort and possibly harmful because resources ought to go where they are likely to yield the greatest results, not where determined by a fairness formula with dubious predictive power.

The connections between a research project and the burdens it creates are certainly less opaque than its connection to eventual benefits to individuals. Yet even in this aspect, the goal of just distribution is difficult to implement in large measure because of the room for disagreement over defining the groups that ought to be treated alike. It would seldom if ever be practical or appropriate to hold a lottery that would place every individual in society at equal risk of being recruited into a research project (Capron 1973). Yet, if all individuals are not treated as inherently the same, defensible grounds need to be found for dividing them into groups.

Again, the principle of justice may be most serviceable as a constraint rather than a goal: Some groupings already exist in society and result in rankings (from the least powerful to the most, from the least well-educated to the best, from the sickest to the healthiest, etc.) to which a researcher selecting subjects can pay attention. The principle of fairness might be taken to require, for example, that subjects for a study of various birth methods ought to be recruited from among the well-insured patients of obstetricians in private practice as well as from the nonpaying patients in the charity wards.

Certain behaviors are plainly inconsistent with an egalitarian view of justice. As American physician Myron Prinzmetal later wrote, describing his training in the United States (as well as Europe) between World War I and World War II:

> New drugs, new experimental surgical procedures were commonly tested on charity patients, who rarely understood what was being done to them. Often they were maimed or killed—experimental "animals" sacrificed in the interests of medical progress. . . . In a word— some patients were not treated like animals, but often worse than animals—for some of them understood (Prinzmetal 1965).

A more stringent interpretation would insist on recruiting well-off and well-educated subjects before turning to those who fall lower on the socio-economic scale, based either on John Rawls' argument that justice favors steps that make the least well-off relatively better off (Rawls 1971), or on the conclusion that Jonas draws from his contention that progress is an optional goal, namely that the appeal to participate in the search for progress ought first to be addressed to those who most identify with the research enterprise. In this view, one has "an inversion of the normal 'market' behavior . . . namely, to accept the lowest quotation last (and excused only by the greatest pressure of need); to pay the highest price first" (Jonas 1969, 235). Jonas thus ties the notion of a just distribution of research risks back into respect for persons by recruiting first those subjects (such as the researchers themselves) whose "service is not just permitted by [them], but willed. That sovereign will of his which embraces the end as his own restores his personhood to the otherwise depersonalizing context" (Jonas 1969, 236).

> [F]or the scientific community to honor [this idea] will mean that it will have to fight a strong temptation to go by routine to the readiest sources of supply—the suggestible, the ignorant, the dependent, the "captive" in various senses. I do not believe that heightened resistance here must cripple research, which cannot be permitted; but it may indeed slow it down by the smaller numbers fed into experimentation in consequences. This price—a possibly slower rate of progress—may have to be paid for the preservation of the most precious capital of higher communal life (Jonas 1969, 237).

Societal decisions to limit or preclude certain types of research subjects (such as prisoners) show that definitions of justifiable research such as Jonas' can affect policy, but in general the principle of justice seems seldom to be implemented in deciding which research projects to undertake or in selecting the subjects among those legally permitted to participate (such as all adult persons capable of giving informed consent).

Justice also has a role in the design of research. In experiments involving the seriously ill or other least well-off groups, Professor Robert Veatch urged "a subject-centered review strategy in which a key question . . . is whether the research design will maximize benefit to the subject (rather than to the researcher, the researcher's institution, or even the pool of knowledge)" (Veatch 1983, 18), indeed, even if it compromises the quality of the research. Veatch argues that justice demands that researchers do not further burden already-burdened patient–subjects by requiring stressful tests or denying access to experimental treatments without randomization.

A timely illustration of this dilemma is the current federal research with the acquired immunodeficiency syndrome (AIDS) patients to discover an effective therapy. Thousands of desperate AIDS patients are enrolling in drug trials despite unknown risks and the fact that the experiments are blind and randomized; half the subjects receive placebos (inert substances), without knowing in which arm of the protocol they are participating. Many other AIDS victims have complained that it was unfair to exclude them from access to these experimental drugs simply because more subjects were not needed according to the design of the clinical trials.

This situation raises two justice issues in the terms raised by Veatch. First, even when use of placebos is preferable in scientific terms (which is not always the case) should a less conclusive design be used—such as comparing groups using different experimental regimens or utilizing data from a matched group of untreated patients as historical controls? Second, should experimental drugs be available outside of formal research programs when they offer the only hope for halting a fatal illness? The government initially justified its policies on the ground that careful research is needed to find an effective therapy; therefore, "the current approach will help the greatest number in the shortest time" (Eckholm 1986), but the Food and Drug Administration (FDA) subsequently revised its rules to permit prescription outside of formal research protocols of certain drugs that have been approved for investigational use. Is sufficient fairness ensured if access to an experiment is randomly available to all? Who should bear the burden here—society (in failing to have research that is scientifically adequate) or fatally ill patients (in either being unable to get into a research program where an unproven drug is being dispensed or in being enrolled in a research program with a 50 percent chance of getting an inert placebo)?

ETHICAL REVIEW PROCEDURES

Ethical and legal guidance for experimentation has tended to evolve from one document to the next, sometimes in surprising ways. For example, the Nuremberg Code declared by the American judges in the process of passing judgment on the Nazi camp physicians in 1946 was itself influenced by the 1931 German government regulations because Boston psychiatrist Leo Alexander, one of the two American medical advisors to the prosecutors of the Nazi physicians, relied on the German standards as well as on those formulated by the American Medical Association after the war in the influential expert testimony that he and Dr. A. C. Ivy provided to the Nuremberg tribunal (Alexander 1966; Conference 1976).

The Nuremberg Code in some ways amounted to a retreat from the German regulations that had emphasized institutional and not merely individual responsibility. The assumption that adequate protection for subjects lay in the conscience of the investigator, professional codes (such as the World Medical Association's Declaration of Helsinki), and the basic requirement of consent predominated in the first twenty years after the War. Indeed, the only piece of national legislation on the subject during this period—the requirement of obtaining informed consent from participants in drug trials added to the Food and Drug Act as a minor part of the sweeping 1962 amendments to that statute (Food and Drug Amendments 1962)—also relied primarily on physicians' consciences and subjects' consent.

The changes in the FDA requirements stimulated its sister agency, the PHS, to examine more closely some concerns about a small percentage of research proposals that the PHS was asked to fund (principally through the NIH) that seemed to involve ethical problems, such as undue risk to subjects. This led in turn to a system of peer review in the Clinical Center at NIH and then to the guidelines for PHS grantees issued by Dr. Shannon in 1966, which marked a return to collective responsibility for the propriety of research projects. The new federal requirements were not quickly or gladly accepted by the research community (Barber et al. 1973), but their necessity was soon borne out for the larger community, as well as for many researchers, first by Dr. Beecher's revelations and then by the Tuskegee scandal and other studies involving prisoners, aborted fetuses, and mentally retarded persons, among others. Following the recitation of such problems during extensive hearings before a Senate subcommittee in 1973, Congress in the 1974 National Research Act (1) directed the Secretary of HEW to require all recipients of departmental research funds to establish Institutional Review Boards (IRBs), and (2) created the National Commission for the Protection of Human Subjects of Biomedical and Behavioral Research, whose duties included recommending changes in the federal rules on human research. The Commission issued a series of reports between 1974 and 1978, as a consequence of which the HHS promulgated a revised set of regulations on January 26, 1981, which provide the basic framework for oversight of research in the United States (HHS 1983; see also Appendix 6.2).

The HHS Institutional Assurance System

Despite the dominance of the HHS model, the federal government actually uses two systems to protect human subjects. The first applies to situations in which a government agency (most notably HHS, through the extramural programs of the NIH) sponsors research with human subjects. HHS regulations stipulate that an institution receiving funds for research provide "written assurance satisfactory to the Secretary that it will comply with the requirements" of 45 C.F.R. Part 46. The heart of these regulations is the existence of an IRB to determine that each research proposal meets federal requirements. In effect, having set the standards for approval of projects (including minimal requirements for diversity of IRB membership), the government delegates the execution of its rules to research institutions based on their assurance that they will comply.

It seems widely agreed that the process of prospective review of research protocols in general, and the IRB as the means of accomplishing this review in particular, are effective in improving the quality of subjects' consent and in avoiding excessively risky research. Yet few data are actually available to support these conclusions. The National Commission's study (1978b) of IRBs occurred before most institutions had much experience with IRBs as constituted under the present rules, and the present methods by which federal agencies monitor research do not provide much information about the actual operation of IRBs, except when a complaint of abuse is raised against a research project (President's Commission 1981, 1983).

Nevertheless, an outline can be given for the regulatory process. First, a researcher devises a plan for testing a hypothesis or otherwise developing generalizable knowledge; before carrying out the investigation with human subjects, the researcher will typically have performed theoretical, laboratory, and animal studies. In addition to the scientific protocol that describes the research plan and objectives in technical terms from which other scientists can judge the proposal's worth, researchers at many institutions must also prepare a second document for the IRB. This plan explains the population to be studied and how and why the human subjects were chosen, salient aspects of research design (with particular attention to the risks and inconveniences for the subjects) and data interpretation (including provisions for monitoring the accumulating data to allow appropriate adjustments or termination if adverse consequences begin to occur), and the potential significance of the research (Cowan 1975). Furthermore, this document includes a copy of the informed consent form that will be read and given to prospective subjects. IRBs devote particular attention to consent forms and frequently request revisions in them (National Commission 1978b; President's Commission 1983).

Once approved by the IRB and other institutional officials, the research proposal is sent to the federal agency from which funding is being sought or to another sponsor, since many private sponsors now expect institutions to use the same review methods for protocols involving human subjects, and many institutional assurances provide for IRB review for research that will not be federally funded, even though such uniformity of process and standards is not actually a regulatory requirement. There it is appraised (typically on a comparative basis against competing proposals) by a group of the investigator's scientific peers (called study sections at the NIH). The IRB's approval is a requirement before the study section may consider funding the proposal. Tension sometimes occurs, however, when the scientific reviewers disagree with an IRB's assessment (for example, if they find the design unduly risky) and want a proposal to be modified for ethical reasons before they will approve it for funding (President's Commission 1983). The Office for Protection from Research Risks (OPRR), which negotiates the institutional assurances on behalf of the NIH, does not actually review each protocol and consent form, but is available to provide information for IRBs and study sections and to investigate cases as needed.

The FDA's Retrospective System

Since the revision of the regulations in 1981, the substance of the FDA's regulations accords with the basic HHS requirements. However, despite the essentially identical process of prior review that will be undergone by a research project subject to FDA jurisdiction, the relationship of the agency to the research institution differs from that of the PHS and the two dozen other federal agencies that fund research with human subjects.

Because the FDA does not usually sponsor research, its oversight of the research institution is indirect. The FDA's protection of human subjects rests on its authority to refuse to approve a new drug or device for general use when the data submitted by the sponsor of the drug or device in support of its approval has been produced through improper research, including re-search that is unacceptable on ethical grounds. Thus, rather than negotiate assurances with institutions and give IRBs prospective approval based on their design and plans as OPRR does, the FDA reviews the adequacy of human subjects protection retrospectively, during its approval process. It is therefore the responsibility of the sponsor to ensure that the protocol com-plies with the regulations and has been properly reviewed by a legitimate IRB (FDA 1981). When FDA inspectors visit the places where research has been conducted in support of drug applications, they check on the compo-sition and functioning of the IRB and the adequacy of its decision making as part of their review of the paper trail that a research protocol leaves in the files of the research institution. The FDA is now taking steps to remedy the gap in its knowledge about what research is being conducted at which institutions with which subjects at any given time, but will continue to rely on the sponsor of the drug or device to keep such records as part of the sponsor's responsibility to monitor testing.

State Regulation of Research with Human Subjects

Several states have adopted statutes that establish policies and procedures for medical and psychological research. New York's law, which applies only to research that is not subject to and in compliance with federal regulations, was enacted in 1975 and draws heavily from the federal rules existing at that time. The statute limits the carrying out of research to licensed physicians or persons "deemed appropriately competent and qualified by a human research review committee" (N.Y. 1985, §§2441(6) and 2443). The requirements for informed consent and for the membership and functioning of the review committee are substantially similar to current HHS rules, except that the reporting and approval requirements tie the institution to the Commissioner of Health in Albany rather than to federal officials (N.Y. 1985, §2444).

California's statute, enacted in 1978, is premised on the Nuremberg Code and Declaration of Helsinki being legally unenforceable standards and hence incapable of meeting "a growing need for protection for citizens of the state from unauthorized, needless, hazardous, or negligently performed medical experiments on human beings" (Calif. 1984, §24171). Research con-ducted at an institution with a valid HHS assurance and in conformance with the federal requirements is exempted from most of the procedural provisions of the California law, but the statute's detailed "experimental subject's bill of rights" and its civil and criminal penalties for negligent or willful failure to obtain informed consent still apply (Calif. 1984, §24178).

Nevertheless, the New Jersey Supreme Court recognized the enforce-ability of professional codes of ethics (*Pierce* 1980). Although the court de-nied Dr. Pierce's suit for damages for the termination of her employment that resulted from her refusal to carry out research she regarded as unethical, the court held that "[e]mployees who are professionals owe a special duty to abide not only by federal and state law, but also by the recognized codes of ethics of their professions" (*Pierce* 1980, 512).

Overall, the states have legislated little on the subject of human research. What legislation exists is consistent, both in the approach (prior review by an IRB of risks and of informed consent) and in the standards applied with the prevailing federal requirements. Of course, like the possibility of a damage action brought by a subject under state tort laws, the very existence of state statutory provisions does add an element of uncertainty and procedural complexity to a field in which legal advice could otherwise be largely based on construing a fairly straightforward set of federal regulations that have not been complicated by numerous or divergent judicial interpretations.

CURRENT ISSUES

Having reviewed the history and principles behind the present structure of decision making about research with human subjects, we now examine some topics that remain as current issues. There are many ways to analyze these issues; the one used here emphasizes the interplay of two central factors— risk and consent—that figure in various combinations in what follows.

Highly Risky Research

Utilitarianism versus Nonmaleficence

An interesting illustration of the unresolved nature of the interplay of risk and consent is provided by research on the artificial heart. One of the major results of the movement after 1966 away from the investigator's conscience/subject's consent model of acceptable research has been to constrict the range of risks to those that appear acceptable to reasonable members of an IRB (Pattullo 1982). Although an IRB might permit an heroic investigator to engage in some highly risky self-experimentation, many modern studies would not lend themselves to the sort of self-experimentation in which the pioneers in physiology and infectious diseases engaged during an earlier era (Forssmann 1964).

Dr. William DeVries could hardly have implanted an artificial heart into his own chest, rather than that of Barney Clark. Yet healthy people did volunteer themselves to the University of Utah team to have artificial hearts implanted (Grady 1984). From a utilitarian viewpoint, it would be ethical to use such subjects (provided that they really give voluntary, informed consent) because so much more could be learned about the artificial heart (and by extension, also about the functioning of other organs once it is possible to observe a normal body in which heart function is totally subject to external manipulation) if it were implanted in a healthy person rather than in the very sick people who are permitted to be selected as patient–subjects under the existing protocol (Jonsen 1984). Yet the obvious excess of risk over benefit *to the subject* makes it highly unlikely that any IRB (or the FDA) would approve such a research design, even though the HHS regulations state that the IRB should be satisfied that "risks to subjects are reasonable in relation to . . . the importance of the knowledge that may reasonably be expected to result" (HHS 1983, §46.111a(2)).

It is interesting to note that the conflict between utility and nonmaleficence is customarily resolved in the opposite fashion—that is, in favor of utility—when it comes to vaccine trials, even when it is not possible to leave the weighing of risks and benefits directly to the prospective subjects, who often are young children. (These subjects are selected both because they are the potential victims of the diseases that the vaccines are intended to prevent and because as a group they have a much lower rate of acquired immunity, which would interfere with the scientific measurements in a vaccine trial.)

The reason for the special concern about vaccine trials is that they expose otherwise healthy subjects to harm. Although the same is true with proven vaccines, vaccination programs are justified on the grounds (1) that since all members of society benefit from immunization, it would be unfair to allow an individual to freeload off the risk taken by others in being vaccinated, and (2) that in being vaccinated individuals confer benefits (in immunity to disease) upon themselves as well as upon the community. In an experimental vaccination program, however, the existence of a benefit remains to be proven nor has the degree of risk yet been determined—indeed, these are among the purposes of the trial. Thus, the justification for a vaccine trial is more utilitarian than for ordinary biomedical research with patient–subjects.

The prevailing strategy is to reduce the risks as much as possible (through studies in animals and in adult volunteers) and then, in effect, to take the plunge by using the experimental vaccine on a small number of children. It may be possible to identify characteristics that would make some children better subjects than others: those who do not experience adverse reactions to other vaccines, or those who are most likely to be exposed to the infectious agent and thus stand the most to gain from the discovery of a vaccine. Finally, compensation to subjects injured in the trial as in any experiment would help to overcome the remaining sense of a communal benefit being purchased at a high price to a few individuals (Congress 1980; President's Commission 1982).

Risky Behavior and Beneficence

What compromises should be made in research design because of investigators' obligations to act beneficently toward subjects? Research in the area of preventing AIDS illustrates the complexity of this ethical issue in several ways. First, there is a tension between the urgent need to reduce the spread of AIDS and the scientific imperative to develop the most effective means of doing so. The best way to gauge the effectiveness of various programs to prevent the spread of AIDS is to measure the rate of conversion of the population to human immune deficiency virus (HIV) seropositivity. To avoid biasing the results, the test for the HIV antibody in the blood should be administered unobtrusively, so as not to alter the experimental conditions. "Ethical considerations, however, require the antibody test to be used 'obtrusively' so as to maximize the test's effectiveness as a spur to risk reduction" (Des Jarlais and Friedman 1987, 6).

A second problem will arise once an AIDS vaccine is ready for testing. The vaccine's effectiveness can only be measured if those who are vaccinated are then exposed to the virus. Yet the virus does not spread randomly through the population; exposure requires direct contact through sexual activities, the sharing of drug paraphernalia, or from pregnant or nursing mother to child. Given the fatal nature of the disease, is it a failure of beneficence for a researcher to test a vaccine on a subject with the expectation—indeed, even the hope—that the subject (who is eligible to be included in the study because he or she has managed to escape HIV infection) will then engage in behavior that risks his or her becoming infected? Is it enough that the subject would have engaged in this behavior anyway, or does the fact of the vaccine research implicate the investigator in the subject's behavior through the failure to do everything in his power ethically and legally to protect the subject from his or her own self-risking activities?

Randomization

At the heart of all concern over human experimentation is the fact that a person in an experiment is being treated differently and exposed to risk that he or she would not encounter absent the experiment. As has already been shown, the two responses to the ethical dilemma that arises once it is decided to go ahead with an experiment anyway are (1) to reduce the actual risk as much as possible through IRB review and the like, and (2) to make the encountering of the risk a matter of the subject's free and informed choice.

A fundamental requisite for ethical experimentation, and hence for IRB approval of a protocol, is appropriate research design because a project that is not scientifically sound is not only wasteful of resources but unnecessarily exposes human beings to risks and inconvenience. Sometimes, however, the attempt to use a scientifically attractive design raises other ethical problems, especially the problem of less than full consent. The use of a randomized design illustrates the difficulties.

To measure the effect of the intervention being investigated, it is usually (though not always) necessary to have a control group whose members do not receive the intervention. Sometimes it is possible to construct such a group from patients who have received, or are receiving, other forms of treatment or who are untreated; if these control subjects can be matched by relevant characteristics with the subjects receiving the experimental intervention, the effects of the latter can be isolated. Such a method is arduous and also fraught with the risk that if all relevant criteria for matching have not been identified, the selection of the control group will be biased in some unrecognized way. For this reason, it is usual to divide potential subjects into at least two groups (i.e., those receiving the experimental intervention and the controls who receive some other treatment or no treatment) for concurrent observation by the investigator.

To avoid conscious or unconscious bias in the assignment of potential subjects to the experimental and control groups, it has become preferred practice to adopt various means of random assignment, particularly in conducting research with patients as subjects. In that case, the design is known as a randomized clinical trial (RCT).

Disclosure of Research Design

The major issues that arise with an RCT are whether and how subjects will be informed of the randomization. The fact of random assignment is plainly an important aspect of research design and is therefore an essential fact to communicate to prospective subjects. It can be argued that the design ought not to be material to the decision making of the subject because the subject should be able to rely on the physician–investigator to watch out for the subject's interests, and once the null hypothesis has been met (see below) it is, as a matter of definition, in each subject's interests to be randomized (Chalmers 1982). Yet a person entering into research (or treatment, for that matter) is not required to make decisions that are objectively welfare-maximizing. Because potential research subjects who have greater (though misguided) faith in their physicians than in the null hypothesis would want to know that the intervention they are undergoing will be determined by a randomizing procedure rather than by their physicians' individualized judgments, the randomization procedures should be included in the informed consent process (Fost 1979).

Beyond this, Charles Fried has argued "that there is a continuing duty on the part of the patient's physician . . . to inform his patient about any significant new information coming out of the experiment that might bear on the patient's choice to remain in the study or to seek other types of therapy" (Fried 1974, 35). The word "significant" can also be problematic. Asking a patient to be randomized can be asking him or her to sacrifice self-interest because data that are not significant to the researcher might very well be significant to the subject. Of course, the investigator should also educate subjects about the danger in drawing conclusions from incomplete data; dissuading a patient from withdrawing prematurely is not just a selfish act (to protect the validity of the research) but also a beneficent act toward the patient–subject. Furthermore, in certain cases, a crossover design (in which subjects are switched from one group to the other during the course of the study) can be employed to minimize the ethical problems; likewise, a data review process can be established to determine whether statistically significant results have been obtained earlier than expected, which allows the research to be terminated and the better treatment offered to all patients (Chalmers et al. 1972).

The Null Hypothesis

Because an RCT involves patients in need of diagnosis and/or treatment, it becomes especially important that one can reasonably maintain a priori that the treatment and control groups will show no difference as a result of the intervention. This position, known as the *null hypothesis*, may seem an odd proposition (why would one test an intervention believed to have no effect when compared with a control group?), but its ethical roots are more apparent if the concept is restated as the proposition that a rational person would not prefer a priori to be in one group rather than the other.

It is important to remember that the null hypothesis is a description of an objective state of affairs and not of the subjective sense of the participants. The personal prejudices of physicians and patients (to believe, for example, that a newly developed treatment will be better than any existing treatment) are not enough to deny the null hypothesis when it rests on valid grounds as it usually does in the absence of actual proof one way or the other; nonetheless, such views would, of course, be good reason for particular patients (or even particular physicians) to decline to participate in a randomized experiment. For example, a patient might have a preference for one arm of the research protocol over the other (e.g., in a comparison of surgery and radiation to treat cancer) or might, as a risk taker in life generally, want to be assigned to the new intervention rather than to the accepted one that is being used as the control.

A current issue involving the null hypothesis arises in the context of studies aimed not at discovering new treatments but at measuring the cost effectiveness of alternative methods. A prevalent complaint today is that many medical interventions have never been shown to be effective and that even among those that are clinically efficacious, data are often missing by which physicians (and their patients) could compare the relative benefits and costs of alternative forms of preventing, diagnosing, and treating a condition. Although such research was initially promoted as a form of technology assessment that might result in better patient care (Congress 1978), increasingly its objective is to conserve resources.[6] Of course, patients collectively have an

---

[6]With the advent of new forms of third-party payment, especially payments provided on a per capita or prospective basis, the medical community is more interested in researching in this field.

interest in avoiding waste in the health-care system; yet this interest, which is comparable to the collective interest in the advance of knowledge, is not, as Jonas pointed out, sufficient to justify the imposition of burdens or risks on individuals without their consent.

Because the design of a research project on the cost-benefit ratio of various treatments aims to find ways of achieving basically equivalent outcomes for patients while trimming costs to the system, not necessarily to find ways to improve the patients' individual outcomes, these studies are an exception to the general rule that the null hypothesis must be reasonable before randomization is justifiable. One arm may be clearly better than the other; therefore, it becomes very important to ensure that patients participating in such research understand the purpose of the study—to discover just how much better the particular intervention is when compared with an alternative and either justify or discontinue the intervention. One method for avoiding the potential exploitation of patients is to make use of the natural experiments that occur as different health providers and insurers adapt to the cost pressures in different ways; however, the uncontrolled variables among the groups often preclude deriving unambiguous or statistically significant results.

Other Features of Research Design

Blind and Double-Blind Studies

It is sometimes impossible to disguise the arm of an experiment to which a subject has been assigned, even though knowledge of this fact may affect the subject's responses and perceptions and the investigator's observations and interpretations. Whenever possible, however, it is preferable to conceal the assignment, that is, make it *blind* to the subject or the observer, or *double-blind* to both. Again, this is a fact that must be disclosed to subjects (Curran 1979). Although an investigator can do nothing to prevent subjects who are anxious to know whether they are in the active or control group from finding this out, acceptance of the blind condition is a valid basis for accepting, or continuing, a subject in a research project.

Placebos

In some research, the control group is given a placebo: an inactive substance, usually compounded to resemble the size, shape, and so forth, of the substance being tested. (Likewise, beyond drug trials, a sham intervention may be used in place of the true intervention.) The purpose is twofold: first, to duplicate for the control group the physical experience of the group receiving the experimental intervention, and second, by leading all subjects to believe that they have an equal chance of actually taking the experimental drug or other intervention, to expose all subjects to the elusive but sometimes very powerful effects (both favorable and unfavorable) that patients' beliefs about an intervention can have on their responses.

Two sets of questions arise about placebos. The first involves the information given to subjects. Plainly, if a subject were told whether or not he or she was receiving a placebo, the whole point of this design would be lost; on the other hand, failure to disclose is a form of deception. Would an acceptable solution be to disclose the fact that a placebo will be used but to keep secret the type of intervention actually used? Subjects who find the possibility of receiving a placebo unacceptable could then decline to participate in the experiment. But is it still deceptive not to tell subjects about the possible side effects of the placebo itself (Connelly 1987)?

The second set of issues around placebos is one of risk more than consent; it concerns the circumstances under which a placebo should not be used. When an effective treatment already exists, the use of a placebo is unacceptable. Ethically, it is justifiable to test a new therapy that promises some advantage (in efficacy, side-effects, cost, etc.) over the existing treatment, but not at the cost of withholding the existing treatment from the control group. In practical terms, the reason for testing a procedure, whether to seek approval of a new drug or to demonstrate a new form of psychological diagnosis, is not to show that it is better than nothing (i.e., has more than a placebo effect), but to find something that is preferable to existing treatments. For both these reasons, when a study is being done with patients, it is usually ethically required to assign the control group to the best available form of treatment rather than to a placebo, although there are factors that can outweigh this presumption (such as when the failure to use any treatment would create at worst a small or transient risk to subjects and when the existing treatment differs too much from the intervention being tested to allow a blind or double-blind study).

It would also be unacceptable to use a placebo when doing so would itself create undue risk for subjects. This is why placebo-controlled studies are much rarer in surgery than in medicine and pharmacology. The danger to subjects from sham operations (including the risks of anesthesia and infection) usually precludes their use, despite their obvious value in avoiding the use of unnecessary or worse surgical procedures which will then potentially expose many people to harm or waste over many years (Beecher 1961).

Special Problems of Nonconsent

Although risk never totally disappears as a topic in human experimentation, some unresolved issues focus more on problems with informed consent as such. These fall into several groups: first, those that arise when investigators are permitted to waive the usual consent requirements for reasons of research design, and second, those that arise because the subjects lack the capacity to give consent.

Waiver

Several instances (e.g., the use of placebos) have already been mentioned in which subjects may not be fully informed about what is being done to them. A desire to deceive is not, of course, limited to scientific investigators. Columnist Bob Greene relates the story of a young woman who, before going to the beach for her summer vacation, made up business cards in a fictious name, claiming to be "vice president for talent of *Gentlemen's Quarterly*." She found that the handsomest men, who would otherwise not have paid her any attention, not only posed for her but treated her like a celebrity in the hopes they would be selected to appear in the magazine. Would the men's feelings be hurt for having been deceived? "I don't think so," she concluded (Greene 1987). Is there a difference between a civilian and a scientist practicing deception of this type?[7]

In some research, investigators have what they regard as more serious reasons to keep subjects uninformed or actively misinformed about the nature, purpose, or even the existence of the research. Largely in response to complaints from social and behavioral scientists that official consent requirements preclude conducting studies in which subjects would alter their behavior if they knew they were being studied or knew the true methods and purposes of the research, the major federal regulations on human subjects research now permit an IRB to alter or even to waive the usual consent rules when (1) the risk to subjects will be minimal; (2) the "rights and welfare" of the subject will not be adversely affected; (3) the project "could not practicably be carried out without the waiver or alteration"; and (4) debriefing of the subjects will occur whenever appropriate (HHS 1983, §46.116d).[8]

Several objections can be raised to waiving consent requirements. First, the existence of a waiver provision, like the existence of the exemption for certain research,[9] may encourage a general disregard of the rules to protect human subjects (Leskovac and Delgado 1987).

More important, the waiver provision undermines the very core of the HHS regulations, which are premised on the respect for persons. The waiver

---

[7]Interestingly, Bob Greene writes that the young woman "told herself that there was a valid reason for what she was doing: 'I've always been interested in the psychology of what goes on in men's minds,' she said. 'What makes them tick. So part of me was thinking that this was a legitimate way to find out'" (Greene 1987). Apparently she believed that behaving like a scientist made her conduct less problematic.

[8]The Food and Drug Administration regulations do not provide for deception waivers, though they do permit use of an unapproved drug or device without consent if that is the best way of dealing with a life-threatening emergency (FDA 1981, §50.23).

[9]Investigators are not required to seek IRB approval of certain activities, such as research on normal educational practices in "commonly accepted educational settings," or surveys or interview procedures, or observation of public behavior, except when the information recorded could link identifiable persons to sensitive actions (such as illegal drug use) that could have adverse criminal, civil, or social consequences (HHS 1983, §46.101b).

provision, in contrast, is baldly utilitarian because it shifts the IRB's "focus from the essence of research ethics—protection of human autonomy—to the important, but secondary, consideration of protecting research subjects from physical or emotional harm" (Leskovac and Delgado 1987, 1154). Assuming that direct risk to the subject is minimal, almost any advance in knowledge will probably be found on utilitarian grounds to justify proceeding with the deception.

For some commentators, any deception or misinformation violates the rights and welfare of subjects and thus the waiver provision could never be applied. Others would differentiate between types of waivers: a waiver to permit an epidemiologist to review existing, and personally identifiable, medical records (where the harm would be a small intrusion on privacy); a waiver to permit the epidemiologist then to contact the persons identified in such records, to link previous data to consequences in their lives (clearly, a more substantial intrusion, not only on private records but on privacy in the sense of personal repose and one's sense of well-being); and a waiver to permit a behavioral scientist to lie to subjects about the purposes of a research project (where the very right of autonomous choice would be denied to the subjects).

One's evaluation of the acceptability of waiver may also turn on the value one finds in the steps that can be taken to mitigate the nondisclosure or deception. Some strategies seek to respect the values behind autonomy by developing substitutes for subjects' previous consent, such as *peer consultants*, members of the same group as the potential subjects who can participate with the investigator in design of the research (Baumrind 1978), or debriefing and after-the-fact veto, including an offer to destroy the data generated by their personal involvement (Capron 1982). Alternatively, to improve research design (another goal to which the usual requirement of informed consent would contribute) investigators could engage the public in discussion of the need for deception to carry out valuable research; public review and approval not only would provide feedback on the particular project but, perhaps even more important, would lessen the risk that deceptive research would weaken public confidence in science or endanger human interactions (Bok 1978). Or, instead of involving the entire public, a group of people who were willing to participate in such research could be used as a deception pool from whom subjects could be drawn (Leskovac and Delgado 1987).

Fetuses and Abortuses

Sometimes the problem with consent lies not in the design of the project but in the inability of the subjects to decide on their own behalf. HHS has recognized the need for extra circumspection in these cases by placing special requirements on researchers. For example, they must obtain approval from a national Ethics Advisory Board or similar group of experts appointed by the Secretary of HHS before the research may be funded (HHS 1983, §§46.204 and 46.407b(ii)).

Perhaps the most troubled area of special protection is that afforded by the federal regulations and the laws of a number of states to fetuses as possible research subjects. Because of its link to the abortion controversy, this area of research has aroused a great deal of public concern, going back at least to the National Research Act of 1974, which made a study of the subject the first assignment for the National Commission.

The simplest provisions are that any research with a dead aborted fetus be performed only with the consent of its mother, as directly required by statute in a number of states (Arkansas 1985, §82-438; Massachusetts 1983, 112 §12Ja(II)), and by implication in all states under the Uniform Anatomical Gift Act (UAGA). Furthermore, the federal regulations prohibit use of a fetus ex utero as a subject "until it has been ascertained whether or not" it is viable; vital functions of a nonviable fetus may neither be artificially maintained nor exposed to the risk of more rapid termination, and a viable fetus is to be treated as an infant and not exposed to anything more than minimal experimental risks that are not necessary for treatment (HHS 1983, §46.209). Statutes in several states forbid any research with a fetus ex utero (Arizona 1986, §36-2302(A); Arkansas 1985, §82-438; Massachusetts 1986, 112, §12Ja(I)).

The direct intersection of the experimentation and abortion issues occurs when an investigator wishes to study the fetus in utero. The HHS rules limit such research to activities intended "to meet the health needs of the particular fetus" and involving the minimal increase in risk necessary to meet these needs, or to activities that generate minimal risk, the purpose of which "is the development of important biomedical knowledge which cannot be obtained by other means" (HHS 1983, §46.208a). Similarly, laws in several states limit experimental interventions to those designed to benefit the fetus (Massachusetts 1986, 112, §12Ja(I); South Dakota 1977, §34-23A-17; Utah 1977, §76-7-310). Does research on prenatal diagnosis fall within the benefit or needs of the fetus category (when the diagnosis may lead to the decision to abort the fetus)? In interpreting a Louisiana statute that prohibits experimentation upon an unborn child unless it is therapeutic to the fetus (Louisiana 1986, §40:1299.35.13), the federal district court simply sidestepped the plaintiff's claim that the statute was so vague that it would inhibit experimentation and held that prenatal diagnosis is not experimental (*Margaret S. v. Edwards* 1980). It seems doubtful that a researcher developing new means of antenatal diagnosis, much less new means of abortion, could take much comfort from this decision if prosecuted for violating one of the state laws prohibiting nonbeneficial research involving the fetus.

Dead or Nearly Dead Subjects

Besides permitting the donation of dead fetuses or their parts for research, the UAGA has general application to dead persons of any age. Unless expressly limited by the donor (i.e., the decedent before death or specified family members after the decedent's death), a body donated under the UAGA may be used for education, research, therapy, and/or transplantation. Although an institution could insist that research using dead bodies be reviewed, IRB review is not required by federal regulations, which apply only to living human subjects.

In the context of organ transplantation, a declaration of death is usually based on the complete cessation of brain functions in bodies whose respiratory and circulatory functions are artificially maintained (Capron 1986, Medical Consultants 1981). It has been suggested that such brain-dead bodies would be good subjects for research (Carson, Frias, and Melker 1981; Martyn 1986, 8). Despite the potential benefits of, and the apparent authority for, such research, the same ethical concerns involved in fetal research arise in research on dead bodies in which the signs of life are being maintained.

Specifically, research regulations and the UAGA fail to protect against two dangers of research on the brain-dead: the disturbing effect such research could have on family members and the violation of "commonly held convictions about respect for the dead" (President's Commission 1983, 40). The President's Commission recommended that those concerns be addressed by expanding the use of IRBs to all research on the deceased, including the brain-dead (1983). The application to the brain-dead of federal research regulations would require full disclosure of the nature, purpose, and duration of the research as well as the benefits and risks, as well as requiring the research protocol to establish the need of the experiment (Martyn 1986). This would give the final right to determine how and whether the body is used to the donors while protecting against infringement of respect for the dead, especially those who in some ways still appear alive (Gaylin 1974).

Beyond potential subjects for research who have lost all brain functions are those who are permanently comatose or anencephalic: both of the latter have intact brain stems (and hence respire spontaneously) but have lost their higher brain functions or, in the case of the anencephalic newborn, never had such capability. Questions may arise about the involvement of such persons in therapeutic research (aimed at finding a means to improve their condition). The difficulties of obtaining consent for research with incompetent subjects are compounded here because the procedures often must be applied on a rapid basis in an emergency room (President's Commission 1983).

The greatest difficulties, however, come with proposals that would involve using persons without higher brain functions as pure subjects (rather than as patient–subjects who might benefit personally from the research). For example, it has been suggested that anencephalic newborns could be useful in physiologic research or as a source of organs for transplantation into other infants and children (Harrison 1986). Approval for the use of this category of subject could be distinguished from using other persons who lack higher brain functions, because an anencephalic infant never had such functions (and will usually die rapidly, even with good support), unlike a fetus (who, if allowed to gestate, will normally develop higher brain functions) or a comatose adult (who may survive for a very long time even after losing all cognitive functions); thus, a foothold may exist against sliding down the slippery slope. Nevertheless, the removal of organs from, or experimentation with, "a living human being, though one born dying" (Meilander 1986, 22) would violate not only generally accepted medical obligations to patients but also homicide statutes, which protect the lives of all live-born persons. Indeed, even steps to prolong the dying of an anencephalic infant in order to facilitate organ removal after death has occurred would go against the spirit of a conclusion of the National Commission that steps not be taken to "alter the duration of life of the nonviable fetus ex utero" (National Commission 1975, 68).

A FINAL WORD

Needless to say, this list of issues has barely skimmed the surface of the interesting problems that are raised by research with human subjects. One whole complicated area—whether, and if so how, to compensate injured research subjects (President's Commission 1982)—has hardly been touched on here, but the resolution of that issue could have profound consequences for the resolution of other issues, such as the use of subjects (e.g., children) without their consent. Moreover, the analysis has been primarily in ethical terms with historical illustrations. Different features might have emerged, or sunk into the shadows, had another analytic light been cast on the topic—such as a sociological analysis emphasizing the role and power relationships of the participants in the research process, or a legal analysis focusing on the ways in which the law is capable or incapable of responding to the interests of various parties and how that, in turn, affects their behavior.

DISCUSSION QUESTIONS

1. If a physician decides to withhold information from a patient about the dangers of the medication the patient is taking as a way to protect the patient from harm, what moral principle underlies the decision? Is such a practice justified? What moral principles would justify opposing such a practice?

2. When a physician decides to try an innovative therapy outside a research protocol, what moral principle would justify such a practice? Should such a practice ever be acceptable outside of a protocol? If so, ought it to be governed by standard rules governing human subjects' research including review by an IRB?

3. In what ways does the principle of justice govern research subject recruitment and research design? Is it ever justified to compromise research design in order to select subjects more fairly or give subjects opportunities to be better off? If so, when?

4. If the ethics of research requires that subjects give a reasonably informed consent, on what grounds, if any, can the following types of information be withheld from subjects: the fact that subjects are randomized? The presence of a placebo in the research design? The presence of deception in the research? The existence of trivial risks that subjects can be expected to know about (such as the pain of an injection)? The fact that medical records will be searched in order to gain research information?

5. Under what circumstances, if any, is it acceptable to conduct research on fetuses: when the pregnant woman is likely to gain? When the fetus has a chance to benefit? When the fetus will not be carried to term? When the fetus has already been aborted?

REFERENCES

Books and Articles

Alexander, L. "Limitations in Experimental Research on Human Beings." *Lex et Scienta* 3 (1966): 8–15.

Barber, B., Lally, J., Makarushka, J., et al. *Research on Human Subjects.* New York: Russell Sage Foundation, 1973.

Baumrind, D. "Nature and Definition of Informed Consent in Research Involving Deception." *The Belmont Report*, Vol. 2 (Appendix), National Commission for the Protection of Human Subjects of Biomedical and Behavioral Research. Washington, DC: Government Printing Office, 1978: 23–42.

Beecher, H. K. "Surgery as Placebo." *JAMA* 176 (1961): 1102–1107.

———. "Ethics and Clinical Research." *N Engl J Med* 274 (1966): 1354–1360.

———. *Research and the Individual: Human Studies*. Boston: Little, Brown, 1970.

Bernard, C. *An Introduction to the Study of Experimental Medicine* (H. C. Greene, Trans.). New York: Macmillan, 1927.

Blumgart, J. "The Medical Framework for Viewing the Problem of Human Experimentation." *Daedalus* 98 (1969): 248–274.

Bok, S. *Lying: Moral Choice in Public and Private Life*. New York: Pantheon Books, 1978.

Brandt, A. M. "Racism and Research: The Case of the Tuskegee Syphilis Study." *Hastings Cent Rep* 8, no. 6 (1978): 21–29.

Capron, A. M. "The Law of Genetic Therapy." In M. Hamilton, Ed., *The New Genetics and the Future of Man*. Grand Rapids: Eerdmans Publishing, 1972: 133–156.

———. "Legal Considerations Affecting Clinical Pharmacological Studies in Children." *Clin Res* 21 (1973): 141–150.

———. "Is Consent Always Necessary in Social Science Research?" In T. L. Beauchamp, R. R. Faden, R. J. Wallace, Jr., and L. Walters, Eds., *Ethical Issues in Social Science Research*. Baltimore: Johns Hopkins University Press, 1982: 215–231.

———. "Determination of Death." In K. Benesch, N. S. Abramson, A. Grenvik, and A. Meisel, Eds., *Medicolegal Aspects of Critical Care*. Rockville, MD: Aspen, 1986: 109–132.

Cardon, P. V., Dommel, F. W., Jr., Trumble, R. "Injuries to Research Subjects: A Survey of Investigators." *N Engl J Med* 295 (1976): 650–654.

Carson, R., Frias, J., Melker, R. "Case Study: Research with Brain-Dead Children." *IRB* 3 (1981): 5–6.

Chalmers, T. C. "The Ethics of Randomization as a Decision-Making Technique, and the Problem of Informed Consent." In T. Beauchamp and L. Walters, Eds., *Contemporary Issues in Bioethics*, 2nd ed. Belmont, CA: Wadsworth, 1982: 538–541.

Chalmers, T. C., Block, J. B., Lee, S. "Controlled Studies in Clinical Cancer Research." *N Engl J Med* 287 (1972): 75–78.

Conference on the Proper Use of the Nazi Analogy in Ethical Debate. "Biomedical Ethics and the Shadow of Nazism." *Hastings Cent Rep* 6 (4) (Suppl.) (1976): 1–16.

Congress of the United States, Office of Technology Assessment. *Assessing the Efficacy and Safety of Medical Technologies*. Washington, DC: Government Printing Office, 1978.

———. *Compensation for Vaccine-Related Injuries*. Washington, DC: Government Printing Office, 1980.

Connelly, R. J. "Deception and the Placebo Effect in Biomedical Research." *IRB* 9, (1987): 5–7.

Cowan, D. "Human Experimentation: The Review Process in Practice." *Case W Res L Rev* 25 (1975): 533–564.

Curran, W. J. "Governmental Regulation of the Use of Human Subjects in Medical Research: The Approach of Two Federal Agencies." *Daedalus* 98 (1969): 542–594.

———. "Reasonableness and Randomization in Clinical Trials: Fundamental Law and Governmental Regulations." *N Engl J Med* 300 (1979): 1273–1275.

Des Jarlais, D. C., Friedman, S. R. "AIDS Prevention Among IV Drug Users: Potential Conflicts between Research Design and Ethics." *IRB* 9 (1987): 6–8.

Deutsch, E. *Das Recht der Klinischen Forschung am Menschen: Zulassigkeit und Folgen der Versuche am Menschen Dargest. Im Vergleich zu den amerikan. Beispeil und die internat. Regelungen.* Frankfurt-am-Main: Lang, 1979.

Eckholm, E. "Should the Rules Be Bent in an Epidemic?" *New York Times*, July 13, 1986: IV-30.

Eisenberg, L. "The Social Imperatives of Medical Research." *Science* 198 (1977): 1105–1110.

Fost, N. "Consent as a Barrier to Research." *N Engl J Med* 300 (1979): 1271–1273.

Fox, R. C. *The Courage to Fail.* Chicago: University of Chicago Press, 1974.

Forssmann, W. "The Role of Heart Catheterization and Angiocardiography in the Development of Modern Medicine." *Nobel Lectures, Physiology or Medicine 1942–1962.* Amsterdam: Elsevier, 1964: 506–512.

Frankel, M. *The Public Health Service Guidelines Governing Research Involving Human Subjects: An Analysis of the Policy-Making Process.* Washington, DC: George Washington University, 1972.

Fried, C. *Medical Experimentation: Personal Integrity and Social Policy.* New York: American Elsevier, 1974.

Gaylin, W. "Harvesting the Dead." *Harpers* 249 (1974): 23–26.

Gomer, R., Powell, J., Roling, B. "Japan's Biological Weapons: 1930–1945." *Bull Atomic Sci* 37 (1981): 43, 45.

Grady, D. "Summary of Discussion on Ethical Perspectives." In M. Shaw, Ed., *After Barney Clark.* Austin: University of Texas Press, 1984: 42–52.

Greene, B. "A Beach Party with the Delaware Hunks." *Chicago Tribune*, February 10, 1987: 5(1).

Harrison, M. "The Anencephalic Newborn as Organ Donor." *Hastings Cent Rep* 16, no. 2 (1986): 21–22.

Holder, A. R. "Can a Court Order Participation in Research?" *IRB* 9 (1987): 8–9.

"How U.S. Used Americans in Radiation Experiments." *San Francisco Chronicle*, October 25, 1986: 2.

Ivy, A. C. "The History and Ethics of the Use of Human Subjects in Medical Experiments." *Science* 108 (1948): 1–8.

Jonas, H. "Philosophical Reflections on Experimenting with Human Subjects." *Daedalus* 98 (1969): 219–247.

Jonsen, A. R. "Do No Harm." *Ann Intern Med* 88 (1978): 827–832.

———. "The Selection of Patients." In M. Shaw, Ed., *After Barney Clark.* Austin: University of Texas Press, 1984: 5–10.

Katz, J. "The Regulation of Human Experimentation in the United States—A Personal Odyssey." *IRB* 9 (1987): 1–6.

Leskovac, H., Delgado, R. "Protecting Autonomy and Personhood in Human Subjects Research." *S Ill Univ L J* 11 (1987): 1147–1158.

Levine, R. J. *Ethics and Regulation of Clinical Research.* Baltimore: Urban & Schwarzenberg, 1986.

Lubasch, A. H. "$700,000 Award Is Made in '53 Secret Test Death." *New York Times,* May 6, 1987: B-3.

Martyn, S. "Using the Brain Dead for Medical Research." *Utah L Rev* (1986): 1–28.

Medical Consultants on the Diagnosis of Death. "Guidelines for the Determination of Death: Report to the President's Commission for the Study of Ethical Problems in Medicine and Biomedical and Behavioral Research." *JAMA* 246 (1981): 2184–2187.

Meilander, G. "The Anencephalic Newborn as Organ Donor." *Hastings Cent Rep* 16, no. 2 (1986): 22–23.

National Advisory Health Council. Stenographic transcript of the Sept. 28, 1965, meeting. (Quoted in Frankel, 1972.)

National Commission for the Protection of Human Subjects of Biomedical and Behavioral Research. *Report and Recommendations: Research on the Fetus.* Washington, DC: Government Printing Office, 1975.

———. *Report and Recommendations: Research Involving Children.* Washington, DC: Government Printing Office, 1977.

———. *The Belmont Report.* Washington, DC: Government Printing Office, 1978a.

———. *Report and Recommendations: Institutional Review Boards.* Washington, DC: Government Printing Office, 1978b.

Pappworth, M. H. *Human Guinea Pigs: Experimentation on Man.* Boston: Beacon Press, 1968.

Pattullo, E. L. "Institutional Review Boards and the Freedom to Take Risks." *N Engl J Med* 307 (1982): 1156–1159.

Powell, J. "A Hidden Chapter in History." *Bull Atomic Sci* 37 (1981): 44–52.

President's Commission for the Study of Ethical Problems in Medicine and Biomedical and Behavioral Research. *Protecting Human Subjects: The Adequacy and Uniformity of Federal Rules and Their Implementation.* Washington, DC: Government Printing Office, 1981.

———. *Compensating for Research Injuries.* Washington, DC: Government Printing Office, 1982.

———. *Implementing Human Research Regulations.* Washington, DC: Government Printing Office, 1983.

Prinzmetal, M. "On the Humane Treatment of Charity Patients." *Medical Tribune,* September 22, 1965: 15.

Rawls, J. *A Theory of Justice.* Cambridge: Harvard University Press, 1971.

Sass, H-M. "Reichsundschreiben 1931: Pre-Nuremberg German Regulations Concerning New Therapy and Human Experimentation." *J Med Philos* 8 (1983): 99–111.

Tuskegee Syphilis Study Ad Hoc Panel to the Department of Health, Education, and Welfare. *Final Report.* Washington, DC: Public Health Service, 1973.

U.S. Senate. *Project MK-ULTRA, The CIA's Program of Research in Behavioral Modification, Joint Hearings Before the Senate Select Comm. on Intelligence and the Subcomm.*

on Health and Scientific Research of the Senate Comm. on Human Resources. 95th Congress, 1st Session 75, 1977.

Veatch, R. M. "Justice and Research Design: The Case for a Semi-Randomization Clinical Trial." *Clin Res* 31 (1983): 12–22.

Veressayev, V. *The Memoirs of a Physician* (S. Linden, trans.). New York: Knopf, 1916.

Warren, J. W., Sobal, J., Tenney, J. H., et al. "Informed Consent by Proxy: An Issue in Research with Elderly Patients." *N Engl J Med* 315 (1986): 1124–1128.

World Medical Association. *Declaration of Helsinki,* 1975.

Statutes, Regulations, and Cases

Arizona. *Revised Statutes Annotated.* St. Paul, MN: West Publishing, 1986.

Arkansas. *Statutes Annotated* (Suppl.). Charlottesville, VA: Michie, 1985.

Barrett v. Hoffman. 521 F.Suppl. 307 (S.D.N.Y.), 1981.

California. *Health and Safety Code.* St. Paul, MN: West Publishing, 1984.

Der Minister der geistlichen. Anweisung an die Vorsteher der Kliniken, Polikliniken under sinstigen Krankenanstakten. *Centralblatt der gesamten Unterrichtsverwaltung in Preussen.* Berlin: Prussian Government, 1901: 188–189.

Food and Drug Amendments. Act of 10 Oct. 1962, Pub. Law No. 87-781, *amending* 21 U.S.C. §355, 1962.

Louisiana. *Revised Statutes Annotated* (Suppl.). St. Paul, MN: West Publishing, 1986.

Margaret S. v. Edwards. 488 F.Suppl. 181 (E.D.La.), 1980.

Massachusetts. *General Laws Annotated.* St. Paul, MN: West Publishing, 1986.

Mink v. University of Chicago. 460 F.Suppl. 713 (N.D. Ill.), 1978.

National Research Act. Pub. Law No. 93-348, 42 USC 289L-3(a), 1974.

Nevin v. United States. 696 F.2d 1229 (9th Cir.), 1983.

New York. *Public Health Law.* Albany: McKinney, 1985.

Pierce v. Ortho Pharmaceutical Corp. 417 A.2d 505 (NJ), 1980.

South Dakota. *Codified Laws Annotated.* Indianapolis: Allen Smith, 1978.

U.S. Department of Health and Human Services. "Protection of Human Subjects." *Code of Federal Regulations* 45, Part 46, issued in *Federal Register* 46 (26 Jan. 1981): 8386–8391 and 48 (4 March 1983): 9269–9270.

U.S. Food and Drug Administration. Protection of Human Subjects; Standards for Institutional Review Boards for Clinical Investigations. *Code of Federal Regulations.* Title 21: Part 56, issued in *Federal Register* 46 (27 Jan. 1981): 8958–8979.

U.S. Public Health Service. *Clinical Research and Investigation Involving Human Beings,* Policy and Procedure Order No. 129, 8 Feb. 1966a.

U.S. Public Health Service. *Clinical Research and Investigation Involving Human Beings,* Policy and Procedure Order No. 129, Revised Supplement No. 2, 12 Dec. 1966b.

Utah. *Criminal Code Annotated.* Indianapolis: Allen Smith, 1982.

APPENDIX 1

THE NUREMBERG CODE

The great weight of evidence before us is to the effect that certain types of medical experiments on human beings, when kept within reasonable well-defined bounds, conform to the ethics of the medical profession generally. The protagonists of the practice of human experimentation justify their views on the basis that such experiments yield results for the good of society that are unprocurable by other methods or means of study. All agree, however, that certain basic principles must be observed in order to satisfy moral, ethical and legal concepts:

1. The voluntary consent of the human subject is absolutely essential.

This means that the person involved should have legal capacity to give consent; should be so situated as to be able to exercise free power of choice, without the intervention of any element of force, fraud, deceit, duress, overreaching, or other ulterior form of constraint or coercion; and should have sufficient knowledge and comprehension of the elements of the subject matter involved as to enable him to make an understanding and enlightened decision. This latter element requires that before the acceptance of an affirmative decision by the experimental subject there should be made known to him the nature, duration, and purpose of the experiment; the method and means by which it is to be conducted; all inconveniences and hazards reasonably to be expected; and the effects upon his health or person which may possibly come from his participation in the experiment.

The duty and responsibility for ascertaining the quality of the consent rests upon each individual who initiates, directs or engages in the experiment. It is a personal duty and responsibility which may not be delegated to another with impunity.

2. The experiment should be such as to yield fruitful results for the good of society, unprocurable by other methods or means of study, and not random and unnecessary in nature.

3. The experiment should be designed and based on the results of animal experimentation and a knowledge of the natural history of the disease or other problem under study that the anticipated results will justify the performance of the experiment.

4. The experiment should be so conducted as to avoid all unnecessary physical and mental suffering and injury.

5. The experiment should be conducted where there is an a priori reason to believe that death or disabling injury will occur except, perhaps, in those experiments where the experimental physicians also serve as subjects.

6. The degree of risk to be taken should never exceed that determined by the humanitarian importance of the problem to be solved by the experiment.

Source: Nuremberg Military Tribunals (1949: 181–82).

7. Proper preparations should be made and adequate facilities provided to protect the experimental subject against even remote possibilities of injury, disability, or death.

8. The experiment should be conducted only by scientifically qualified persons. The highest degree of skill and care should be required through all stages of the experiment of those who conduct or engage in the experiment.

9. During the course of the experiment the human subject should be at liberty to bring the experiment to an end if he has reached the physical or mental state where continuation of the experiment seems to him to be impossible.

10. During the course of the experiment the scientist in charge must be prepared to terminate the experiment at any stage, if he has probable cause to believe, in the exercise of the good faith, superior skill and careful judgment required of him that a continuation of the experiment is likely to result in injury, disability, or death to the experimental subject. . . .

APPENDIX 2

DEPARTMENT OF HEALTH AND HUMAN SERVICES, BASIC HHS POLICY FOR PROTECTION OF HUMAN RESEARCH SUBJECTS

§46.101   To What Do These Regulations Apply?

(a) Except as provided in paragraph (b) of this section, this subpart applies to all research involving human subjects conducted by the Department of Health and Human Services or funded in whole or in part by a Department grant, contract, cooperative agreement or fellowship.

(1) This includes research conducted by Department employees, except each Principal Operating Component head may adopt such nonsubstantive, procedural modifications as may be appropriate from an administrative standpoint.

(2) It also includes research conducted or funded by the Department of Health and Human Services outside the United States, but in appropriate circumstances, the Secretary may, under paragraph (e) of this section waive the applicability of some or all of the requirements of these regulations for research of this type.

(b) Research activities in which the only involvement of human subjects will be in one or more of the following categories are exempt from these regulations unless the research is covered by other subparts of this part:

(1) Research conducted in established or commonly accepted educational settings, involving normal educational practices, such as (i) research on regular and special education instructional strategies, or (ii) research on the effectiveness of or the comparison among instructional techniques, curricula, or classroom management methods.

Source: This HHS policy is excerpted from 46 *Federal Register* 8386, January 26, 1981; 48 *Federal Register* 9269, March 4, 1983.

(2) Research involving the use of educational tests (cognitive, diagnostic, aptitude, achievement), if information taken from these sources is recorded in such a manner that subjects cannot be identified, directly or through identifiers linked to the subjects.

(3) Research involving survey or interview procedures, except where all of the following conditions exist: (i) responses are recorded in such a manner that the human subjects can be identified, directly or through identifiers linked to the subjects, (ii) the subject's responses, if they became known outside the research, could reasonably place the subject at risk of criminal or civil liability or be damaging to the subject's financial standing or employability, and (iii) the research deals with sensitive aspects of the subject's own behavior, such as illegal conduct, drug use, sexual behavior, or use of alcohol. All research involving survey or interview procedures is exempt, without exception, when the respondents are elected or appointed public officials or candidates for public office.

(4) Research involving the observation (including observation by participants) of public behavior, except where all of the following conditions exist: (i) observations are recorded in such a manner that the human subjects can be identified, directly or through identifiers linked to the subjects, (ii) the observations recorded about the individual, if they became known outside the research, could reasonably place the subject at risk of criminal or civil liability or be damaging to the subject's financial standing or employability, and (iii) the research deals with sensitive aspects of the subject's own behavior such as illegal conduct, drug use, sexual behavior, or use of alcohol.

(5) Research involving the collection or study of existing data, documents, records, pathological specimens, or diagnostic specimens, if these sources are publicly available or if the information is recorded by the investigator in such a manner that subjects cannot be identified, directly or through identifiers linked to the subjects.

(6) Unless specifically required by statute (and except to the extent specified in paragraph (i)), research and demonstration projects which are conducted by or subject to the approval of the Department of Health and Human Services, and which are designed to study, evaluate, or otherwise examine: (i) programs under the Social Security Act, or other public benefit or service programs; (ii) procedures for obtaining benefits or services under those programs; (iii) possible changes in or alternatives to those programs or procedures; or (iv) possible changes in methods or levels of payment for benefits or services under those programs.

(c) The Secretary has final authority to determine whether a particular activity is covered by these regulations.

(d) The Secretary may require that specific research activities or classes of research activities conducted or funded by the Department, but not otherwise covered by these regulations, comply with some or all of these regulations.

(e) The Secretary may also waive applicability of these regulations to specific research activities or classes of research activities, otherwise covered by these regulations. Notices of these actions will be published in the *Federal Register* as they occur.

(f) No individual may receive Department funding for research covered by these regulations unless the individual is affiliated with or sponsored by an institution which assumes responsibility for the research under an assurance satisfying the requirements of this part, or the individual makes other arrangements with the Department.

(g) Compliance with these regulations will in no way render inapplicable pertinent federal, state, or local laws or regulations.

(h) Each subpart of these regulations contains a separate section describing to what the subpart applies. Research which is covered by more than one subpart shall comply with all applicable subparts.

(i) If, following review of proposed research activities that are exempt from these regulations under paragraph (b)(6), the Secretary determines that a research or demonstration project presents a danger to the physical, mental, or emotional well-being of a participant or subject of the research or demonstration project, then federal funds may not be expended for such a project without the written, informed consent of each participant or subject.

§46.102 Definitions

(e) "Research" means a systematic investigation designed to develop or contribute to generalizable knowledge. Activities which meet this definition constitute "research" for purposes of these regulations, whether or not they are supported or funded under a program which is considered research for other purposes. For example, some "demonstration" and "service" programs may include research activities.

(f) "Human subject" means a living individual about whom an investigator (whether professional or student) conducting research obtains (1) data through intervention or interaction with the individual, or (2) identifiable private information. "Intervention" includes both physical procedures by which data are gathered (for example, venipuncture) and manipulations of the subject or the subject's environment that are performed for research purposes. "Interaction" includes communication or interpersonal contact between investigator and subject. "Private information" includes information about behavior that occurs in a context in which an individual can reasonably expect that no observation or recording is taking place, and information which has been provided for specific purposes by an individual and which the individual can reasonably expect will not be made public (for example, a medical record). Private information must be individually identifiable (i.e., the identity of the subject is or may readily be ascertained by the investigator or associated with the information) in order for obtaining the information to constitute research involving human subjects.

(g) "Minimal risk" means that the risks of harm anticipated in the proposed research are not greater, considering probability and magnitude, than those ordinarily encountered in daily life or during the performance of routine physical or psychological examinations or tests.

§46.103 Assurances

(a) Each institution engaged in research covered by these regulations shall provide written assurance satisfactory to the Secretary that it will comply with the requirements set forth in these regulations.

(b) The Department will conduct or fund research covered by these regulations only if the institution has an assurance approved as provided in this section, and only if the institution has certified to the Secretary that the research has been reviewed and approved by an IRB provided for in the assurance, and will be subject to continuing review by the IRB. This assurance shall at a minimum include:

(1) A statement of principles governing the institution in the discharge of its responsibilities for protecting the rights and welfare of human subjects of research conducted at or sponsored by the institution, regardless of source of funding. This may include an appropriate existing code, declaration, or statement of ethical principles, or a statement formulated by the institution itself. This requirement does not preempt provisions of these regulations applicable to department-funded research and is not applicable to any research in an exempt category listed in §46.101.

(2) Designation of one or more IRBs established in accordance with the requirements of this subpart, and for which provisions are made for meeting space and sufficient staff to support the IRB's review and recordkeeping duties.

(3) A list of the IRB members identified by name; earned degrees; representative capacity; indications of experience such as board certifications, licenses, etc., sufficient to describe each member's chief anticipated contributions to IRB deliberations; and any employment or other relationship between each member and the institution; for example: full-time employee, part-time employee, member of governing panel or board, stockholder, paid or unpaid consultant. Changes in IRB membership shall be reported to the Secretary.

(4) Written procedures which the IRB will follow (i) for conducting its initial and continuing review of research and for reporting its findings and actions to the investigator and the institution; (ii) for determining which projects require review more often than annually and which projects need verification from sources other than the investigators that no material changes have occurred since previous IRB review; (iii) for insuring prompt reporting to the IRB of proposed changes in a research activity, and for insuring that changes in approved research, during the period for which IRB approval has already been given, may not be initiated without IRB review and approval except where necessary to eliminate apparent immediate hazards to the subject; and (iv) for insuring prompt reporting to the IRB and to the Secretary of unanticipated problems involving risks to subjects or others.

§46.107   IRB Membership

(a) Each IRB shall have at least five members, with varying backgrounds to promote complete and adequate review of research activities commonly conducted by the institution. The IRB shall be sufficiently qualified through the experience and expertise of its members, and the diversity of the members' backgrounds including consideration of the racial and cultural backgrounds of members and sensitivity to such issues as community attitudes, to promote respect for its advice and counsel in safeguarding the rights and welfare of human subjects. In addition to possessing the professional competence necessary to review specific research activities, the IRB shall be able to ascertain the acceptability of proposed research in terms of institutional commitments and regulations, applicable law, and standards of professional conduct and practice. The IRB shall therefore include persons knowledgeable in these areas. If an IRB regularly reviews research that involves a vulnerable category of subjects, including but not limited to subjects covered by other subparts of this part, the IRB shall include one or more individuals who are primarily concerned with the welfare of these subjects.

(b) No IRB may consist entirely of men or entirely of women, or entirely of members of one profession.

(c) Each IRB shall include at least one member whose primary concerns are in nonscientific areas; for example: lawyers, ethicists, members of the clergy.

(d) Each IRB shall include at least one member who is not otherwise affiliated with the institution and who is not part of the immediate family of a person who is affiliated with the institution.

(e) No IRB may have a member participating in the IRB's initial or continuing review of any project in which the member has a conflicting interest, except to provide information requested by the IRB.

(f) An IRB may, in its discretion, invite individuals with competence in special areas to assist in the review of complex issues which require expertise beyond or in addition to that available on the IRB. These individuals may not vote with the IRB.

§46.111   Criteria for IRB Approval of Research

(a) In order to approve research covered by these regulations the IRB shall determine that all of the following requirements are satisfied:

(1) Risks to subjects are minimized: (i) By using procedures which are consistent with sound research design and which do not unnecessarily expose subjects to risk, and (ii) whenever appropriate, by using procedures already being performed on the subjects for diagnostic or treatment purposes.

(2) Risks to subjects are reasonable in relation to anticipated benefits, if any, to subjects, and the importance of the knowledge that may reasonably be expected to result. In evaluating risks and benefits, the IRB should consider only those risks and benefits that may result from the research (as distinguished from risks and benefits of therapies subjects would receive even if not participating in the research). The IRB should not consider possible long-range effects of applying knowledge gained in the research (for example, the possible effects of the research on public policy) as among those research risks that fall within the purview of its responsibility.

(3) Selection of subjects is equitable. In making this assessment the IRB should take into account the purposes of the research and the setting in which the research will be conducted.

(4) Informed consent will be sought from each prospective subject or the subject's legally authorized representative, in accordance with, and to the extent required by §46.116.

(5) Informed consent will be appropriately documented, in accordance with, and to the extent required by §46.117.

(6) Where appropriate, the research plan makes adequate provision for monitoring the data collected to insure the safety of subjects.

(7) Where appropriate, there are adequate provisions to protect the privacy of subjects and to maintain the confidentiality of data.

(b) Where some or all of the subjects are likely to be vulnerable to coercion or undue influence, such as persons with acute or severe physical or mental illness, or persons who are economically or educationally disadvantaged, appropriate additional safeguards have been included in the study to protect the rights and welfare of these subjects.

§46.116   General Requirements for Informed Consent

Except as provided elsewhere in this or other subparts, no investigator may involve a human being as a subject in research covered by these regulations unless the investigator has obtained the legally effective informed consent of the subject or the subject's legally authorized representative. An investigator shall seek such consent only under circumstances that provide the prospective subject or the representative sufficient opportunity to consider whether or not to participate and that minimize the possibility of coercion or undue influence. The information that is given to the subject or the representative shall be in language understandable to the subject or the representative. No informed consent, whether oral or written, may include any exculpatory language through which the subject or the representative is made to waive or appear to waive any of the subject's legal rights, or releases or appears to release the investigator, the sponsor, the institution or its agents from liability for negligence.

(a) Basic elements of informed consent. Except as provided in paragraph (c) or (d) of this section, in seeking informed consent the following information shall be provided to each subject:

(1) A statement that the study involves research, an explanation of the purposes of the research and the expected duration of the subject's participation, a description of the procedures to be followed, and identification of any procedures which are experimental;

(2) A description of any reasonably foreseeable risks or discomforts to the subject;

(3) A description of any benefits to the subject or to others which may reasonably be expected from the research;

(4) A disclosure of appropriate alternative procedures or courses of treatment, if any, that might be advantageous to the subject;

(5) A statement describing the extent, if any, to which confidentiality of records identifying the subject will be maintained;

(6) For research involving more than minimal risk, an explanation as to whether any compensation and an explanation as to whether any medical treatments are available if injury occurs and, if so, what they consist of, or where further information may be obtained;

(7) An explanation of whom to contact for answers to pertinent questions about the research and research subjects' rights, and whom to contact in the event of a research-related injury to the subject; and

(8) A statement that participation is voluntary, refusal to participate will involve no penalty or loss of benefits to which the subject is otherwise entitled, and the subject may discontinue participation at any time without penalty or loss of benefits to which the subject is otherwise entitled.

(b) Additional elements of informed consent. When appropriate, one or more of the following elements of information shall also be provided to each subject:

(1) A statement that the particular treatment or procedure may involve risks to the subject (or to the embryo or fetus, if the subject is or may become pregnant) which are currently unforeseeable;

(2) Anticipated circumstances under which the subject's participation may be terminated by the investigator without regard to the subject's consent;

(3) Any additional costs to the subject that may result from participation in the research;

(4) The consequences of a subject's decision to withdraw from the research and procedures for orderly termination of participation by the subject;

(5) A statement that significant new findings developed during the course of the research which may relate to the subject's willingness to continue participation will be provided to the subject; and

(6) The approximate number of subjects involved in the study.

(c) An IRB may approve a consent procedure which does not include, or which alters, some or all of the elements of informed consent set forth above, or waive the requirement to obtain informed consent provided the IRB finds and documents that:

(1) The research or demonstration project is to be conducted by or subject to the approval of state or local government officials and is designed to study, evaluate, or otherwise examine: (i) programs under the Social Security Act, or other public benefit or service programs; (ii) procedures for obtaining benefits or services under those programs; (iii) possible changes in or alternatives to those programs or procedures; or (iv) possible changes in methods or levels of payment for benefits or services under those programs; and

(2) The research could not practicably be carried out without the waiver or alteration.

(d) an IRB may approve a consent procedure which does not include, or which alters, some or all of the elements of informed consent set forth above, or waive the requirements to obtain informed consent provided the IRB finds and documents that:

(1) The research involves no more than minimal risk to the subjects;

(2) The waiver or alteration will not adversely affect the rights and welfare of the subjects;

(3) The research could not practicably be carried out without the waiver or alteration; and

(4) whenever appropriate, the subjects will be provided with additional pertinent information after participation.

(e) The informed consent requirements in these regulations are not intended to preempt any applicable federal, state, or local laws which require additional information to be disclosed in order for informed consent to be legally effective.

(f) Nothing in these regulations is intended to limit the authority of a physician to provide emergency medical care, to the extent the physician is permitted to do so under applicable federal, state, or local law.

§46.117   Documentation of Informed Consent

(a) Except as provided in paragraph (c) of this section, informed consent shall be documented by the use of a written consent form approved by the IRB and signed by the subject or the subject's legally authorized representative. A copy shall be given to the person signing the form.

(c) An IRB may waive the requirement for the investigator to obtain a signed consent form for some or all subjects if it finds either:

(1) That the only record linking the subject and the research would be the consent document and the principal risk would be potential harm resulting from a breach of confidentiality. Each subject will be asked whether the subject wants documentation linking the subject with the research, and the subject's wishes will govern; or

(2) That the research presents no more than minimal risk of harm to subjects and involves no procedures for which written consent is normally required outside of the research context.

In cases where the documentation requirement is waived, the IRB may require the investigator to provide subjects with a written statement regarding the research.

7

Informed Consent

TOM L. BEAUCHAMP

SUMMARY

This chapter begins with a discussion of the history of informed consent in medical ethics and research ethics. Even in the early writings of the Hippocratic period, the view was held that monitoring medical information in encounters with patients was a basic moral responsibility of physicians. However, these writings had virtually nothing to say about informed consent and thus have contributed little to our understanding of the concept. Informed consent obligations and requirements have emerged from influential cases, potential developments, regulatory interventions, government-appointed ethics commissions, and the occurrence of intraprofessional events since the end of World War II.

The second section of the chapter discusses the concept and elements of informed consent. It presents several assumptions regarding the notion of informed consent that are commonly held by patients, physicians, and other health-care professionals. Five key elements are fundamental to the concept of informed consent: disclosure, comprehension, voluntariness, competence, and consent. On the basis of these elements a definition of informed consent is discussed. One can confidently presume that an act is an informed consent if a patient or subject agrees to an intervention on the basis of an understanding of relevant information, the consent is not controlled by influences that engineer the outcome, and the consent given was intended to be a consent and therefore qualified as a permission for an intervention.

The mere listing of these elements and their subsequent transformation into a definition of informed consent may be problematic and confusing. Formulating a definition of informed consent is complicated primarily because there exists at least two common, entrenched and irreducibly different meanings of informed consent. Broadly, these meanings can be categorized as autonomous choice and institutional consent.

The next topic of discussion in this chapter involves the doctrine of informed consent that is derived from the common law. The focus is primarily on disclosure and liability for injury. This doctrine has been more influential as an authoritative statement and source of reflection than any other body of thought on the subject.

Next, the chapter turns to the quality of the consent obtained. Questions include: How well is the information delivered? How well does the patient–subject understand? And how freely is consent given? The author examines the even more difficult issue of obtaining consent from an incompetent or otherwise vulnerable subject.

Finally, various justifications for not obtaining consent are examined. These might include patient incompetence and therapeutic privilege (the notion that consent be foregone to protect the patient or subject from harm).

The practice of obtaining informed consent has its history in medicine and biomedical research, in which the disclosure of information and the withholding of information are aspects of the daily encounters between patients and physicians. Although discussions of disclosure and justified nondisclosure have played a role in the history of medical ethics, the term *informed consent* emerged only in the 1950s, and discussions of the concept as it is used today began only about 1972. Concomitantly, a revolution was occurring in standards of appropriate patient–physician interaction. Medical ethics moved from a narrow focus on the physician's or researcher's obligation to disclose information to the quality of a patient's or subject's understanding of information and the right to authorize or refuse a biomedical intervention.

HISTORICAL BACKGROUND

Many writers have proposed that managing medical information in encounters with patients is a basic moral responsibility of physicians. Some pioneering ventures are found in classic historical documents in the history of medicine such as the Hippocratic writings (5–4 B.C.), Percival's *Medical Ethics* (1803), the first Code of Ethics (1846–1847) of the American Medical Association (AMA) as well as in the historically significant didactic writings on medical ethics in the eighteenth and nineteenth centuries, sometimes referred to as the "learned" tradition, comprising discursive study of medical ethics through treatises and books.

These codes and writings present a disappointing history from the perspective of informed consent. Hippocratic writings did not hint at obligations of veracity or disclosure, and throughout the ancient, medieval, and early modern periods, medical ethics developed predominantly within the profession of medicine. With few exceptions, no serious consideration was given to issues of consent or self-determination by patients and research subjects. The central concern was how to make disclosures without harming patients by revealing their conditions too abruptly and starkly. The emphasis on the principle "first, do no harm" promoted the idea that a health-care professional is obligated not to make disclosures because to do so would be to risk a harmful outcome.

The Nineteenth Century

Thomas Percival's historic *Medical Ethics* (1803) stands in this same tradition. It makes no more mention of consent solicitation and respect for decision making by patients than had previous codes and treatises. Percival struggled with the issue of truth telling, but he believed that the patient's right to the truth must yield to the obligation to benefit the patient in cases of conflict, and thus he recommended benevolent deception. The AMA accepted virtually without modification the Percival paradigm in its 1847 Code of Ethics (American Medical Association 1847). This code, and most codes of medical ethics before and after, do not include rules of veracity. For more than a century thereafter, American and British medical ethics developed under Percival's vision.

Although the nineteenth century saw no hint of a rule or practice of informed consent in clinical medicine, consent procedures were not entirely absent. Evidence exists in records of surgery that seeking consent and rudimentary rules for obtaining consent have existed since at least the middle of the nineteenth century (Pernick 1982). However, the consents obtained do not appear to have been meaningful by contemporary standards of informed consent because they had little to do with the patient's right to decide after being informed. Before the 1950s, practices of obtaining consent for surgery were pragmatic responses to a combination of concerns about medical reputation, malpractice suits, and practicality in medical institutions. It is physically difficult and interpersonally awkward to perform surgery on a patient without obtaining the patient's permission. Such practices of obtaining permission, however, did not constitute practices of obtaining informed consent, although they did provide a modest nineteenth-century grounding for this twentieth-century concept.

The situation is similar in research involving human subjects. Little evidence exists that, until recently, requirements of informed consent had a significant hold on the practice of investigators. In the nineteenth century, for example, it was common for research to be conducted on slaves and servants without consent on the part of the subject. By contrast, at the turn of the century, American Army surgeon Walter Reed's yellow fever experiments involved formal procedures for obtaining the consent of potential subjects. Although deficient by contemporary standards of disclosure and consent, these procedures recognized the right of the individual to refuse or authorize participation in the research. The extent to which this principle became ingrained in the ethics of research by the mid-twentieth century remains a matter of historical controversy.

Early Twentieth-Century Legal History

The legal history of disclosure obligations and rights of self-determination for patients evolved gradually. In the doctrine of legal precedent, each decision, relying on earlier court opinions, joins a chain of authority that incorporates the relevant language and reasoning from the cited cases. In this way, a few early consent cases built on each other to produce a legal doctrine. The best known and ultimately the most influential of these early cases is *Schloendorff v. Society of New York Hospitals* (1914). *Schloendorff* used rights of self-determination to justify imposing an obligation to obtain a patient's consent. Subsequent cases that followed and relied upon *Schloendorff* implicitly adopted its reasoning. In this way, self-determination came to be the primary justification for legal requirements that consent be obtained from patients.

Mid-Twentieth-Century Changes

During the 1950s and 1960s, the traditional duty to obtain consent evolved into a new, explicit duty to disclose certain forms of information and then to obtain consent. This development needed a new term, and so "informed" was tacked onto "consent," creating the expression *informed consent*, in the landmark decision in *Salgo v. Leland Stanford, Jr. University Board of Trustees* (1957). The *Salgo* court latched tenaciously onto the problem of whether the consent had been adequately informed. The court thus created the language and the substance of informed consent by invoking the same right of self-determination that had heretofore applied only to a less robust consent requirement.

Not surprisingly, the number of articles in the medical literature on issues of consent increased substantially following this and other precedent legal cases. Indifference to consent procedures seems to have changed by the late 1960s, when most physicians appear to have recognized some moral and legal duty to obtain consent for certain procedures and to provide some kind of disclosure. An explosion of commentary on informed consent emerged in the medical literature of the early 1970s, but much of this commentary was negative: Physicians saw the demands of informed consent as impossible to fulfill and, at least in some cases, inconsistent with good patient care.

The histories of informed consent in research and in clinical medicine were at this time developing largely as separate pieces in a larger mosaic of biomedical ethics. These pieces have never been well integrated even when they developed simultaneously. Research ethics before World War II was no more influential on research practices than was the parallel history of clinical medicine on clinical practices. But events that unquestionably influenced thought about informed consent occurred at the Nuremberg trials. The Nuremberg Military Tribunals unambiguously condemned the sinister political motivation of Nazi experiments. A list of ten principles constituted the Nuremberg Code. Principle One of the Code states, without qualification, that the primary consideration in research is the subject's voluntary consent, which is "absolutely essential" (*United States v. Karl Brandt* 1947).

The Nuremberg Code served as a model for many professional and governmental codes formulated in the 1950s and 1960s, and several additional incidents involving consent violations that subsequently moved the discussion of post-Nuremberg problems into the public arena. Thus began a rich and complex interplay of influences on research ethics: scholarly publications, journalism, public outrage, legislation, and case law. In the United

States, one of the first incidents to achieve notoriety in research ethics involved a study conducted at the Jewish Chronic Disease Hospital (JCDH) in Brooklyn, New York. In July 1963, Dr. Chester Southam of the Sloan-Kettering Institute for Cancer Research persuaded the hospital's medical director, Emmanuel E. Mandel, to permit research involving injection of a suspension of foreign, live cancer cells into 22 patients at the JCDH. The objective was to discover whether a decline in the body's capacity to reject cancer transplants was caused by their cancer or by debilitation. Patients without cancer were needed to supply the answer. Southam had convinced Mandel that although the research was nontherapeutic, such research was routinely done without consent. Some patients were informed orally that they were involved in an experiment, but it was not disclosed that they were being given injections of cancer cells. No written consent was attempted, and some subjects were incompetent to give informed consent. In 1966 the Board of Regents of the State University of New York censured Drs. Southam and Mandel for their role in the research. They were found guilty of fraud, deceit, and unprofessional conduct (*Hyman v. Jewish Chronic Disease Hospital* 1965).

The most notorious case of prolonged and knowing violation of subjects' rights in the United States was a Public Health Service (PHS) study initiated in the early 1930s. Originally designed as one of the first syphilis control demonstrations in the United States, the stated purpose of the Tuskegee Study (as it is now called) was to compare the health and longevity of an untreated syphilitic population with a nonsyphilitic but otherwise similar population. These subjects, all African American males, knew neither the name nor the nature of their disease. Their participation in a nontherapeutic experiment also went undisclosed. They were informed only that they were receiving free treatment for "bad blood," a term local African Americans associated with a host of unrelated ailments, but which the white physicians allegedly assumed was a local euphemism for syphilis (Jones 1981).

It was remarkable that, although this study was reviewed several times between 1932 and 1970 by PHS officials and medical societies, and reported in 13 articles in prestigious medical and public health journals, it continued uninterrupted and without serious challenge. It was not until 1972 that the Department of Health, Education, and Welfare (DHEW) appointed an ad hoc advisory panel to review the study and the Department's policies and procedures for the protection of human subjects. The panel found that neither DHEW nor any other government agency had a uniform or adequate policy for reviewing experimental procedures or securing subjects' consents.

Late Twentieth-Century Changes

The events of the mid-twentieth century do not explain why informed consent became the focus of so much attention in both case law and biomedical ethics. Many hypotheses can be invoked to explain the developments. The most likely explanation is that law, ethics, and medicine were all affected by issues and concerns in the wider society regarding individual liberties and social equality. These issues were made dramatic by an increasingly technological, powerful, and impersonal medical care. The issues raised by civil rights, women's rights, the consumer movement, and the rights of prisoners and the mentally ill often included health care components and helped reinforce public acceptance of rights applied to health care. Informed consent was swept along with this body of social concerns, which propelled the new bioethics throughout the 1970s.

Three 1972 court decisions stand as informed consent landmarks: *Canterbury v. Spence, Cobbs v. Grant*, and *Wilkinson v. Vesey. Canterbury* had a particularly massive influence in demanding a more patient-oriented standard of disclosure. In *Canterbury*, surgery on the patient's back and a subsequent accident in the hospital led to further injuries and unexpected paralysis, the possibility of which had not yet been disclosed. Judge Spottswood Robinson's opinion focused on the needs of the reasonable person and the right to self-determination. As for sufficiency of information, the court held: "The patient's right of self-decision shapes the boundaries of the duty to reveal. That right can be effectively exercised only if the patient possesses enough information to enable an intelligent choice."

Among the most important publications in the medical literature to appear during this period was a statement in 1981 by the Judicial Council of the AMA. For the first time, the AMA recognized informed consent as a basic social policy necessary to enable patients to make their own choices, even if their physicians disagree. The AMA's statement is a testament to the impact of the law of informed consent on medical ethics.

The 1980s saw the publication of several books devoted to the subject of informed consent, as well as hundreds of journal articles, and the passage of procedure-specific, informed consent laws and regulations. These events gave testimony to the importance of informed consent in moral and legal thinking about medicine in the United States. By themselves, however, they tell us little about physicians' or researchers' actual consent practices or opinions, or about how informed consent was viewed or experienced by patients and subjects.

THE CONCEPT AND ELEMENTS
OF INFORMED CONSENT

Informed consent began to play a central role in clinical and research ethics when problems of the autonomy of subjects gradually grew more insistent in twentieth-century practice and research and when the idea of respecting autonomy gained equal recognition as a form of justification with protecting against risk. The practice of obtaining consent is a social phenomenon, and no analysis of the concept of informed consent will succeed if it ignores the contexts in which informed consent arose. However, considerable vagueness has attended the term informed consent in these contexts and has left a need to sharpen the concept.

Presumptions about the Concept

The claim that something is an informed consent or that an informed consent has been obtained cannot always be taken at face value. Before we can confidently infer that what appears to have been or was called an informed consent is a bona fide instance of informed consent, we need to know what to look for. The inquiry requires criteria of what qualifies as informed consent.

If an overdemanding criterion, such as "full disclosure and complete understanding," is adopted, an informed consent becomes impossible to obtain. Conversely, if an underdemanding criterion, such as "the patient signed the form" is used, an informed consent becomes too easy to obtain and the term loses all moral significance. Many interactions between a physician and a patient or between an investigator and a subject that have been called informed consents have been so labeled only because they rested on underdemanding criteria; they are inappropriately referred to as informed consents. For example, a physician's truthful disclosure to a patient has often been declared the essence of informed consent, as if a patient's silence after disclosure constituted an informed consent. The existence of such inadequate understanding of informed consent can be explained in part by empirical information about physicians' beliefs concerning informed consent.

Contemporary Presumptions in Medicine

Some data about the meaning of informed consent are found in a survey of physicians conducted by Louis Harris (Harris 1982), which asked physicians "What does the term informed consent mean to you?" In their answers, only 26 percent of physicians indicated that informed consent had anything to do with a patient's giving permission, consenting, or agreeing to treatment; only 9 percent indicated that it involved the patient's making a choice or stating a preference about his or her treatment. Similar results have been found in recent surveys of Japanese physicians' beliefs about informed consent (Hattori 1991; Kai 1993; Mizushima 1990; Takahashi 1990).

Like the views expressed by lawyers and courts, most doctors (according to the surveys) appeared to recognize only disclosure as the criterion of informed consent. That is, they viewed informed consent as explaining to a patient the nature of his or her medical condition and a recommended treatment plan. If physicians regard informed consent as nothing more than an event of conveying information to patients, rather than a process of discussion and obtaining permission from the patient, claims that doctors regularly obtain consents from their patients before initiating medical procedures are vague and unreliable unless one knows in some detail the procedures they used to obtain consent.

Matters may be worse than they appear. Perhaps physicians who responded to the surveys understood informed consent entirely in terms of the patient's signature on a form, or perhaps they understood informed consent as a form of disclosure. This interpretation fits with the results of several studies of informed consent that have failed to find any sizeable evidence of informed consent in clinical medicine and that have found little evidence that the consents being obtained are meaningful exercises of informed choice by patients (Quaid 1990; Scherer and Reppucci 1988; Siminoff et al. 1989; Siminoff and Fetting 1991).

The Authority of Oaths, Codes, and Treatises

Similar problems exist regarding what can be reasonably inferred from oaths, prayers, codes of ethics, published lectures, and general pamphlets and treatises on medical conduct, usually written by individual physicians or medical societies for their colleagues. In the absence of more direct data about actual consent practices, these documents have been relied on heavily in writings on informed consent as sources that provide information about the history of informed consent and related matters of clinical medical ethics. However, it is often difficult to determine whether the statements that appear in these documents are primarily exhortatory, descriptive, or self-protective. Some writings describe, for educational purposes, conduct that was in accordance with prevailing professional standards. Other documents aim at reforming professional conduct by prescribing what should be established practice. Still others seem constructed to protect the physician from suspicions of misconduct or from legal liability.

The Elements of Informed Consent

Legal, philosophical, regulatory, medical, and psychological literatures have often tried to define or analyze informed consent in terms of its elements. The following elements have been identified as fundamental to the concept: (1) disclosure, (2) comprehension, (3) voluntariness, (4) competence, and (5) consent (Levine 1978; Meisel and Roth 1981; National Commission 1978). The postulate is that a person gives an informed consent to an intervention only if the person is competent to act, receives a thorough disclosure about the procedure, comprehends the disclosed information, acts voluntarily, and consents.

This definition is attractive because of its consistency with standard usage of the term informed consent in medicine and law. However, medical convention and malpractice law tend to distort the meaning of informed consent in ways that need correction. Analyses using the above five elements and the conventional usage in law and medicine are best suited for cataloguing the analytical *parts* of informed consent and for delineating moral and legal *requirements* of informed consent, not for conceptually analyzing the meaning of informed consent. Neither requirements nor parts amount to a definition.

For instance, the U.S. Supreme Court addressed the definition of informed consent in *Planned Parenthood of Central Missouri v. Danforth* as follows: "One might well wonder . . . what 'informed consent' of a patient is. . . . We are content to accept, as the meaning [of informed consent], the giving of information to the patient as to just what would be done and as to its consequences" (1976, 67, *n*. 8). The exclusive element of informed consent here listed is *disclosure*, which recalls the assumptions made by physicians in the Harris poll. However, nothing about an informed consent requires disclosure as part of its *meaning*. A patient or subject already knowledgeable about a proposed intervention could give a thorough informed consent without having received a disclosure from a second party. Similarly, other conditions in the above list of conditions are not necessary. For example, persons who are legally incompetent (see element 4) sometimes give informed consents, and in some instances even psychologically incompetent persons (also often the referent of element 4) may be able to consent meaningfully to or refuse a particular intervention. The above norms delineate an *obligation to make disclosures* so that a consent can be informed, rather than a *meaning of informed consent*. Even all five of the above elements merged as a set do not satisfactorily capture the meaning of informed consent.

The following seven categories express the analytical components of informed consent more adequately than the above five categories, but this sevenfold list still does not adequately express the *meaning* of informed consent (Beauchamp and Childress 1994):

I. Threshold elements (preconditions)

    1. Competence (to understand and decide)
    2. Voluntariness (in deciding)

II. Information elements

    3. Disclosure (of material information)
    4. Recommendation (of a plan)
    5. Understanding (of 3. and 4.)

III. Consent elements

    6. Decision (in favor of a plan)
    7. Authorization (of the chosen plan)

The language of material information in item 3 is pivotal for an adequate analysis of the elements of disclosure and understanding item 5. Critics of legal requirements of informed consent have often held that procedures sometimes have so many risks and benefits that they cannot be disclosed and explained, but material risks are simply the risks a reasonable patient needs to understand to decide among the alternatives. Only these risks and benefits need to be disclosed and understood.

Informed consent *requirements* can be constructed to correspond to each of the above *elements*. That is, specific disclosure requirements, comprehension requirements, noninfluence requirements, competence requirements, authorization requirements, and the like, can be fashioned. These requirements would specify the conditions that must be satisfied for a consent to be *valid*; but an adequate meaning of informed consent is still lacking.

Two Meanings of Informed Consent

The question What is an informed consent? is complicated because at least two common, entrenched, and irreducibly different meanings of informed consent have been at work in its history. That is, the term is analyzable in different ways because different conceptions of informed consent have emerged. In one sense, an informed consent is an *autonomous authorization* by individual patients or subjects. In the second sense, informed consent is analyzable in terms of *institutional and policy rules of consent* that collectively form the social practice of informed consent in institutional contexts (Faden and Beauchamp 1986).

In the first meaning, an *autonomous authorization* requires more than merely acquiescing in, yielding to, or complying with an arrangement or a proposal made by a physician or investigator. A person gives an informed consent in this first sense if and only if the person, with substantial understanding and in substantial absence of control by others, intentionally authorizes a health-care professional to do something. A person who intentionally refuses to authorize an intervention, but otherwise satisfies these conditions, gives an *informed refusal*. The first sense derives from philosophical premises that informed consent is fundamentally a matter of protecting and enabling autonomous or self-determining choice.

In the second meaning, informed consent refers only to a legally or institutionally effective approval given by a patient or subject. An approval is therefore effective or valid if it conforms to the rules that govern specific institutions, whatever the operative rules may be. In this sense, unlike the first, conditions and requirements of informed consent are relative to a social and institutional context and need not be autonomous authorizations. This meaning is driven by demands in the legal and health-care systems for a generally applicable and efficient consent mechanism by which responsibilities and violations can be readily and fairly assessed.

Under these two contrasting understandings of informed consent, a patient or subject can give an informed consent in the first sense, but not in the second sense, and vice versa. For example, if the person consenting is a minor and therefore not of legal age, he or she cannot give an effective or valid consent under the prevailing institutional rules; a consent is invalid even if the minor gives the consent autonomously and responsibly. ("Mature minor" laws sometimes make an exception and give minors the right to authorize medical treatments in a limited range of circumstances.)

Informed consent in the second sense, as institutional consent, has until very recently constituted the mainstream conception in the regulatory rules of federal agencies as well as in health-care institutions. The documents governing consent in these contexts derive from some concept about what the rules must be to promote effective authorizations in these institutions, but the rules were only rarely premised on a conception of autonomous authorization that had more than a superficial quality. However, literature in bioethics has increasingly suggested that any justifiable analysis of informed consent must be rooted in autonomous choice by patients and subjects.

In principle, although less clearly in practice, the conditions of informed consent as autonomous authorization can function as model standards for fashioning the institutional and policy requirements of informed consent— a model of autonomous choice thus serves as the benchmark against which the moral adequacy of prevailing rules and practices might be evaluated.

Autonomous Choice

It has often been said that the justification of requirements of informed consent (in the first sense) is the principle of respect for autonomy. However, the goal of ensuring that persons make autonomous choices has proved to be difficult to implement. Historically, little can be said other than that a clear societal consensus has developed that there must be adequate protection of patients' and subjects' decision-making rights, especially their rights of autonomy. Therefore, we need to examine the meaning of autonomy in addition to the meaning of informed consent.

In the literature on informed consent, *autonomy* and *respect for autonomy* are terms loosely associated with several ideas, such as privacy, voluntariness, self-mastery, choosing freely, the freedom to choose, choosing one's own moral position, and accepting responsibility for one's choices. Because of such conceptual uncertainty, both the concept of autonomy and its connection to informed consent need careful analysis.

In moral philosophy, personal autonomy has come to refer to personal self-governance: personal rule of the self by adequate understanding while remaining free from controlling interferences by others and from personal limitations that prevent choice. Many issues about consent concern failures to respect autonomy, which range from manipulative underdisclosure of pertinent information to nonrecognition of a refusal of medical interventions. To respect an autonomous agent is to recognize with due appreciation the person's capacities and perspective, including his or her right to hold certain views and to take certain actions based on personal values and beliefs. Accordingly, an informed consent made on the basis of autonomous authorization suggests a well-informed agent with the competence to authorize or refuse authorization of a medical or research intervention.

It has sometimes been claimed that informed consent, so understood, has a mythical quality because true informed consent is never obtained under such a high ideal—that is, most patients and subjects cannot comprehend enough information or appreciate its relevance sufficiently to make decisions about medical care or about participation in research. This objection, however, springs from a serious misunderstanding of the nature and goals of informed consent, in part because of unwarranted standards of full disclosure and full understanding. The ideal of complete disclosure of all possibly relevant knowledge needs to be replaced by a more acceptable account of how patients and subjects understand relevant information. Merely because one's actions fail to be *fully* informed, voluntary, or autonomous is no indication that they are never *adequately* informed or autonomous. No one would autonomously sign contracts, have automobiles repaired, file income tax returns, and the like, if this were the case.

This argument does not deny that some individuals have a knowledge base that is so impoverished that autonomous decision making about alien or novel situations is exceedingly difficult. But even in difficult situations there may be no reason to foreclose the possibility of a person being able to make an adequate decision. Successful communication of novel, alien, and specialized information to laypersons can be accomplished by drawing analogies between the information and more ordinary events with which the patient or subject is familiar. Similarly, professionals can express probabilities in both numeric and nonnumeric terms and help the patient or subject to assign meanings to the probabilities through comparison with more familiar risks and previous experiences.

THE LAW AND ITS LIMITS

The law of informed consent has been more influential as an authoritative set of statements and source of reflection than has any other body of thought on the subject. *The doctrine of informed consent,* as it is sometimes called, is the legal doctrine; informed consent has often been treated as synonymous with the legal doctrine, which derives from the common law and includes the entire body of law dealing with the obligation to obtain consent. The legal vision is focused on *disclosure* and on *liability for injury.* There are good reasons why the law turns on such a narrow basis and also why it is ill-equipped to serve beyond these boundaries.

Theory of Liability

The primary basis for the legal doctrine is tort law. A *tort* is a civil injury to one's person or property that is inflicted by another person and that is measured in terms of, and is compensated by, money damages. Tort law imposes duties on members of society, and one who fails to fulfill a legal duty is liable to compensation for the misdeed (in the civil law). The theory of liability under which a case is tried determines the duty that must be fulfilled. In recent informed consent cases, negligence is the theory of liability almost always applied. However, the informed consent doctrine originally developed and flourished as applied to cases of battery, a different theory of liability. Currently, no unified legal theory underlies all informed consent cases.

Under *battery theory* the defendant is held liable for any intended (i.e., not careless or accidental) action that results in physical contact for which the plaintiff has given no permission. A defendant need not have an evil intent, nor must injury result; the unpermitted contact is itself considered wrongful. Under negligence theory, by contrast, unintentional, careless action or omission is the source of liability. The carelessness occurs in regard to some activity in which the defendant has a duty to take care or to behave reasonably toward others, and an injury measurable in monetary terms is caused by failure to discharge the duty (Schloendorff 1914; Berkey 1969; Meisel 1977).

The Duty of Disclosure

Two competing disclosure standards have evolved as attempts to resolve problems regarding the nature and amount of the information that must be disclosed: the professional practice standard and the reasonable person standard. (A third standard, the subjective standard, has also been discussed in legal commentary.) The *professional practice standard* holds that both the range of the duty to disclose and the criteria of adequate disclosure are properly determined by the customary practices of a professional community. These practices establish the standards of care for disclosure and care alike. The patient, subject, or reasonable person lacking expert knowledge is considered unqualified to decide what should be disclosed.

Although the professional practice standard remains the primary standard in informed consent law, it contains inadequacies and whether a customary standard of disclosure actually exists for much of medical practice may be doubtful. A basic problem is that negligent care might be perpetuated if relevant professionals throughout the profession offer inferior information; another doubtful premise is that physicians have sufficient expertise to be able to judge in many cases what information their patients need. However, the principal objection to this standard is its failure to promote decisional autonomy, the protection of which is generally accepted as the primary function and moral justification of informed consent requirements.

By contrast, the *reasonable person standard* focuses on the information a reasonable person needs to know about procedures, risks, alternatives, and consequences. The legal test of an adequate disclosure is the materiality (significance) of information to the decision making of the patient. Thus, the right to decide what information is material and due is shifted away from the physician to the reasonable patient. The reasonable person standard requires a physician to divulge any fact that is material to a reasonable person's decision, but no requirement exists to meet the unreasonable demand of a patient.

The reasonable person standard is as vulnerable to criticism as the professional-based standard. Whether the reasonable person standard serves the interests of patients who know little about their informational needs or the medical system is doubtful. The interpretation of the standard for clinical practice is also difficult because it specifies no precise duty for physicians. Both the concept of material information and the central concept of the reasonable person are left at an intuitive level. Therefore, whether the reasonable person standard more adequately protects the patient's right to choose than does the professional practice standard is doubtful.

These arguments are not intended to eliminate standards of disclosure. In the absence of a disclosure initiated by the professional, patients or subjects often cannot formulate their concerns and ask meaningful questions. A patient or subject needs to understand what an informed professional judges to be of value for most patients or subjects as material information, and what it means for consent to be an authorization to proceed. The problem is not whether we need adequate disclosures but whether a legal vehicle can be expected to provide an adequate standard of disclosure for clinical practice.

The larger problem with these standards, for our purposes, is that they are not of major assistance in formulating a concept of informed consent for clinical medicine and research. Because courts are captivated by the context of after-the-fact resolution of narrow and concrete questions of duty, responsibility, blame, injury, and damages in specific cases, the law has no systematic way of affecting *contemporary* medical practice other than by a somewhat muted threat of prosecution for legal wrongdoing. For all these reasons, the heart of issues about informed consent is not legal but moral. Informed consent has less to do with the liability of professionals and more to do with the autonomous choices of patients and subjects.

THE QUALITY OF CONSENT

Problems about the quality and adequacy of consent probably cannot be resolved unless conventional disclosure rules are redirected toward the quality of understanding present in a consent. This approach focuses on the need for communication, dispensing with liability-oriented discussions about proper legal standards of disclosure. The key to effective communication is to invite participation by patients or subjects in an exchange of information and dialogue. Asking questions, eliciting the concerns and interests of the patient or subject, and establishing a climate that encourages the patient or subject to ask questions seem more important for medical ethics than do requirements of disclosure in law.

If the proper climate is not introduced into the context of consent, a request from a professional that the patient or subject ask for information is as likely to result in silence as to elicit the desired result of a meaningful informational exchange and consent. Patients find it difficult to approach physicians with questions or concerns, and even when they do not understand their physicians, many still do not ask questions. The extent to which a passive attitude characterizes research subjects is less clear. Although still understudied, it is a good guess that relatively little educating of this quality occurs at present in clinical practice or in research in the United States.

VULNERABLE SUBJECTS AND COMPLIANT PATIENTS

Patients and subjects are entitled to expect that physicians and research investigators who request interventions do so free of coercion and manipulation. Much discussion about the morality of asking subjects and patients to consent centers not on how informed the subjects are, but on how *free* they are. For example, this topic dominated the deliberations of the National Commission for the Protection of Human Subjects over the involvement of prisoners in drug research. The Commission raised the question whether prisoners are, in the words of the Nuremberg Code, "so situated as to be able to exercise free power of choice" (National Commission 1976, 5–7). The Commission answered that "although prisoners who participate in research affirm that they do so freely, the conditions of social and economic deprivation in which they live compromise their freedom. The Commission believes, therefore, that the appropriate expression of respect consists in protection from exploitation" (National Commission 1976, 5–7).

The Commission went on to recommend a ban on drug research with prisoners, on grounds that in coercive institutions free choice would be too often compromised. Six years later this argument continued. Robert Levine, who had served on the staff of the Commission, argued—as had a minority of Commissioners—that prisoners are actually better off, not worse off, by their involvement in research, and that exclusion from research was a far worse restriction of free choice (Levine 1982). Many were dubious, however, that such abstract statements take account of the realities of manipulation and coercion in the prison (Dubler 1982).

A similar controversy occurred in the 1980s when Dr. Mortimer Lipsett at the NIH explored the question whether phase I clinical trials of cancer chemotherapies involve a special class of subjects deserving special protections. He presented the problem as follows:

> The President's Commission for the Study of Ethical Problems in Medicine and Biomedical and Behavioral Research developed and extended the concept of the vulnerable subject in medical research. Children, prisoners, and the mentally disabled were defined as

vulnerable because a variety of constraints and inducements effectively removed their capacity to function autonomously. Similarly, patients with advanced cancer are faced with inducements that may sway their judgment of the risk-benefit ratio. Should such patients be treated as vulnerable research subjects necessitating extraordinary supervision by third parties? (Lipsett 1982, 941–942)

Lipsett answered that every patient entering such a therapeutic trial is vulnerable by virtue of the disease state and the unique opportunity to receive a promising drug, but he maintained that the problem could be and was being overcome by "painstaking consultation and preparation" involving families, IRBs, third-party consultation, and the like. He concluded that, as conducted, the phase I clinical trials of "cancer chemotherapies are ethical and necessary" (Lipsett 1982, 941–942).

Some published responses to Lipsett were less sanguine. Alexander Capron, who had been staff director of the President's Commission, and Terrence Ackerman and Carson Strong, argued that the notion of therapeutic intent in the trials is easily subject to misunderstanding by patients, who may be misled by the hope of a favorable effect, especially when the prospect for therapeutic efficacy is as exceedingly remote as it often is at the dosage level offered. They maintained that patients should be given a realistic picture of how they are contributing to medical knowledge. They noted the dangers of manipulating subjects and of subjecting them to affective factors that impair understanding and judgment. In general, they challenged the view that present safeguards are sufficient to preclude exploitation (Capron 1983; Ackerman and Strong 1983).

Underlying these discussions is a theoretically difficult and partially unresolved set of problems about free choice, coercion, and manipulation. Certain forms of withholding information, playing on emotion, or presenting constraints can rob a person of the capacity of free choice through manipulation or coercion. Deceptive and misleading statements limit freedom by restricting the range of choice and by getting a person to do what the person otherwise would not do (cf. Bok 1992). The National Commission was worried about *coercion* in the case of prisoners; by contrast, those engaged in the discussion of phase I trials and cancer chemotherapies were interested in *manipulation*.

A continuum of controlling influences is present in our daily lives, running from coercion, which is at the most controlling end of the continuum (compare the National Commission's model of prisoners), to persuasion and education, which are not controlling at all, even though they are influences. Influence thus does not necessarily imply constraint, governance, force, or compulsion, although these concepts are essential to certain kinds of influence. Important decisions are usually made in contexts replete with influences in the form of competing claims and interests, social demands and expectations, and straightforward or devious attempts by others to bring about the outcome they desire. Some of these influences are unavoidable, and some may be desirable. Clearly, not all of them interfere with or deprive persons of autonomous belief and action, as when patients are persuaded by sound reasons to do something.

Coercion—which involves a threat of harm so severe that a person is unable to resist acting to avoid it—is always completely controlling. It entirely negates freedom because it entirely controls action. Persuasion, by contrast, is the intentional and successful attempt to induce a person, through appeals to reason, to freely accept the beliefs, attitudes, values, intentions, or actions advocated by the persuader. Like informing, persuading is entirely compatible with free choice.

The most sweeping and difficult area of influence is manipulation, a broad, general category that runs from highly controlling to altogether noncontrolling influences. The essence of manipulation is getting people to do what the manipulator intends without resort to coercion or to reasoned argument. In a paradigm case of manipulation in contexts of informed consent, information is managed so that the person does not know what the manipulator intends. Whether such uses of information necessarily compromise or restrict free choice is an unresolved and untidy issue, but one plausible view is that some manipulations, such as the use of rewards such as reduced medical fees for being involved in research, are compatible with free choice, whereas others, such as deceptive offers of hope where there is none, are not compatible with free choice.

In contexts of informed consent, the central question is not whether we are entirely free of manipulative influences, but whether we are *sufficiently* free to remain autonomous—free to perform our own actions—as opposed to being controlled by the actions of another. The thorniest of all problems about autonomy and manipulation is not that of punishment and threat but the effect of rewards and offers. This category refers to the intentional use of offers of rewards to bring about a desired response. For example, during the Tuskegee syphilis experiments various methods were used to stimulate and sustain the interest of subjects in continued participation. They were offered free burial assistance and insurance, free transportation, and a free stop in town on the return trip. They were also rewarded with free medicines and free hot meals on the days of the examination. The deprived socioeconomic condition of these subjects made them easily manipulable by those means.

This general range of problems is compounded still further by what is sometimes called the problem of coercive situations. Most accounts of coercion require that coercion be intentional by the coercer, but coercive situations suggest nonintentional coercion—the person is controlled by the situation, not by the design of another person. Sometimes people unintentionally make other persons feel threatened, and sometimes situations of illness and economic necessity present threats of serious harm that a person feels compelled to prevent at all costs. The earlier example of using prisoners in experimentation is again applicable if we assume that a prisoner is left without any viable alternative to participation in research because of the risks of the alternatives in the circumstance or because of what may appear to be threats presented by prison officials. Alvin Bronstein, Director of the National Prison Project, once stated the problem for informed consent as "You cannot create . . . [a prison] institution in which informed consent without coercion is feasible" (1975, 130–131).

Beyond a prison, in circumstances of severe physical or health deprivation, a person might accept an offer or sign a contract that the person would refuse under less stringent circumstances. Cancer patients provide good examples—the prospect that they will die if they reject an objectionable, toxic drug seems to coerce a choice of the drug no less than would an intentional threat. The psychological effect on the person forced to choose may be identical, and the person can appropriately say in both cases, "There was no real choice; I would have been crazy to refuse." But if, as we usually believe, a contract signed under another person's threat is invalid (and the consent behind the signing an invalid consent), can we not say that a person who agrees to drug experimentation in a coercive situation has made an invalid contract (and has given an invalid consent)?

It is a mistake to suppose that persons in such coercive situations cannot act *autonomously*. A loss of alternatives cannot be equated with coercion. It is, then, a confusion to move from a correct claim about a loss of options caused by desperate circumstances to a fallaciously drawn conclusion that there has been a loss of autonomy because of a coercive situation. Nevertheless, even if knowledgeable intent to threaten is not present, one may feel just as forced to a choice and may just as heartily wish to avoid it, and this is why the worry is often presented in the language of vulnerable subjects. Their situation does make them vulnerable, even desperately vulnerable, and may subject them to control by their emotions and anxieties to an abnormal degree.

Despite the tense and pressured nature of such circumstances, most patients *can*, if properly managed, consent freely. What is doubtful is how often a free informed consent *does in fact occur*.

COMPETENCE TO CONSENT

We noticed earlier that competence is commonly listed as a necessary condition of informed consent. In legal and policy contexts, reference to competent persons is far more common than reference to autonomous persons. Competence judgments function as a gatekeeping device for informed consent. That is, competence judgments function to distinguish persons from whom consent should be solicited from those from whom consent need not or should not be solicited. In health care, competence judgments distinguish the class of individuals whose autonomous decisions must be respected from those individuals whose decisions need to be checked and perhaps overridden by a surrogate (Buchanan and Brock 1989).

Competence can be either a factual or a categorical determination. Minors, for example, are incompetent in law, whereas adults can generally be declared legally incompetent only on the basis of some factual determination. The issue of legal capacity is more complex for adult patients, for whom an individual determination normally must be made. If a person is incompetent, the physician is usually required, unless there is an emergency, to secure some form of third-party consent from a guardian or other legally empowered representative. Placement of the label incompetent on a patient or subject automatically introduces the possibility of coercive treatment and the presumption that there is no need to obtain consent. *Competence* commonly functions to denote persons whose consents, refusals, and statements of preference will be accepted as binding; *incompetence* denotes those who are to be placed under the guidance and control of another.

JUSTIFICATIONS FOR NOT OBTAINING CONSENT

Several standard exceptions to requirements of informed consent exist in law and ethics. All courts passing judgment on the issue have ruled that a patient's right to self-determination is not absolute. Five exceptions to the informed consent requirement are generally recognized: the public health emergency, the medical emergency, the incompetent patient, the therapeutic privilege, and the patient waiver (Meisel 1979). All but the therapeutic privilege have been widely accepted in law and ethics. However, the therapeutic privilege has elicited a particularly furious exchange over whether autonomy rights can be validly set aside.

The *therapeutic privilege* allows a physician to withhold information on the basis of sound medical judgment that to divulge the information would be potentially harmful to a depressed, emotionally drained, or unstable patient. Several harmful outcomes have been cited, including endangering life, causing irrational decisions, and producing anxiety or stress (*Canterbury v. Spence* 1972; van Oosten 1991). In clinical settings, this privilege has long been used to justify not obtaining consent.

If framed broadly, the therapeutic privilege can permit physicians to withhold information if disclosure would cause *any* countertherapeutic deterioration, however slight, in the physical, psychological, or emotional condition of the patient. If framed narrowly, it can permit the physician to withhold information only if the patient's knowledge of the information would have serious, health-related consequences—for example, by jeopardizing the success of the treatment or harming the patient psychologically by impairing decision making.

The narrowest formulation is that the therapeutic privilege can be validly invoked only if the physician has good reason to believe that disclosure would render the patient incompetent to consent to or refuse the treatment, that is, would render the decision nonautonomous. To invoke the therapeutic privilege under such circumstances does not conflict with respect for autonomy because an autonomous decision could not be made. However, broader formulations of the privilege that require only medical contraindication do operate at the expense of autonomy. These formulations may unjustifiably endanger autonomous choice, as when use of the privilege is based on the belief that an autonomous patient would refuse an indicated therapy for medically inappropriate reasons.

Unless the therapeutic privilege is tightly and operationally formulated, the medical profession can use it to deprive the unreasonable but competent patient of the right to make decisions, especially if the physician sees his or her commitment to the patient's best interest as the overriding consideration. Loose standards can permit physicians to climb to safety over a straw bridge of speculation about the psychological consequences of information. In short, there is a significant potential for abuse of the privilege because of its inconsistency with the patient's rights to know and to decline treatment (Faden and Beauchamp 1986).

In 1986 U.S. Supreme Court Justice Byron White vigorously attacked the idea that concerns about increasing a person's anxiety about a procedure provide grounds for an exception to rules of informed consent: "It is the very nature of informed consent provisions that they may produce some anxiety in the patient and influence her in her choice. This is in fact their reason for existence, and . . . it is an entirely salutary reason" (*Thornburgh v. American College of Obstetricians*, 2199–2200). White is suggesting that the legal status of the doctrine of therapeutic privilege is no longer as secure as it once was.

In addition to the five standard exceptions to informed consent, several circumstances encountered in contemporary medicine suggest a need to relax requirements of informed consent. For example, in observational studies that examine behavior without the subject's knowledge and in analysis of secondary data, we often need only to avoid invasions of privacy and the presentation of significant risk to subjects, without procuring consents. In other cases, third-party consent may be acceptable when access to a person is impractical, the subject is incompetent, or (in very rare cases) when cultural customs suggest a third-party consent that is adequately protective. In some cases of low-risk research, subjects of research need not be contacted at all. In some cases disclosures and warnings may be substituted for obtaining explicit informed consents.

It does not follow from any of the analyses above that institutional policies of informed consent must rank the protection of decision making above all other values. The preservation of autonomous choice is the first but not the only institutional commitment. For example, a patient's need for education and counseling must be balanced against the interests of other patients and of society in maintaining a productive and efficient health-care system. Accordingly, institutional policies must consider what is fair and reasonable to require of health-care professionals and researchers and what the effect would be of alternative consent requirements on efficiency and effectiveness in the delivery of health care and the advancement of science.

CONCLUSION

Jay Katz has argued that the history of the physician–patient relationship from ancient times to the present reveals how inattentive physicians have been to their patients' rights and needs. Katz is equally unrelenting in his criticisms of court decisions and legal scholarship. He regards the declarations of courts as filled with overly optimistic rhetoric. The problem, in his view, is that the law has little to do with fostering real communication in the clinic and tends to line up with the professional judgments of physicians in the crucial test cases (Katz 1984, 1987).

Katz is correct in judging that informed consent has always been an alien notion in the history of medicine and medical ethics and that informed consent has still not severely modified the physician–patient relationship. At the same time, the scene in American medicine is undergoing what may prove to be an extensive transformation through the implementation of the idea of informed consent. Patients are giving more informed consents and more attention is being paid in institutions to the quality of those consents. It is indisputable that research ethics and policies have been dramatically affected by requirements of informed consent.

Before we condemn the defects in the writings and practices of the past, we should remember that the history of informed consent is still unfolding and that our failures may be no less apparent to future generations than are the failures that we find with the past.

DISCUSSION QUESTIONS

1. Is the purpose of consent to benefit the individual or to promote autonomous choice? What should happen when providing information may do more harm than good?

2. Is consent more important in research in which the subject cannot benefit or in therapeutic medicine? In which circumstance is consent harder to obtain?

3. Are there any good reasons for obtaining consent for interventions in research or therapy that can do no harm to patients or subjects?

4. If patients want some information about therapy, but clinicians, customarily, tend not to provide it, is there any moral reason for providing it?

5. Should physicians have a duty to provide information that individual patients desire even if most reasonable patients would not desire it? If so, under what circumstances?

REFERENCES

Ackerman, Terrence F., Strong, Carson M. "Letters." *JAMA* 249 (Feb. 18, 1983): 882–883.

American Medical Association. *Proceedings of the National Medical Conventions, New York, May 1846 and Philadelphia, May 1847.* Philadelphia: American Medical Association, 1847.

Beauchamp, Tom L., Childress, James F. *Principles of Biomedical Ethics*, 4th ed. New York: Oxford University Press, 1994.

Bok, Sissela. "Informed Consent in Tests of Patient Reliability." *JAMA* 267 (Feb. 26, 1992): 1118–1119.

Bronstein, Alvin. "Remarks." In National Academy of Sciences, *Experiments and Research with Humans: Values in Conflict.* Washington, DC: National Academy, 1975: 130–131.

Buchanan, Allen E., Brock, Dan W. *Deciding for Others: The Ethics of Surrogate Decision Making.* Cambridge: Cambridge University Press, 1989.

Capron, Alexander M. "Letters." *JAMA* 249 (Feb. 18, 1983): 882–883.

Dubler, Nancy. "The Burdens of Research in Prisons." *IRB* 4 (Nov. 1982): 9–10.

Faden, Ruth R., Beauchamp, Tom L. *A History and Theory of Informed Consent.* New York: Oxford University Press, 1986.

Harris, Louis, et al. "Views of Informed Consent and Decisionmaking: Parallel Surveys of Physicians and the Public." In President's Commission for the Study of Ethical Problems in Medicine and Biomedical and Behavioral Research, *Making Health Care Decisions*, Vol. 2. Washington, DC: Government Printing Office, 1982: 17–316.

Hattori, Hiroyuki, et al. "The Patient's Right to Information in Japan—Legal Rules and Doctor's Opinions." *Soc Sci Med* 32 (1991): 1007–1016.

Hippocrates. In W. H. S. Jones (Trans.), *Hippocrates.* Cambridge: Harvard University Press, 1931.

Jones, James H. *Bad Blood*, 2nd ed. New York: Maxwell Macmillan, 1993.

Kai, Ichiro, et al. "Communication between Patients and Physicians about Terminal Care: A Survey in Japan." *Soc Sci Med* 36 (1993): 1151–1159.

Katz, Jay. "Physician-Patient Encounters 'On a Darkling Plain.'" *West New Engl L Rev* 9 (1987): 207–226.

———. *The Silent World of Doctor and Patient.* New York: The Free Press, 1984.

Levine, Robert J. "The Nature and Definition of Informed Consent in Various Research Settings." *The Belmont Report* (Appendix) Vol. I. Washington, DC: DHEW Publication No. (OS) 78-0013, 1978: 3-1–3-91.

———. "Research Involving Prisoners: Why Not?" *IRB* 4 (May 1982): 6.

Lipsett, Mortimer B. "On the Nature and Ethics of Phase I Clinical Trials of Cancer Chemotherapies." *JAMA* 248 (Aug. 27, 1982): 941–942.

Meisel, Alan. "The Expansion of Liability for Medical Accidents: From Negligence to Strict Liability by Way of Informed Consent." *Nebr L Rev* 56 (1977): 51–152.

———. "The 'Exceptions' to the Informed Consent Doctrine: Striking a Balance Between Competing Values in Medical Decisionmaking." *Wisc L Rev* (1979): 413–488.

Meisel, Alan, Roth, Loren H. "Toward an Informed Discussion on Informed Consent: A Review and Critique of the Empirical Studies." *Ariz L Rev* 25 (1983): 265–346.

———. "What We Do and Do Not Know About Informed Consent." *JAMA* 246 (Nov. 1981): 2473–2477.

Mizushima, Yutaka, et al. "A Survey Regarding the Disclosure of the Diagnosis of Cancer in Toyama Prefecture, Japan." *Japan J Med* 29 (1990): 146–155.

National Commission for the Protection of Human Subjects of Biomedical and Behavioral Research. *The Belmont Report.* Washington, DC: DHEW Publication No. (OS) 78-0012, 1978.

National Commission for the Protection of Human Subjects. *Research Involving Prisoners.* Washington, DC: DHEW Publication No. (OS) 76-131, 1976.

Percival, Thomas. *Medical Ethics; or a Code of Institutes and Precepts, Adapted to the Professional Conduct of Physicians and Surgeons.* Manchester: S. Russell, 1803. (Available as Chauncey D. Leake, Ed., *Percival's Medical Ethics*, Huntington, NY: Robert E. Krieger Publishing Company, 1975.)

Pernick, Martin S. "The Patient's Role in Medical Decisionmaking: A Social History of Informed Consent in Medical Therapy." In President's Commission for the Study of Ethical Problems in Medicine and Biomedical and Behavioral Research, *Making Health Care Decisions*, Vol. 3. Washington, DC: Government Printing Office, 1982.

President's Commission for the Study of Ethical Problems in Medicine and Biomedical and Behavioral Research. *Deciding to Forego Life-Sustaining Treatment.* Washington, DC: Government Printing Office, March 1983.

President's Commission for the Study of Ethical Problems in Medicine and Biomedical and Behavioral Research. *Making Health Care Decisions*, Vols. 1–3. Washington, DC: Government Printing Office, 1982.

Quaid, Kimberly A., et al. "Informed Consent for a Prescription Drug: Impact of Disclosed Information on Patient Understanding and Medical Outcomes." *Patient Educ Counsel* 15 (1990): 249–259.

Scherer, David G., Reppucci, N. D. "Adolescents' Capacities to Provide Voluntary Informed Consent." *Law Hum Behav* 12 (1988): 123–141.

Siminoff, L. A., Fetting, J. H., Abeloff, M. D. "Doctor-Patient Communication about Breast Cancer Adjuvant Therapy." *J Clin Oncol* 7 (1989): 1192–1200.

Siminoff, L. A., Fetting, J. H. "Factors Affecting Treatment Decisions for a Life-Threatening Illness: The Case of Medical Treatment for Breast Cancer." *Soc Sci Med* 32 (1991): 813–818.

Takahashi, Yoshimoto. "Informing a Patient of Malignant Illness: Commentary from a Cross-Cultural Viewpoint." *Death Stud* 14 (1990): 83–91.

van Oosten, F. F. W. "The So-Called 'Therapeutic Privilege' or 'Contra-Indication': Its Nature and Role in Non-Disclosure Cases." *Med Law* 10 (1991): 31–41.

Cases

Berkey v. Anderson, 1 Cal. App. 3d 790, 82 Cal. Rptr. 67 (1969).

Canterbury v. Spence, 464 F.2d 772 (D.C. Cir. 1972).

Cobbs v. Grant, 104 Cal. Rptr. 505, 502 P.2d 1 (1972).

Hyman v. Jewish Chronic Disease Hospital, 251 N.Y. 2d 818 (1964); 206 N.E. 2d 338 (1965).

Planned Parenthood of Central Missouri v. Danforth, 428 U.S. 52, 67 n.8 (1976).

Salgo v. Leland Stanford Jr. University Board of Trustees, 317 P.2d 170 (1957).

Schloendorff v. Society of New York Hospitals, 211 N.Y. 125, 105 N.E. 92, (1914).

U.S. Supreme Court. *Thornburgh v. American College of Obstetricians*, 106 S.Ct. 2169 (1986) (White, J., dissenting).

U.S. Supreme Court. *Planned Parenthood of Central Missouri v. Danforth*, 423 U.S. 52 (1976).

United States v. Karl Brandt, Trials of War Criminals Before the Nuremberg Military Tribunals under Control Council Law No. 10, Vols. 1 and 2. *The Medical Case* Military Tribunal I, 1947. Washington, DC: Government Printing Office, 1948–1949.

Wilkinson v. Vesey, 295 A.2d 676 (R.I. 1972).

8

Reproductive Technologies and Genetics

LeRoy Walters

SUMMARY

This chapter covers three major topics: reproductive technologies, genetic testing and screening, and genetic engineering and therapy. On the issue of reproductive technologies, several key issues are explored. The first section considers the challenges that reproductive technologies present for the traditional notion of the family and genetic lineage and analyzes what is now meant by the term *family*. It also examines issues surrounding the appropriate role of government and the effects of new reproductive technologies on the lives of citizens. The chapter discusses metaphysical, legal, and ethical dilemmas presented by assisted insemination, in vitro fertilization, embryo freezing and storage, and the future applications of technology for sex selection, diagnosis of disease, and research. The dilemmas and ethical and public-policy questions surrounding surrogate motherhood are also explored.

The discussion of genetic testing and screening introduces the technical and legal background of techniques such as neonatal, prenatal, and other types of testing and screening and summarizes current efforts to map and sequence the human genome. The discussion that follows analyzes the major ethical and public-policy issues surrounding genetic testing and screening, including freedom and coercion in genetic testing, the confidentiality or disclosure of test results, access to genetic testing services, and the probable benefits and harms of genetic testing and screening programs.

In the final section, the issues surrounding human gene therapy and genetic engineering are explored. The chapter first distinguishes several possible types of genetic intervention. Various ethical and public-policy questions are also discussed in terms of both present and future implications. In addition, some obstacles and alternatives to genetic intervention are explored, and the question of enhancing human characteristics is considered.

The new science of gene mapping and gene sequencing may lead to breathtaking and unanticipated possibilities as well as potentially serious harms. It is therefore prudent to consider these technological possibilities and their potential social impact well before they are upon us.

REPRODUCTIVE TECHNOLOGIES

Before considering specific reproductive technologies such as assisted insemination and in vitro fertilization, we will examine some of the background assumptions that cut across the various technologies.

Background Assumptions

The Naturalness or Artificiality of the New Technologies

If one believes that nothing artificial should intrude into the sexual relations between human beings, that belief will have profound implications for one's attitude toward contraceptive techniques and reproductive technologies. One critic of the new reproductive technologies has formulated his objection as follows:

> Is there possibly some wisdom in that mystery of nature which joins the pleasure of sex, the communication of love, and the desire for children in the very activity by which we continue the chain of human existence? . . .
>
> My point is simply this: there are more and less human ways of bringing a child into this world. I am arguing that the laboratory production of human beings is no longer *human* procreation, that making babies in laboratories—even "perfect" babies—means a degradation of parenthood (Kass 1972, 49).

Diametrically opposed to this antitechnological viewpoint is the perspective of those who regard the rational control of nature as one of the major achievements of human beings. According to this view, liberation from some of the unpredictable aspects of human reproduction is a major boon to the human species.

> Should we leave the fruits of human reproduction to take shape at random, keeping our children dependent on the accidents of romance and genetic endowment, of [the] sexual lottery or what one physician calls "the meiotic roulette of his parents' chromosomes?" Or should we be responsible about it, that is, exercise our rational and human choice, no longer submissively trusting to the blind worship of raw nature? (Fletcher 1974, 36).

A third position tends to mediate between these radically different views. In agreement with the first, it accepts reproduction without technological assistance as natural and good. However, this third position also argues that the development and use of new methods of contraception or reproduction can be morally justifiable, depending on the circumstances and on the reasons adduced. According to this view, it is natural for human beings to create culture in an effort to cope with some of the uncertainties and inconveniences of the natural world. Technology is an important part of that culture (Callahan 1972, 100–101).

The Moral Status of the Early Human Embryo

To speak of the moral status of anything is to use a shorthand expression for more complex formulations like "What are our moral obligations to X?" or "What moral rights does X possess?" Analogously, one can speak of the legal status of an adult, a newborn infant, or a human embryo.

There are three principal viewpoints on the moral status of the *early human embryo*—here defined as the embryo within the first 14 days of postfertilization development. The first viewpoint asserts that human embryos are entitled to protection as human beings from the time of fertilization forward. Thus, any research or other manipulation, such as freezing, that damages an embryo or interferes with its prospects for transfer to a uterus and subsequent development is ethically unacceptable. This perspective on embryonic status is based on two kinds of factual evidence. First, the embryonic genotype is established at the time of fertilization. Second, given the proper environment, early embryos have the potential to become full-term fetuses, children, and adults.

A second viewpoint denies that early human embryos have any moral status. According to this view, adult human beings have no moral obligations to early human embryos. This viewpoint also appeals to scientific evidence, especially the fact that only about 30 to 40 percent of embryos produced through human sexual intercourse develop to maturity in utero and are delivered as live infants (Leridon 1973; Chard 1991). It also notes that the biological individuality of the early embryo is established only toward the end of the first 14 days of development: Before that time, one embryo can divide into twins or, more rarely, two embryos with different genotypes cam combine into a single hybrid embryo. This position also argues that an undifferentiated entity like the early embryo, which has no organs, no limbs, and no sentience, cannot have moral status.

Again there is a mediating position. This viewpoint accords some moral status to the early embryo, on grounds of its potential. This feature differentiates the early embryo from other human tissues or cells. However, the third view acknowledges that our prima facie moral obligation to early human embryos can be outweighed by other moral duties, for example, the duty to develop new and better methods of providing care to infertile couples.

The Role of the Family and Genetic Lineage

The practice of donating gametes or early embryos has occasioned debate among commentators on the new reproductive technologies. One view is that even though the new reproductive technologies are not unnatural, they should be employed only within the family unit. Proponents of this view argue that if a couple cannot conceive a child by means of their own sperm and egg cell, even with medical assistance, they should accept their infertility and explore other alternatives such as adopting a child. According to this view, adoption is qualitatively different from the deliberate and premeditated introduction of "foreign" gamete and embryos into the family unit because adopting parents rescue an already-existing child from a situation of homelessness. The opposing viewpoint on gamete and embryo donation is that these practices are morally justified when employed by a couple for good reasons, such as untreatable infertility or the presence of a genetic abnormality in one or both partners. The use of the new reproductive technologies is thus seen as a useful adjunct that allows couples to approximate, as closely as possible, the usual experience of reproduction.

Another controversial issue is the meaning of the term *family*. The traditional understanding of family was that it included a husband, a wife, and one or more children. This traditional understanding has been called into question not by the new reproductive technologies but by several social developments of the twentieth century—especially divorce rates that are approaching 50 percent in the United States and the increasing number of children born to single women. The general debate about the meaning of family is carried over into discussions of the new reproductive technologies as members of nontraditional families—unmarried heterosexual couples, single men or women, and homosexual couples—request technical assistance in reproduction.

The Appropriate Role of Government

The classical Western view of the proper role of government, articulated by philosophers like Plato, was that government should promote virtue in its citizens, who were viewed in some sense as part of an organic whole, the state. In modern times, most Western political philosophers have rejected this view. The closest modern parallel to the Platonic view is that governments should ensure that citizens act in accordance with the principles of morality. According to this view, governments are justified in intervening to prevent private immoral behavior, such as illicit sexual activity, because such behavior undermines the public good (Devlin 1965, 14–15).

A second view sees the primary role of government as protecting individual liberties and preventing individuals from inflicting harm on others. This view often includes the "clear and present danger" tests sometimes used in debates about freedom of speech—namely, that only serious, imminent harms are of sufficient importance to warrant government intrusion (Feinberg 1973, 41–45). On this view, government would not normally intervene in the private sexual activities or reproductive efforts of consenting adults except, perhaps, to prevent tangible, highly-probable physical or psychological harm to potential offspring.

A third view would limit individual liberty not only to protect citizens from harm but also to ensure that every citizen enjoys at least a certain minimum of welfare—that is, income, food, clothing, shelter, and health care (Daniels 1985; Rawls 1973). Applied to the new reproductive technologies, this view of government might include infertility treatment within the scope of the minimum health-care services that every citizen should be guaranteed by society.

Assisted Insemination

Assisted insemination (previously, artificial insemination) is widely used in animal husbandry, especially in the breeding of cattle. The technique was first demonstrated unequivocally in toads in 1779 by Lazaro Spallanzani, Italian priest and physiologist. The first known successful assisted insemination of a human female occurred in 1790 when John Hunter, Scottish anatomist and surgeon, inseminated the wife of a linen draper with her husband's sperm (Corea 1985, 35). Almost a century later William Panacost, a medical-school professor in Philadelphia, performed assisted insemination with donor sperm. When a wealthy Philadelphia couple requested his help in overcoming their infertility, Panacost asked the best-looking member of his medical-school class to volunteer as a semen donor. The insemination was performed in the doctor's office under general anesthesia, and neither the husband nor the wife was informed about the method employed to initiate the pregnancy (Andrews 1985a, 148).

Two types of assisted insemination are usually distinguished: assisted insemination with the husband's semen (AIH) and assisted insemination with a donor's semen (AID) (U.S. Office of Technology Assessment 1988a; Canada 1993, 425–495). AIH is often considered a therapeutic intervention when a couple has tried unsuccessfully for several years to conceive a child by means of sexual intercourse. One or more factors may be responsible for the couple's infertility, among them the husband's impotence, a low sperm count, or an immunological incompatibility between the husband's sperm and the wife's cervical or vaginal secretions. The freezing of semen samples for possible future AIH is also considered by some couples when the husband is about to undergo surgery, drug treatment, or radiation treatment that may cause sterility or damage the sperm cells.

The technique of AIH is quite straightforward. One or more semen samples are produced by the husband through masturbation. After treatment by various laboratory techniques, the samples or the sperm from the samples are placed by a health-care professional into the vagina, cervical canal, or uterus of the wife (American Fertility Society 1994, 41S–42S). No patterns of handicapped offspring have been observed after the use of AIH.

The major ethical objections raised against AIH by some critics is that it separates the lovemaking and procreative aspects of human sexual activity (Pius XII 1956; Catholic Church 1987). This objection seems to be based on an ideal of natural reproduction and on a rejection of some kinds of technological interventions into the reproductive process. Defenders of AIH respond by arguing that nature, not the husband and wife, causes the separation of lovemaking and reproduction for couples who are involuntarily infertile. Proponents of AIH also assert that couples who resort to AIH merely extend the sphere of their lovemaking to include the physician's office and the technological assistance of a third party (McCormick 1978, 1458; 1985, 399).

AID is usually considered as an option by a couple when the husband or male partner has no viable sperm in his semen, when there is a rhesus (Rh) incompatibility between man and woman, or when the man does not want to transmit a genetic defect to offspring (American Fertility Society 1994, 43S–45S). As noted above, donor semen has been used by some physicians in treating infertile couples since the late nineteenth century. The technique precisely parallels AIH, except that the provider of semen in AID is not the women's spouse.

Because AID involves the introduction of third-party gametes, the use of this technique is a more complicated matter both ethically and legally. Some critics of AID have suggested that the practice undermines the family or that it could have negative psychological effects on the man or the potential child. These are empirical questions that can be systematically studied. The meager data currently available indicate no pattern of psychological harm if the man has consented to AID and if resulting children are informed of the circumstances of their conception in a reasonable way (Andrews 1985a, 168).

From the standpoint of safety to the woman and to the potential child, the most important issue of AID is appropriate screening of the semen donor, who is often technically a "vendor" rather than a donor. In several tragic cases, fatal genetic diseases in children have resulted from improper screening of the biological father. Communicable diseases, including infection with the human immunodeficiency virus (HIV) that causes acquired immunodeficiency syndrome (AIDS), have also been transmitted from semen donors to recipient women (Stewart et al. 1985). At a minimum, the prospective donor's family history should be taken, and he should be tested for evidence of infectious disease. Whether his chromosomes should also be examined through karyotyping is currently a matter of debate. Careful, permanent records about the donor's health status should be maintained in a confidential file, to which medical practitioners should have access if later follow-up with the donor becomes necessary (American Fertility Society 1994, 44S–45S).

As currently practiced in the United States, AID often includes a commercial dimension. If fresh semen from a nonrelative is used for AID, the donor is usually a student who receives $25 to $50 per acceptable specimen. If frozen semen is employed, it is most likely to be purchased from one of approximately 30 commercial sperm banks in the United States (U.S. Office of Technology Assessment 1988a, 33). One can debate whether a paid donor is being compensated for his time and inconvenience or for the gametes themselves.

Some critics of AID object to what they call the commercialization of the reproductive process when semen donors are paid and sperm banks become profit-making enterprises. They argue that the collection and distribution of sperm should be conducted in the same voluntary, nonprofit way that whole blood and transplantable organs are. France, for example, has established a centralized, national system for sperm donors. Fertile males who have already fathered healthy children are urged to consider donating semen to the national sperm banking system, as a fulfillment of a civic duty (United Kingdom 1984, 27–28).

In Vitro Fertilization

Clinical Applications

The birth of Louise Brown in Lancashire, England, on July 25, 1978, inaugurated a new era in the history of the reproductive technologies. Louise had been conceived, not inside her mother's body, but in a Petri dish, where eggs from her mother were mixed with sperm from her father, and where fertilization took place.

In vitro fertilization (IVF) is most often proposed when the members of a married couple are unable to reproduce because of obstructions in the wife's reproductive tract or because of the husband's low sperm count. Typically, the egg cells used in IVF are surgically removed from the wife's ovaries, and the semen is provided by the husband. In most cases, no early embryos are frozen, and one or more developing embryos are transferred to the uterus of the wife (Canada 1993, 497–580; American Fertility Society 1994, 35S–37S).

The possible risks of clinical IVF to offspring were, in the 1970s, the object of a rather vigorous debate. By the early 1990s, however, a series of more than 25,000 births after IVF showed no clear evidence of an increased incidence of congenital defects. The long-term consequences of IVF on children conceived by means of this technique have not yet been assessed.

The major ethical reservation about clinical IVF in cases involving only the reproductive cells of the husband and wife is that this technical procedure separates lovemaking from procreation. This reservation and its counter-argument exactly parallel the discussion in the case of AIH.

Several emerging and potential future uses of clinical IVF have occasioned considerable debate. These uses include the freezing and storage of early human embryos, the donation or sale of human embryos, early gender selection, and early diagnosis of genetic or chromosomal abnormalities (American College of Obstetricians and Gynecologists 1986; U.S. Office of Technology Assessment 1988b; American Fertility Society 1994).

The freezing and storage of early human embryos is increasingly employed in conjunction with clinical IVF. This technique is also widely used in animal husbandry, especially in the cattle-breeding industry. There are several reasons why the freezing and storage of early human embryos is useful to an infertile couple. An infertile woman is often given hormonal stimulation so that her ovaries produce multiple eggs in a given cycle. After fertilization with her husband's sperm, the woman's multiple eggs may develop into multiple early embryos, perhaps even five or six embryos. The freezing and storage of some of these embryos may help to solve the "surplus-embryo" problem. Rather than transferring all five or six embryos at one time—thus risking the possibility of a triplet or quadruplet pregnancy—the couple may elect to transfer only two or three and save the remaining embryos for a later cycle. Further, the freezing and storage of embryos spares the wife the trauma of another surgical procedure for retrieving eggs in a subsequent ovulatory cycle.

At the same time, however, human embryo freezing raises metaphysical, ethical, and legal problems. The metaphysical problem is what status to ascribe to an undifferentiated human entity that can be preserved for years in a state of suspended animation. The ethical and legal problems center on the question whether frozen, stored embryos should be regarded as in some sense the "property" of the couple whose reproductive cells combined to produce the embryos. A famous case in Australia, the Rios case, sparked a lively public debate about what should be done with frozen early embryos that were suddenly "orphaned" by the death of their future "parents" in a plane crash (Sellar 1984). More recently, a disagreement over the disposition of frozen embryos that seemed analogous to a traditional custody dispute arose between the genetic parents of the embryos. The dispute was resolved by the Tennessee Supreme Court (Tennessee 1992).

The freezing or storing of embryos also facilitates the donation or sale of human embryos to third parties. The question of embryo donation or sale closely parallels the question of semen donation or sale discussed above. In the future, human egg freezing and storage may also become technically feasible. The same issues of third-party involvement, donor screening, and public policy on donation or sale that we examined in connection with AID also arise regarding the freezing and storage of human embryos. In addition, many would argue that the ethical stakes are higher in the case of an embryo that may one day develop into a human adult than with a sperm or egg cell.

Noninvasive techniques for determining whether early human embryos are destined to be males or females have recently been developed. If these techniques are used to help a couple avoid transmitting a sex-linked genetic disorder to their children, the use of the techniques would seem, in the view of most commentators, to be morally justifiable. This strategy has the advantages, compared with prenatal diagnosis and selective abortion, of sparing women physical trauma and of intervening when the embryo is relatively undeveloped. However, the use of gender-selection techniques for purely social reasons, such as the desire to "have a boy first," raises subtle, and hotly debated, questions about sex discrimination and possible long-term effects on the sex ratio (Canada 1993, 908–915; American Fertility Society 1994, 64S–66S).

Another recent application of IVF and freezing and storage techniques is early (preimplantation) diagnosis of genetic or chromosomal abnormalities.

The technique employed removes one or more cells from the developing embryo for diagnostic purposes and freezes the remaining cells. Various tests are then performed on the removed cells. If a particular embryo is found to be free of detectable defects, it can be transferred to the uterus of the woman in a subsequent ovulatory cycle. Any embryo found to be affected by a genetic or chromosomal abnormality is presumably not transferred but discarded. Again, in this case, preimplantation intervention seems morally preferable to intervention on the basis of prenatal diagnosis after a pregnancy is already well established. However, the consequences, for the later development of potential children, of removing embryonic cells still need to be evaluated in careful scientific studies (Simpson and Carson 1992; Institute of Medicine 1994, 35–36, 42; American Fertility Society 1994, 64S–66S).

Research

Laboratory research with early human embryos has been proposed as a way to gain important information about fertilization, the prevention of fertilization (contraception), and the causes of birth defects in children. However, critics of laboratory research with early human embryos argue that such research is not compatible with the kind of respect that should be shown to developing entities that may have the potential to become human beings.

Contrasting viewpoints of the ethics of human embryo research are clearly based on differing conceptions of the moral status of the early human embryo (Robertson 1986; Robertson 1994, 198–202; American Fertility Society 1994, 78S–80S). The public-policy debate on this question has raged in several countries with no clear resolution. Most public bodies charged with reaching a judgment on human embryo research have found the research to be ethically acceptable, in principle, if the research is intended to develop important knowledge that cannot be gained in any other way (Ontario 1985; United Kingdom 1984; U.S. Ethics Advisory Board 1979; Victoria 1984; Canada 1993; U.S. National Institutes of Health 1994).

Surrogate Parenthood

Surrogate parenthood arrangements are generally proposed when a woman who wishes to bear and raise a child is medically incapable of carrying a pregnancy. She may, for example, have been born without a uterus. Or she may be afflicted with a medical condition that would make pregnancy a life-threatening condition for her (American College of Obstetricians and Gynecologists 1990; U.S. Office of Technology Assessment 1988b, 267–290; Canada 1993, 661–693; American Fertility Society 1994, 67S–77S).

The first documented attempt to employ a surrogate motherhood arrangement in the United States occurred in 1976 under the direction of Michigan attorney Noel Keane (Keane and Breo 1981). In the early years of this new social practice, the relatively old technology of assisted insemination donor (AID) was employed, using sperm provided by the husband of the future social mother. Thus, in the usual ("full") surrogate motherhood arrangement, the child results from the union of the surrogate mother's egg and the social father's sperm. In 1985 the first instance of surrogate motherhood assisted by in vitro fertilization occurred. In this arrangement, the future social mother was able to produce fertilizable eggs but medically unable to carry a pregnancy. Her eggs were fertilized in vitro with sperm from her husband, and the resulting embryos were then transferred to the uterus of a surrogate mother (Utian et al. 1985). In this latter arrangement, which is sometimes called *partial surrogacy*, the gestational mother is often called a *surrogate carrier* because she makes no genetic contribution to the child.

While surrogate motherhood in the United States has usually involved a professional who formalizes the arrangements between the surrogate and the social parents, as well as arranging for the payment of a fee to the surrogate mother, a formal and commercial relationship is not a necessary part of surrogate motherhood. In some subcultures, a fertile wife readily conceives and bears an extra child for her sister if the sister is infertile. Further, there have been anecdotal reports of noncommercial surrogacy arrangements in which a fertile woman bore a child for an infertile friend or coworker. In fact, some commentators on surrogate motherhood have argued that the earliest pretechnological surrogate arrangement occurred in biblical times, for example, when Sarah suggested that Abraham conceive a child with her maid Hagar because Sarah herself was infertile (Genesis 16:1–15).

Four principal ethical and public-policy questions have been raised about surrogate motherhood arrangements.

1. If the surrogate mother decides during the pregnancy or at the time of delivery to keep the child that she had agreed to bear for a couple, who should have parental rights?
2. To what extent should the adopting couple be able to control the lifestyle of the surrogate mother during the pregnancy?
3. If the child is born with physical or mental handicaps, are the adopting parents nonetheless obligated to accept the child as their own?
4. If the surrogate mother receives payment, for what is the payment made, and how can exploitative or coercive relationships be avoided?

All these questions suggest that the duration and intensity of third-party involvement in surrogate motherhood arrangements raise special problems. In the case of semen or egg donation, or even embryo donation, the act of donation can be completed in a few minutes, at most. However, surrogate mothers are pregnant for approximately nine months, interact physically with the fetus, give birth to a child, and perhaps even develop a relationship with the future social parents. This extended period of de facto interdependence among surrogate mother, fetus, and adopting parents, plus the uncertainties inherent in any pregnancy, carries with it the risk that complications will arise in some surrogate motherhood arrangements (Capron and Radin 1988; Annas 1992; California 1993; Robertson 1994, 130–145).

Given these likely complications, should surrogate motherhood arrangements be legally prohibited? The answer to this question has varied from country to country. The United Kingdom and the state of Victoria in Australia have legally banned commercial surrogate motherhood arrangements (King 1986, 131–132). In 1985 the Ontario Law Reform Commission recommended that surrogate motherhood arrangements be permitted only with the active participation of a court in the entire transaction (1985, 242–262). However, the 1993 report by the Canadian Royal Commission on New Reproductive Technologies recommended that the payment of a surrogate mother and the brokering of a commercial surrogacy agreement should be prohibited by the criminal law (1993, 689–691). In the United States, the two most thorough analyses of surrogate motherhood by professional committees have described potential problems in the practice, but have stopped short of recommending legal prohibition even of commercial surrogacy (American College of Obstetricians and Gynecologists 1990; American Fertility Society 1994, 67S–77S). The 1994 report of the American Fertility Society Ethics Committees concluded:

> The Committee has serious ethical reservations about surrogacy that cannot be fully resolved until appropriate data are available for assessment of the risks and possible benefits of this alternative. In light of these reservations, some members of the committee judged that surrogacy cold not be ethically recommended. Others concluded that it could be cautiously recommended while research on the key issues continued (1994, 77S).

In the future, it is possible that an artificial placenta or artificial uterus will be developed that will make extracorporeal gestation possible. Such a device, if demonstrated to be safe and efficacious, might make the current practice of surrogate motherhood obsolete. However, this new technology would raise additional ethical questions in its own right (Fletcher 1974, 163–165).

GENETIC TESTING AND SCREENING

We live in the golden age of medical genetics. Even before the 1950s Gregor Mendel's classic work on various modes of inheritance was available as a theoretical framework for understanding how genetic disease is transmitted. However, Watson and Crick's description of the molecular structure of DNA in 1953 and the rapid advances based on the use of recombinant DNA techniques in the 1960s and 1970s opened up entirely new possibilities for genetic diagnosis and therapy.

The principal benefits of medical genetics through the early 1990s have been diagnostic and predictive rather than therapeutic. We now understand much more clearly the genetic dimensions of many human diseases, including conditions that in the past were not thought to include genetic components, for example, breast cancer and coronary heart disease. For a minority of gene-mediated diseases, some helpful therapy can currently be offered to patients. For the most part, however, the medical treatment of genetic disease is a future goal.

Genetic disorders exact an enormous toll of human suffering. In the latest edition of the standard catalog of Mendelian disorders in humans, 5710 distinguishable genetic or chromosomal conditions are described (McKusick 1992). Genetic disorders are the second leading cause of death among 1- to 4-year-olds in the United States and the third leading cause of death in 15- to 17-year-olds. It is estimated that 25 to 30 percent of admissions to U.S. acute-care hospitals for persons under 18 years of age are for genetic conditions; about 13 percent of adult admissions are genetically related conditions. In addition, 20 to 25 percent of persons institutionalized because of mental retardation have genetically caused diseases (Antenatal Diagnosis 1979, I-27–I-30). These 1979 estimates probably understated the genetic contribution to the human disease burden; in many cases, recent research has clarified the role of inheritance in nongenetic diseases.

In this chapter, *genetic testing* is defined as the use of diagnostic procedures or determination of the presence or absence of one or more genetic traits or conditions in an individual. *Genetic screening* refers to the use of genetic tests in programs that are intended to reach a large number of persons who have a particular genetic trait or condition. Thus, genetic screening always involves genetic testing, but genetic testing may not always involve a systematic, organized genetic screening program.

As currently practiced, genetic testing usually occurs at one of four stages of life: (1) in the neonatal period; (2) prenatally; (3) when couples are considering marriage or reproduction; or (4) when a person, on the basis of family history, recognizes that he or she has a higher-than-average risk of developing a genetic disease. In the future, the technique of gene mapping and the sequencing of the human genome may significantly extend medicine's current diagnostic capabilities.

Neonatal Screening

Historically, the capacity to test newborns for phenylketonuria (PKU)—a so-called inborn error of metabolism—was the first to be used in a mass screening program. In 1962, using a test developed by Dr. Robert Guthrie, Massachusetts tried a voluntary screening program for PKU. The following year, Massachusetts adopted the first law requiring PKU screening for newborns in the United States (U.S. President's Commission 1983, 13).

From these modest beginnings, newborn screening expanded until all 50 states and the District of Columbia had newborn screening programs by 1990 (Institute of Medicine 1994, 68–69).

The list of genetic conditions screened for has also expanded. Many states now attempt to detect hypothyroidism, sickle-cell anemia, galactosemia, homocystinuria, and maple-syrup urine disease, as well as PKU (Institute of Medicine 1994, 5). Because most U.S. screening programs are mandatory, most newborn infants are in fact tested. Thus, just over 4 million babies receive heel sticks and are tested each year in the United States.

Prenatal Diagnosis

The second type of genetic testing developed, historically, was prenatal diagnosis. In 1966 a report was published of the first study of chromosomes taken from cultured cells withdrawn from the amniotic sac by amniocentesis. During the next 2 years, successful prenatal diagnosis of a chromosomal disorder and an inborn error of metabolism was reported in scientific publications (U.S. President's Commission 1983, 23). Since the early 1960s, other diagnostic methods have also become available for the prenatal detection of genetic or chromosomal abnormalities. These include ultrasonography (which provides echolike pictures of the developing fetus), the withdrawal of a blood sample from the umbilical cord with the aid of fetoscopy, the testing of blood samples from pregnant women, and the removal of fetal cells from chorionic villi inside the uterus toward the end of the first trimester of pregnancy. By 1994 prenatal diagnosis was available for hundreds of conditions ranging from anomalies that cause profound retardation and early death (e.g., trisomies 13 and 18, Tay-Sachs disease) to disorders that "affect daily living and shorten life span but do not cause serious mental incapacity" (e.g., cystic fibrosis and hemophilia) (Institute of Medicine 1994, 75).

In recent years, another type of prenatal diagnosis has become available in conjunction with in vitro fertilization—preimplantation diagnosis (American Fertility Society 1994, 64S–66S). Typically one cell of a four- or eight-cell embryo is removed, the DNA from the cell is amplified in the laboratory, and a variety of tests are performed on the DNA. Conditions that can be diagnosed at this early stage of embryonic development include Duchenne muscular dystrophy, cystic fibrosis, hemophilia, fragile X syndrome, and Down syndrome (Handyside et al. 1992; Simpson and Carson 1992; Institute of Medicine 1994, 82). Preimplantation diagnosis can also determine the future gender of an embryo if a couple wishes to avoid a sex-linked disorder (Handyside 1990). Because preimplantation diagnosis is performed only in conjunction with in vitro fertilization, it has limited applicability.

Carrier Testing and Screening

The third type of genetic testing and screening is most frequently used when couples are considering marriage and reproduction. In the United States, the earliest carrier screening programs focused on two diseases, Tay-Sachs disease, which affects primarily people of Ashkenazi Jewish descent, and sickle-cell anemia, which is most prevalent among members of the African American population (U.S. President's Commission 1983, 17–23). More recently, with the identification of multiple mutations that cause cystic fibrosis, the question of population screening for cystic fibrosis—at least among persons of European ancestry—has been intensively debated (Collins 1992; U.S. Office of Technology Assessment 1992a; Institute of Medicine 1994, 73–74). In the Mediterranean region, similar programs have been developed for thalassemia, a hemoglobin disorder that is in some respects similar to sickle-cell disease (Cao 1989).

In carrier testing, a genetic counselor helps couples to understand their relative risk of transmitting a genetic defect to their children. Typically, both members of the couple provide cell samples, which are then studied in the laboratory. The results of the laboratory tests help the genetic counselor to explain a series of probabilities to the couple. For example, if only one member of the couple carries the gene for a recessive genetic disease, the couple is not at risk of producing a child afflicted with the disease but has a one-in-two chance of producing a carrier. However, if both members of a couple carry the gene for a recessive genetic disease that is not sex-linked, the couple has a 25 percent chance of producing an unaffected child, a 50 percent chance of producing a carrier, and a 25 percent chance of producing a child who will have the disease.

Predictive or Presymptomatic Testing and Screening

The fourth type of genetic testing has emerged only during the late 1980s and early 1990s. It allows persons with a family history of certain diseases to learn in advance whether they themselves are at high risk to develop those diseases later in life. Because the testing is performed before any symptoms of the disease occur, it is called *presymptomatic*, or *predictive*, *genetic testing*.

Huntington disease is one of the best-known single-gene disorders for which such testing can be done. This disease, which afflicted singer Woody Guthrie, usually strikes its victims between the ages of 35 and 45 years. An inexorable course of deterioration follows for 10 to 20 years. The person afflicted with Huntington disease gradually loses control of motor functions and cognitive capacities. Frequently, the person's psyche is affected as well, with resultant depression, apathy, or obsessive-compulsive disorder (Institute of Medicine 1994, 88–89). At present, no effective treatment exists for Huntington disease. However, in early 1993 the gene that causes this devastating disease was identified, and a reliable test for the gene is now available (Huntington Disease Collaborative Research Group 1993; Institute of Medicine 1994, 88–89).

Huntington disease is one example of single-gene disorders for which presymptomatic testing will be relatively straightforward, from a technical standpoint, at least, when the gene is precisely identified. Other single-gene disorders are early-onset Alzheimer's disease, an iron-storage disease called hemochromatosis, polycystic kidney disease, familial hypercholesteremia, and mutations in the p53 gene that helps to suppress various types of cancers. Other so-called genetic disorders involve environmental factors as well as inheritance—coronary heart disease, high blood pressure, diabetes, rheumatoid arthritis, certain types of cancers, and some psychiatric disorders (Institute of Medicine 1994, 86–99).

Gene Mapping and the Sequencing of the Human Genome

Human beings usually have 23 pairs of chromosomes in the nuclei of every cell. In turn, the chromosomes contain the genes that code for proteins and other products that our bodies need to function, as well as intervening stretches of DNA whose function is not yet well understood. The smallest coding units within the genes and intervening sequences are called bases. It is estimated that our 23 pairs of chromosomes contain 50,000 to 100,000 genes and 3 to 3.5 billion base pairs. Scientists are eager to learn more about the structure and function of human genes and chromosomes, which, all taken together, are called the *human genome*. Thus, researchers plan first to map the genome, then to sequence areas of special interest, and finally to sequence (or decipher the genetic letters contained in) all 3 to 3.5 billion base pairs that comprise our genome (Cooperative Human Linkage Center 1994; Cox et al. 1994; Knoppers and Chadwick 1994).

A geographical analogy may be helpful for understanding how gene mapping and sequencing will be done. If you wanted to make a physical map of the United States, you might first use a satellite photograph to get an overview of the whole country. This satellite photo would correspond to locating the 23 pairs of human chromosomes. You might divide the country into 1000 regions, each comprising a certain number of square miles. For this more detailed map you might use photographs taken from airplanes. Similarly, scientists will divide the human genome into major regions, each of which will consist of perhaps 40,000 base pairs. In our geography project, there might be certain regions that required special attention even at this stage of mapping, for example, major metropolitan areas or areas with potentially dangerous geological faults. In a parallel way, scientists have already discovered that certain disease-related genes are located in particular regions of particular chromosomes. They will therefore subject these regions to special scrutiny at this stage of mapping. The final stage in the geography project might be a highly detailed map that indicates individual streets or even individual buildings on those streets. This fine level of detail would correspond to knowing the sequence in which some or all of the 3 to 3.5 billion base pairs are arranged in human chromosomes.

The massive project of gene mapping and sequencing will initially provide detailed knowledge about where important genes are located and how they function. The first application of this new knowledge will probably be diagnostic—tests will be developed for large numbers of diseases, and these tests will be used in genetic testing and screening. At the same time, however, gene mapping and sequencing may help scientists and clinicians to develop ways to correct or compensate for some genetic defects.

Ethical and Public-Policy Issues

Much has been written about the ethical and public-policy issues surrounding genetic testing and screening. Four issues have been central to this discussion: (1) freedom and coercion in genetic testing and screening, (2) the confidentiality or disclosure of test results, (3) access to genetic testing services, and (4) the probable benefits and harms of genetic testing and screening programs.

Freedom and Coercion

All programs of prenatal diagnosis and nearly all programs of carrier screening have been voluntary. In contrast, virtually all newborn screening programs are mandated by state governments. The major rationale for mandatory newborn screening programs is that such programs protect the helpless from serious, avoidable harm through the use of low-risk, minimally intrusive diagnostic procedures (U.S. President's Commission 1983, 51). The arguments in favor of newborn screening for treatable conditions are so strong, in fact, that most parents want such screening to be preformed on their newborns. A study of Maryland's voluntary newborn screening program for PKU found, for example, that the prenatal refusal rate was only .05 percent—one refusal for every 1999 acceptances (Faden et al. 1982). One can view this result in two ways. On the one hand, the result indicates that so-called mandatory newborn screening programs are probably not perceived as coercive by a large majority of parents. On the other hand, the high rate of voluntary parental compliance suggests that laws or regulations mandating newborn screening may not be necessary; at the very least, the social costs of initiating any kind of mandatory program need to be weighed against the benefits conferred to a tiny minority of newborns and their families. One approach to voluntary programs of genetic screening is to require health-care professionals to *offer* genetic testing to the parents of all newborns (Institute of Medicine 1994, 100–101).

A second type of mandatory program can be distinguished from the unconditionally mandated screening imposed by a state. We might call such testing "contingently mandatory." For example, an employer might require all applicants for employment to undergo a battery of genetic diagnostic tests. The tests would not be mandatory—a person could decide not to apply to work for a company that had such a screening policy. However, the tests would be mandatory for all who did apply. Similar questions may arise if health insurance companies begin requiring batteries of genetic tests before they write individual insurance policies (U.S. Office of Technology Assessment 1992b; U.S. NIH-DOE Working Group 1993; Institute of Medicine 1994, 271–273, 281–282). The debates that currently surround drug testing in the workplace and testing for antibody to HIV in a variety of settings suggest that contingently mandatory genetic testing may become an important public-policy issue in the future.

In its report on genetic counseling and screening, the President's Commission on Bioethics reached the following conclusion:

> In sum, the fundamental value of genetic screening and counseling is their ability to enhance the opportunities for individuals to obtain information about their personal health and to make autonomous and noncoerced choices based on that information (U.S. President's Commission 1983, 55).

This conclusion clearly states an autonomy-oriented approach to genetic testing and screening. However, moral freedom is generally accompanied by moral responsibility. Thus, a complementary and balancing thesis is that individuals and couples have a moral duty to learn what they can about the likelihood that they will transmit genetic conditions to their offspring and to take reasonable steps—steps that are compatible with their other ethical convictions—to avoid causing preventable harm to their descendants. This "ethics of genetic duty" (Ramsey 1977, 57) need not, and in the author's view should not, be enacted into law. It does, however, qualify the ethic of autonomy in the genetic and reproductive spheres.

Confidentiality and Disclosure

If a genetic condition is detected through mandatory or voluntary testing or screening, there remains a further question: Who, besides the individual and his or her health-care provider, should have access to the information about the genetic condition? This question arises primarily in two contexts—an extended familial context and a business context. In the extended family context, individuals or couples who learn that they have a genetic disease or carry a genetic trait may face decisions about whether to inform their parents, their siblings, their children, and more distant relatives. For example, if an individual discovers that he has the gene for a late-onset, genetically dominant disorder such as Huntington disease, he will also realize that each of his siblings will have a 50 percent chance of having the gene and, if one or more siblings have the gene, a 50 percent chance of transmitting the gene to each of their children. Most individuals in this situation would probably want to warn their siblings voluntarily, especially because no one is causally or morally responsible for the genetic conditions with which he or she is born. However, if an individual refuses to disclose such information voluntarily and serious harm to others is likely to result from the nondisclosure, a case can be made for breaching the normal duty to protect the confidentiality of information about a patient's genetic condition (U.S. President's Commission 1983, 44–45; Wertz and Fletcher 1989, 16–17, 509; Institute of Medicine 1994, 23, 165–166, 264–267).

The business context for questions about confidentiality in medical genetics is likely to involve employers or insurers. For example, health insurance companies might charge a higher premium for, or even refuse to insure at all, an individual who is afflicted with a certain kind of genetic condition. Similarly, an employer might be reluctant to hire and train an individual if the employer knew that the employee were at high risk of premature death from a lethal genetic disease. These are highly complicated issues that cannot be solved with simple formulas. Employers and insurance companies have a legitimate interest in controlling their costs, but there is the possibility that individuals will be unfairly discriminated against because of medical conditions over which they have no control. The result for these individuals may be loss of access to employment or to the health-care system.

The President's Commission on Bioethics argued that, because of "the potential for misuse as well as unintended social or economic injury, information about genetic conditions should be disclosed to insurers or employers only with the explicit consent of the person tested" (1983, 44; Institute of Medicine 1994, 267–273). This argument may be an important element in an overall public policy about confidentiality and genetic testing, but it should be supplemented by a more thorough analysis of society's responsibility, or lack or responsibility, to provide access to employment and health care to every member of society. Specific mechanisms, at the state or federal level, for spreading the financial risks of caring for members of high-risk groups should also be addressed (National Academy of Sciences 1986, 168–173).

Access to Genetic Testing Services

Problems of access to genetic testing services can arise in at least two ways. First, because health insurance systems are often oriented toward the performance of procedures, insurance carriers sometimes reimburse health-care professionals or policyholders for tests but not for the counseling and interpretation that should accompany the tests. The result may be either the loss of critical information or a major unanticipated expense (Institute of Medicine 1994, 234–246).

Second, in some cases an individual may not know what further tests may be required if the results of an initial test are positive or suspicious. For example, maternal serum alpha-fetoprotein (MSAFP) screening usually involves only a single test of a blood sample from a pregnant woman. However, an initial positive test may lead to a repeat blood (serum) test, detailed ultrasonography, amniocentesis, and a decision about selective abortion. Pregnant women who are uninsured or underinsured may be able to afford the initial and repeat serum tests but be unable to bear the expense of the later, more sophisticated tests in the series. The State of California has sought to confront this kind of access problem by providing a statewide and state-run program that charges a nominal flat fee—in 1994 the figure was $57—to every pregnant woman who enrolls for MSAFP testing. The $57 fee guarantees access to all necessary diagnostic tests (Steinbrook 1986; California 1994).

Benefits and Harms of Genetic Testing and Screening

The principal benefits of genetic testing and screening programs are knowledge, the ability to avoid transmitting genetic disease to offspring, and, in some cases, the ability to secure timely treatment for a genetic condition. However, genetic testing and screening programs can also cause harm—through coercion, through leading to exclusion from the work force or the health-care system, and through providing incomplete information of partial services.

Two other dimensions of the benefit–harm issue deserve brief consideration. The first is that a positive genetic test, even if it does not lead to economic loss, may result in the stigmatization of the individual tested. Sometimes the stigmatization is based on erroneous information, as was the case in the early 1970s when carriers of the sickle-cell trait, who did not have sickle-cell anemia, were subjected to several baseless restrictions (Andrews 1985b, 147–148). The stigmatization may also result from informing children of their genetic problems or carrier status when they are not yet able to cope with the information.

However, in a curious way, the new techniques of gene mapping and gene sequencing may help to "democratize" genetic disease. We all know, theoretically, that we have certain genetic tendencies and may in fact carry several potentially lethal genes. In addition, our chromosomes include a set of dormant but nonetheless potentially dangerous cancer-causing genes called proto-oncogenes. As more is learned about the human genome, and as diagnostic tests for more genetic diseases and traits become available, it may become clearer that visible and invisible genetic problems are simply an omnipresent aspect of the human condition.

The technique of prenatal diagnosis and selective abortion also raises special ethical questions. Some commentators argue that abortion is always wrong, even if performed for so-called fetal indications (Ramsey 1970, 114). Other commentators have raised the question of whether it is psychologically possible to advocate the selective abortion of fetuses discovered to have genetic defects while at the same time pressing for nondiscriminatory treatment of the already-born who are handicapped (Hauerwas 1986, 159–181; Motulsky and Murray 1983). This quandary may be resolved, in part, by the development of new and better methods of intrauterine intervention, both medically and surgically (Fletcher 1983a; Walters 1986a; Annas and Elias 1990). However, some conditions that are detectable prenatally may never be amenable to corrective treatment.

HUMAN GENE THERAPY AND GENETIC ENGINEERING

Types of Genetic Intervention

Four major kinds of genetic intervention in humans may one day become technically feasible. These types of possible intervention can be represented schematically (Table 8.1). The first type of genetic intervention would aim to cure a condition that is generally acknowledged to be a disease by genetically altering the nonreproductive cells of a patient. For example, if the bone-marrow cells of a patient suffering from sickle-cell anemia were able to be treated, the patient would be cured of the disease. However, this cure would not be transmitted to the patient's descendants. In the second type of genetic intervention, both somatic (nonreproductive) and reproductive cells would be treated; thus, the changes of the genetic cure would be passed on to the patient's descendants. (Depending on the type of genetic alteration and the stage of development at which it was performed, it is possible that disease would be prevented in only some of the patient's descendants.)

The distinction between cure or prevention of disease and enhancement of capabilities may not always be clear. However, a plausible example of enhancement would be doubling the efficiency of an individual's long-term memory. If this enhancement were based on somatic-cell alterations, one would have the third type of genetic intervention. If the enhancement also affected the reproductive cells of the subject—who would perhaps not be called a patient—improved long-term-memory efficiency would also be passed on to at least some of the subject's descendants. This germ-line enhancement of a human capability would be an example of the fourth type of genetic intervention.

The first type 1 gene therapy study performed in the United States was initiated in September 1990. The target disease in this pioneering study was severe combined immune deficiency—a condition in which both major components of the immune system are incapacitated. Children afflicted with this rare, single-gene disorder often die of infections before reaching the age of 2 years. David, the so-called bubble boy in Houston, Texas, suffered from a variant of this devastating disease (Drummond 1985).

In the initial gene-therapy study, researchers at the National Institutes of Health began by removing some of the white blood cells (T cells) from their pediatric patients through a procedure called plasmapheresis. They then employed a retroviral vector, or vehicle, to deliver copies of the properly

TABLE 8.1 Type of Genetic Intervention

	Somatic	Germ-Line
Cure or prevention of disease	1	2
Enhancement of capabilities	3	4

functioning gene into as many of the T cells as possible. There the gene began to function, producing the enzyme that was missing in the patients' bodies. The genetically modified cells were then returned to the patients' bodies in the hope that they would survive for at least several months and produce the enzyme that is essential for the functioning of the immune system. In the first two young women treated for severe combined immune deficiency by means of this technique, the therapeutic results have been quite dramatic (Anderson 1992; Culver 1993; Thompson 1994).

By late 1995, 99 additional gene therapy studies had been reviewed and approved in the United States. Similar studies have also been initiated in the United Kingdom, France, the Netherlands, Italy, and China (Anderson 1992). In about two-thirds of the U.S. studies, the target diseases have been cancers of various kinds. Other target diseases have included cystic fibrosis, HIV infection and AIDS, Gaucher's disease, and rheumatoid arthritis.

Type 2 genetic intervention, germ-line gene therapy, has not been attempted in human beings. However, researchers have been able to introduce genetic changes into the reproductive cells of laboratory animals by adding new DNA to early embryos of the animals. In studies involving mice, for example, genes have been added to one-cell mouse embryos after the sperm had penetrated the egg but before the genetic material from the sperm and egg had joined within the same nucleus. In successful experiments, the added genes are then incorporated into the embryo. As the embryo grows and the number of embryonic cells increases, the added genes become part of every new embryonic cell. Later, when the sperm or egg cells of the mouse develop, the added genes are included in approximately half of the reproductive cells. Thus, when the mouse reproduces, some of its progeny receive the added genes, and so on through the generations. Genetic defects have been corrected in the germ line in laboratory experiments with fruit flies and mice (Rubin and Spradling 1982; Hammer et al. 1984; Costantini et al. 1986; Gordon 1990).

The closest approximation to enhancement studies in laboratory animals has been the attempt to produce very large mice by means of genetic intervention. In widely publicized studies, a team of researchers introduced the gene for either rat growth hormone or human growth hormone into one-cell mouse embryos. A small fraction of the embryos developed to maturity; some of the mature mice expressed the added gene and, as a result, grew to be significantly larger than their siblings. Several offspring of these "supermice" were also abnormally large—thus demonstrating that the genetic change had indeed been transmitted through the germ line (Palmiter et al. 1982, 1983).

Ethical and Public-Policy Questions

For the short-term future, only somatic-cell gene therapy for the cure of disease—type 1 gene therapy—will be proposed for use with human patients. Because the changes effected through somatic-cell gene therapy will not be passed on to future generations, many commentators think that this technique will not be qualitatively different from other biomedical innovations, such as kidney transplants (U.S. Office of Technology Assessment 1984, 1, 7, 28; U.S. President's Commission 1982, 45, 61).

The major ethical questions surrounding type 1 gene therapy parallel those raised about any biomedical innovation. In a document entitled "Points to Consider," the National Institites of Health (NIH) committee that reviews gene therapy proposals in the United States raised seven central questions (U.S. NIH 1994):

1. What is the disease to be treated, and why is it a good candidate for gene therapy?
2. What alternative treatments are available?
3. What are the major potential harms that could be caused by the intervention?
4. What are the major potential benefits of the intervention?
5. If more patients apply to participate in a gene therapy study than can be enrolled, how will fairness be achieved in the selection process?
6. How will researchers seek to ensure that participants in the gene therapy study give consent that is both informed and voluntary?
7. How will the privacy and confidentiality of patients be protected?

A special public-review process for somatic-cell gene therapy has been established in the United States. After a gene-therapy proposal has been reviewed and approved by an institution's local research-review committee (often called an *institutional review board*), the proposal is forwarded to the Recombinant DNA Advisory Committee at NIH. If the committee approves the proposal, it is forwarded to the NIH Director for final approval. Thus, for publicly funded research, everyone interested in the topic of gene therapy is able to know about the researchers, the institution, and the disease to be treated before gene therapy is performed (Walters 1986b, 226; Walters 1991).

Type 2 gene therapy—germ-line gene therapy for the cure of disease—may raise qualitatively new kinds of ethical questions because the genetic alterations performed in this case are likely to be passed on to at least some of the subject's descendants (Fletcher 1983b; Fowler et al. 1989; Juengst 1991). As noted above, the germ-line approach to the treatment and prevention of disease in fruit flies and mice is modestly successful in some laboratory experiments. Why would germ-line gene therapy be proposed for the cure or prevention of human disease? One rationale might be that the cells in some parts of the body can be reached and effectively treated only if gene therapy is administered very early, probably at the embryonic stage of development. For example, certain diseases of the brain may fall into this category (U.S. Office of Technology Assessment 1984, 24). In an experiment aimed at treating otherwise-unreachable brain cells, the researcher's primary intention would no doubt be to prevent the brain-based disease from occurring in the future person; a side effect of the early intervention would be to produce a genetic alteration in the reproductive cells of the future person, as well.

A second possible rationale for the germ-line approach is the argument from efficiency. Correcting a defect once, through germ-line therapy, and having the correction passed on to the subject's descendants might seem more reasonable than repeating somatic-cell gene therapy generation after generation in a family afflicted by a genetic disease. However, given the current method of gene addition as the likely means of performing gene therapy, only some of the subject's descendants would receive the properly functioning added gene; others would receive the malfunctioning gene. Only if a technique for *replacing* malfunctioning genes with properly functioning genes is developed will germ-line gene therapy have the desired effect of eliminating a genetic disease from a particular family line.

The major current obstacles to germ-line gene therapy through, for example, the treatment of early human embryos, are technical rather than ethical. One technical obstacle is that the large majority of mouse embryos into which added DNA is microinjected do not survive the injection procedure, do not implant, do not survive because of a new lethal mutation, or do not express the added gene or genes. Further, if one were thinking of therapeutic interventions with human embryos at the time of fertilization, one would not usually know whether a particular embryo were destined to be afflicted with a genetic disease. For example, in a case in which both parents are carriers of a recessive genetic trait, any embryo produced by those parents has a 25 percent chance of being completely unaffected, a 50 percent chance of being a carrier of the genetic trait, and a 25 percent chance of having the genetic disease. In other words, any given embryo of those parents has a 75 percent chance of *not having* the genetic disease— poor odds for early genetic intervention, especially if the intervention has a moderate or high probability of harming embryos that would otherwise not manifest the disease.

A possible alternative to genetic intervention with early human embryos has been employed since 1990, namely, preimplantation genetic testing or screening. With this method, a cell is removed from a 4- or 8-cell embryo, or even a later embryo (a blastocyst) for diagnostic purposes. The remaining cells of the embryo are frozen and stored. Various genetic tests are then run on the amplified DNA of the removed cells. If the results of the test show an embryo to be free of the genetic disease about which the potential parents were concerned, the remainder of the embryo that has been frozen is thawed at the appropriate time and transferred to the uterus of the wife. If the diagnostic tests indicate that an embryo will develop the genetic disease in the future, the embryo will probably not be transferred but will, instead, be discarded.

It is possible that ways to overcome the current technical obstacles to germ-line therapy will be found, and that safe and effective ways to repair either sperm or egg cells or early embryonic cells will be developed. In that case, germ-line genetic intervention for the prevention of genetic disease in some or all of one's descendants will become technically feasible. We will then have to face the question of deciding whether we ought to do what we now can do (Wivel and Walters 1993). Although the action of intervening in a way that intentionally and directly affects multiple future generations is momentous, it is difficult to see why this type of preventive strategy should not at least be considered. Reducing the probability that a couple will pass on genetic problems to their descendants—assuming that the couple freely consents to the intervention—could provide benefits to the couple, to their descendants, and to society as a whole.

The question of enhancing human characteristics, whether by somatic-cell or germ-line intervention, is surely controversial. Many commentators on gene therapy and genetic engineering have argued that the negative quest to cure or prevent disease, even through the germ line, is ethically acceptable, but that attempts to improve the capabilities of human beings by genetic means are ethically unacceptable (Anderson 1989). These commentators would presumably not be opposed to attempts by an individual to improve him- or herself (or his or her children) through good diet, adequate exercise, and advanced training. Objection is registered specifically to genetic modes of improvement.

Several specific arguments have been raised against the genetic enhancement of human beings. One is that such an endeavor is a manifestation of hubris, or, in religious language, an attempt to play God. A second objection is that such a program would inevitably lead to *eugenics*, an attempt by society or the state to coerce everyone to participate in the genetic improvement program. A third objection is that such a program would be utopian; it would seek to develop a perfect human being or a perfect society. A final objection is that different cultures have different ideals and that therefore human beings would not be able to agree on which traits are better or worse for human beings.

The most provocative and sustained philosophical defense of human enhancement by genetic means is presented in Jonathan Glover's book, *What Sort of People Should There Be?* Glover proposes a voluntary program of genetic improvement that could be freely accepted or rejected by parents (1984, 29). He argues that such a program need not be utopian; it would simply aim for modest improvements in human capabilities, one family at a time (1984, 185). There are two respects, in particular, in which human beings seem to Glover to be a good candidates for improvement: intellectual ability and moral character. On the intellectual front, Glover believes that enhancement might produce not simply a boost in IQ but also the capacity to think in new ways (1984, 180). In the ethical sphere, Glover notes our emotional and imaginative limitations, as well as the restricted range of our sympathies. In his view, humans have, in some respects, retained a tribal ethic while achieving great feats technologically, especially in the military sphere (1984, 181–84; Muller 1959).

The types of genetic enhancements that Glover envisions may never be technically feasible. If so, we and our descendants will never face momentous choices about the kinds of persons we wish to be, genetically speaking. On the other hand, the new science of gene mapping and gene sequencing may lead to breathtaking and unanticipated possibilities of the kind Glover describes. It may therefore be prudent to consider the technological possibilities and their potential social impact well before they are upon us.

DISCUSSION QUESTIONS

1. Should human characteristics be enhanced by genetic means if such a technique becomes possible?

2. Does it make any moral difference whether genetic changes are made in somatic or germ-line cells?

3. Should couples be free to use prenatal genetic diagnosis and abortion to assess and terminate pregnancy in cases in which fetuses have characteristics of which the couple disapproves? Does this include minor medical problems? Sickle-cell trait? XYY syndrome? A fetus of a sex not desired by the couple?

4. What are the moral differences between the use of reproductive technologies such as assisted insemination and in vitro fertilization within a marriage and outside a marriage? Should persons have the liberty to produce pregnancies involving third parties? What is the moral difference, if any, between assisted insemination by donor and surrogate motherhood? Do these procedures unfairly or coercively induce lower-income persons to contribute to reproduction for the sake of other persons?

5. How do the new reproductive technologies challenge the traditional notion of the family? What other social developments are also calling the family into question? What are the advantages and disadvantages of nontraditional families?

REFERENCES

American College of Obstetricians and Gynecologists Committee on Ethics. *Ethical Issues in Surrogate Motherhood*. Washington, DC: American College of Obstetricians and Gynecologists, November 1990.

———. *Ethical Issues in Human In Vitro Fertilization and Embryo Placement*. Washington, DC: American College of Obstetricians and Gynecologists, July 1986.

American Fertility Society, Ethics Committee. "Ethical Considerations of the New Reproductive Technologies." *Fertil Steril* 62(Suppl. 1) (1994): i–125S.

Anderson, W. French. "Human Gene Therapy: Why Draw a Line?" *J Med Philos* 14 (1989): 681–693.

———. "Human Gene Therapy." *Science* 256 (1992): 808–813.

Andrews, Lori B. *New Conceptions: A Consumer's Guide to the Newest Infertility Treatments*. New York: Ballantine Books, 1985a.

———. *State Laws and Regulations Governing Newborn Screening*. Chicago: American Bar Foundation, 1985b.

Annas, George J. "Using Genes to Define Motherhood—the California Solution." *N Engl J Med* 326 (1992): 417–420.

Annas, George J., Elias, Sherman. "Legal and Ethical Implications of Fetal Diagnosis and Gene Therapy." *Am J Med Genet* 35 (1990): 215–218.

Antenatal Diagnosis: Report of a Consensus Development Conference Sponsored by the National Institutes of Health and Human Development. Bethesda, MD: National Institutes of Health, December 1979.

California Department of Health Services, Genetic Disease Branch. *The California Alpha Fetoprotein Screening Program*. Berkeley: Genetic Disease Branch, 1994.

California Supreme Court in Bankruptcy. *Johnson v. Calvert*. Decided May 20, 1993. *P Rep*, 2d Series, 851: 776–801.

Callahan, Daniel. "New Beginnings in Life: A Philosopher's Response." In Michael Hamilton, Ed., *The New Genetics and the Future of Man*, Grand Rapids, MI: Eerdmans, 1972: 90–106.

Canada, Royal Commission on New Reproductive Technologies. *Proceed with Care: Final Report* (2 vols.). Ottawa: Minister of Government Services Canada, 1993.

Cao, Antonio. "The Prevention of Thalassemia in Sardinia." *Clin Genet* 36 (1989): 277–285.

Capron, Alexander Morgan, Radin, Margaret Jane. "Choosing Family Law over Contract Law as a Paradigm for Surrogate Motherhood." *Law Med Health Care* 16 (1988): 34–43.

Catholic Church, Congregation for the Doctrine of the Faith. *Instruction on Respect for Human Life in Its Origins and on the Dignity of Procreation*. Rome: The Congregation, 1987.

Chard, T. "Frequency of Implantation and Early Pregnancy Loss in Natural Cycles." *Baillieres Clin Obstet Gynaecol* 5 (1991): 179–189.

Collins, Francis. "Cystic Fibrosis: Molecular Biology and Therapeutic Implications." *Science* 256 (1992): 774–779.

Cooperative Human Linkage Center. "A Comprehensive Human Linkage Map with Centimorgan Density." *Science* 265 (1994): 2049–2054.

Corea, Gena. *The Mother Machine: From Artificial Insemination to Artificial Wombs*. New York: Harper & Row, 1985.

Costantini, Frank, Chanda, Kiran, Magram, Jeanne. "Correction of Murine Beta-Thalassemia by Gene Transfer into the Germ Line." *Science* 223 (1986): 1192–1194.

Cox, David R., et al. "Assessing Mapping Progress in the Human Genome Project." *Science* 265 (1994): 2031–2032.

Culver, Kenneth W. "Splice of Life: Genetic Therapy Comes of Age." *Science* 33 (1993): 18–24.

Daniels, Norman. *Just Health Care*. New York: Cambridge University Press, 1985.

Delvin, Patrick. *The Enforcement of Morals*. New York: Oxford University Press, 1965.

Drummond, Rennie. "Bubble Boy" [Editorial]. *JAMA* 253 (1985): 78–80.

Faden, Ruth, et al. "A Survey to Evaluate Parental Consent as Public Policy for Neonatal Screening." *Am J Public Health* 72 (1982): 1347–1352.

Feinberg, Joel. *Social Philosophy*. Englewood Cliffs, NJ: Prentice Hall, 1973.

Fletcher, John C. "Emerging Ethical Issues in Fetal Therapy." In Kare Berg and Knut Erik Tranøy, Eds., *Research Ethics*. New York: Alan R. Liss, 1983a: 293–318.

———. "Moral Problems and Ethical Issues in Prospective Human Gene Therapy." *Va L Rev* 69 (1983b): 515–546.

Fletcher, Joseph. *The Ethics of Genetic Control: Ending Reproductive Roulette*. Garden City, NY: Anchor Press/Doubleday, 1974.

Fowler, Gregory, Juengst, Eric T., Zimmerman, Burke K. "Germ-Line Gene Therapy and the Clinical Ethos of Medical Genetics." *Theoretical Med* 10 (1989): 151–165.

Glover, Jonathan. *What Sort of People Should There Be? Genetic Engineering, Brain Control and Their Impact on our Future World*. New York: Penguin Books, 1984.

Gordon, Jon W. "Micromanipulation of Embryos and Germ Cells: An Approach to Gene Therapy." *Am J Med Genet* 35 (1990): 206–214.

Haddow, James E., et al. "Prenatal Screening for Down's Syndrome with Use of Maternal Serum Markers." *N Engl J Med* 327 (1992): 588–593.

Hammer, Robert E., Palmiter, Richard D., Brinster, Ralph L. "Partial Correction of Murine Hereditary Growth Disorder by Germ-Line Incorporation of a New Gene." *Nature* 311 (1984): 65–67.

Handyside, Alan H., Lesko, John G., Tarín, Juan J., et al. "Birth of a Normal Girl after In Vitro Fertilization and Preimplantation Diagnostic Testing for Cystic Fibrosis." *N Engl J Med* 327 (1992): 905–909.

Handyside, A. H., Kontogianni, E. H., Hardy, K., Winston, R. M. L. "Pregnancies from Biopsied Human Preimplantation Embryos Sexed by Y-Specific DNA Amplification." *Nature* 344 (1990): 768–770.

Hauerwas, Stanley. *Suffering Presence: Theological Reflections on Medicine, the Mentally Handicapped, and the Church*. Notre Dame, IN: University of Notre Dame Press, 1986.

Huntington Disease Collaborative Research Group. "A Novel Gene Containing a Trinucleotide Repeat That Is Expanded and Unstable on Huntington's Disease Chromosomes." *Cell* 72 (1993): 971–983.

Institute of Medicine, Committee on Assessing Genetic Risks. In Lori B. Andrews, Jane E. Fullarton, Neil A. Holtzman, and Arno G. Motulsky, Eds., *Assessing Genetic Risks: Implications for Health and Social Policy.* Washington, DC: National Academy Press, 1994.

Juengst, Eric T., Ed. "Human Germ-Line Engineering." *J Med Philos* 16 (1991): 587–694.

Kass, Leon R. "Making Babies—The New Biology and the 'Old' Morality." *Public Interest* 26 (1972): 18–56.

Keane, Noel P., Breo, Dennis L. *The Surrogate Mother*. New York: Dodd, Mead, 1981.

King, Patricia L. "Reproductive Technologies." In *BioLaw: A Legal and Ethical Reporter on Medicine, Health Care, and Bioengineering Resource Manual.* Frederick, MD: University Publications of America, 1986: 113–148.

Knoppers, Martha Maria, Chadwick, Ruth. "The Human Genome Project: Under an International Ethical Microscope." *Science* 265 (1994): 2035–2036.

Leridon, H. "Démographie des échecs de la reproduction." In André Boué and Charles Thibault, Eds., *Les Accidents Chromosomiques de la Reproduction.* Paris: Centre International de l'Enfance, 1973: 13–27.

McCormick, Richard A. "Reproductive Technologies: Ethical Issues." In Warren T. Reich, Ed., *Encyclopedia of Bioethics.* New York: Free Press/Macmillan, 1978: 1454–1464.

———. "Therapy or Tampering? The Ethics of Reproductive Technology." *America* 153 (1985): 396–403.

McKusick, Victor A. *Mendelian Inheritance in Man: Catalogs of Autosomal Dominant, Autosomal Recessive, and X-Linked Phenotypes*, 10th ed. Baltimore: Johns Hopkins University Press, 1992.

Motulsky, Arno G., Murray, Jeffry. "Will Prenatal Diagnosis with Selective Abortion Affect Society's Attitude Toward the Handicapped?" In Kare Berg and Knut Erik Tranøy, Eds., *Research Ethics.* New York: Alan R. Liss, 1983: 277–291.

Muller, Hermann J. "The Guidance of Human Evolution." *Perspect Biol Med* 3 (1959): 1–43.

National Academy of Sciences and Institute of Medicine. *Confronting AIDS: Directions for Public Health, Health Care, Research.* Washington, DC: National Academy Press, 1986.

Ontario Law Reform Commission. *Report on Human Artificial Reproduction and Related Matters.* Toronto: Ministry of the Attorney General, 1985.

Palmiter, Richard D., Brinster, Ralph L., Hammer, Robert E., et al. "Dramatic Growth of Mice That Develop from Eggs Microinjected with Metallothionein-Growth Hormone Fusion Genes." *Nature* 300 (1982): 611–615.

Palmiter, Richard D., Norstedt, Gunnar, Gelinas, Richard E., et al. "Metallothionein-Human GH Fusion Genes Stimulate Growth of Mice." *Science* 222 (1983): 809–814.

Pius XII. 1956. "Address of His Holiness, Pope Pius XII, to the Second World Congress on Fertility and Sterility." In G. Tesauro, Ed., *Proceedings of the Second World*

Congress on Fertility and Sterility. Naples, Italy, May 18–26, 1956. Naples: Institute of Clinical Obstetrics and Gynecology, University of Naples, 1957–1958: 38–46.

Press, Nancy Anne, Browner, C. H. "'Collective Fictions': Similarities in Reasons for Accepting Maternal Serum Alpha-Fetoprotein Screening among Women of Diverse Ethnic and Social Class Backgrounds." *Fetal Diagn Ther* 8(Suppl. 1) (1993): 97–106.

Ramsey, Paul. *Fabricated Man: The Ethics of Genetic Control*. New Haven: Yale University Press, 1970.

Rawls, John. *A Theory of Justice*. Cambridge: Belknap, 1973.

Robertson, John A. *Children of Choice: Freedom and the New Reproductive Technologies*. Princeton: Princeton University Press, 1994.

———. "Embryo Research." *Univ West Ont L Rev* 24 (1986): 15–37.

Rubin, Gerald M., Spradling, Allan C. "Genetic Transformation of *Drosophila* with Transposable Element Vectors." *Science* 218 (1982): 348–353.

Sellar, Jeffrey. "Australian IVF: Orphan Embryos." *Nature* 309 (1984): 738.

Simpson, Joe Leigh, Carson, Sandra Ann. "Preimplantation Genetic Diagnosis" [Editorial]. *N Engl J Med* 327 (1992): 951–953.

Steinbrook, Robert. "In California, Voluntary Mass Prenatal Screening." *Hastings Cent Rep* 16 (Oct. 1986): 5–7.

Stewart, G. J., Tyler, J. P. P., Cunningham, A. L., et al. "Transmission of Human T-Cell Lymphotropic Virus Type III (HTLV-III) by Artificial Insemination by Donor." *Lancet* 2 (1985): 581–584.

Tennessee Supreme Court at Knoxville. *Davis v. Davis*. Decided June 1, 1992. *S W Rep*, 2d Series, 842: 588–604.

Thompson, Larry. *Correcting the Code: Inventing the Genetic Cure for the Human Body*. New York: Simon & Schuster, 1994.

Townes, Philip L. "Newborn Screening: A Potpourri of Policies" [Editorial]. *Am J Public Health* 76 (1986): 1191–1192.

United Kingdom Collaborative Study on Alpha-Fetoprotein in Relation to Neural Tube Defects. "Maternal Serum Alpha-Fetoprotein Measurement in Antenatal Screening for Anencephaly and Spina Bifida in Early Pregnancy." *Lancet* 1 (1977): 1323–1332.

United Kingdom, Department of Health and Social Security. *Report of the Committee of Inquiry into Human Fertilisation and Embryology*. London: Her Majesty's Stationery Office, July 1984.

U.S. Office of Technology Assessment. *Artificial Insemination: Practice in the United States*. Washington, DC: Office of Technology Assessment, August 1988a.

———. *Cystic Fibrosis and DNA Tests: Implications of Carrier Screening*. Washington, DC: Office of Technology Assessment, August 1992a.

———. *Human Gene Therapy: Background Paper*. Washington, DC: Office of Technology Assessment, December 1984.

———. *Infertility: Medical and Social Choices*. Washington, DC: Office of Technology Assessment, May 1988b.

———. *Genetic Tests and Health Insurance: Results of a Survey—Background Paper*. Washington, DC: Office of Technology Assessment, October 1992b.

U.S. Department of Health, Education, and Welfare, Ethics Advisory Board. *HEW Support of Research Involving Human in Vitro Fertilization and Embryo Transfer*. Washington, DC: Department of Health, Education, and Welfare, May 1979.

U.S. National Institutes of Health, Human Embryo Research Panel. *Report*. Bethesda, MD: National Institutes of Health, September 27, 1994.

U.S. National Institutes of Health, Recombinant DNA Advisory Committee. "Points to Consider in the Design and Submission of Protocols for the Transfer of Recombinant DNA into the Genome of One or More Human Subjects." *Federal Register* 59 (1994): 34528–34534, 40169–40174.

U.S. National Institutes of Health and Department of Energy, Task Force on Genetic Information and Health Insurance. *Genetic Information and Health Insurance*. Bethesda, MD: National Center for Human Genome Research, May 1993.

U.S. President's Commission for the Study of Ethical Problems in Medicine and Biomedical and Behavioral Research. *Screening and Counseling for Genetic Conditions*. Washington, DC: Government Printing Office, February 1983.

———. *Splicing Life: The Social and Ethical Issues of Genetic Engineering with Human Beings*. Washington, DC: Government Printing Office, November 1982.

Utian, Wulf H., Sheean, Leon, Goldfarb, James M., Kiwi, Robert. "Successful Pregnancy after In Vitro Fertilization and Embryo Transfer from an Infertile Woman to a Surrogate." *N Engl J Med* 313 (1985): 1351–1352.

Victoria, Australia, Committee to Consider the Social, Ethical, and Legal Issues Arising from In Vitro Fertilization. *Report on the Disposition of Embryos Produced by In Vitro Fertilization*. Melbourne: F. D. Atkinson Government Printer, August 1984.

Walters, LeRoy. "Ethical Issues in Intrauterine Diagnosis and Therapy." *Fetal Ther* 1 (1986a): 32–37.

———. "The Ethics of Human Gene Therapy." *Nature* 320 (1986b): 225–227.

———. "Human Gene Therapy: Ethics and Public Policy." *Hum Gene Ther* 2 (1991): 115–122.

Wertz, Dorothy C., Fletcher, John C., Eds. *Ethics and Human Genetics: A Cross-Cultural Perspective*. New York: Springer-Verlag, 1989.

Wivel, Nelson A., Walters, LeRoy. "Germ-Line Gene Modification and Disease Prevention: Some Medical and Ethical Perspectives." *Science* 262 (1993): 533–538.

9

Ethical Issues
in Organ Transplantation

ALBERT R. JONSEN

SUMMARY

Organ transplantation poses serious moral questions about the intrinsic morality of transplantation, the determination of the death of the source of a cadaveric organ, the right of persons to donate their own organs, the selection of recipients for scarce organs, and the procurement and allocation of organs as a scarce social resource.

Some people question the intrinsic morality of organ transplantation. Does a person have the right to give up, for any reason, an important bodily part? Is it morally legitimate to remove a vital organ from one person and place the organ in another person's body? Is it morally right for a donor to consent to the deliberate excision of an important bodily part? Particular features of the Roman Catholic and Judaic faiths, such as whether there is an ethical duty to risk one's own life or well-being for the benefit of another, are relevant to the morality of organ transplantation.

Regarding the procurement of organs, the first issue is the need for free and informed consent. Another is the determination of death. When does death really occur, legally and medically? Although death was once determined on the basis of heart–lung criteria, it now is based on brain-death criteria. The shift has important implications for the supply of organs.

Several factors determine the size of the organ pool. Ethical and policy issues surround each factor. This chapter reviews proposals to increase the organ supply. Because determining who should receive scarce organs is often difficult, approaches for determining the recipients of organs are discussed. Some ethical problems that arise as medical technology constantly approaches new frontiers are also discussed.

On December 3, 1967, in the Schur Groot Hospital, Capetown, South Africa, Dr. Christiaan Barnard transplanted a living heart from the thoracic cavity of a presumably dead person into the chest of a patient suffering from end-stage cardiac disease. That patient lived for 18 days. Again, on January 2, 1968, Barnard attempted the same procedure to save the life of Dr. Philip Blaiberg, who lived 18 months. These events, heralded as "the miracle of Capetown," ushered in the age of transplantation. It can be said, with only slight exaggeration, that the same events ushered in the age of bioethics. Discussion of bioethical problems stimulated by the allocation of renal dialysis, by abortion, and by advances in genetics took place with some intensity for several years. But the first transplantation of a human heart focused the attention of the world and of scholars on the science and practice of organ transplant and the ethical problems that immediately came to mind (Wolstenholme and O'Connor 1968).

The public fascination with the sight of one human being kept alive by the heart of another and the scientific curiosity over the problem of immunological rejection of foreign tissue did much to focus attention on the miracle of Capetown. But public and scientific interest are not enough to create an ethical problem. There was something in organ transplantation that seemed to sound the depths of human ethical concern. That depth—the fundamental question of ethics—is the question of the nature and degree of one human person's obligation to another. In all transplantation of major organs between individuals of the same species, a part of one person is useful for the survival of another. Whether the source of the organ is a person who died, as it always is for heart transplantation, or whether the one who grants an organ is a living donor, as is often the case with renal transplantation, the question can be asked, Does one human owe this to another? This echoes the ancient question, Am I my brother's keeper? The conjunction between an extraordinary medical technology and a profound ethical question stimulated the questions and answers that comprise the new complex discipline of bioethics. In a certain sense, the question lies at the heart of all bioethical questions about all forms of technology and medicine.

Organ transplantation began in 1954 at Boston's Peter Bent Brigham Hospital when a surgical team, led by Dr. Joseph Murray (awarded the Nobel Prize in 1990), performed the first successful kidney transplant. The principal medical obstacle to transplantation is the human immunological system—it rejects foreign tissue. Great strides in understanding immunological rejection and in its medical manipulation have broken through, although not eliminated, that barrier. The result has been a notable expansion of major organ transplantation. Kidneys began the expansion, followed by hearts, lungs, pancreases, livers, and bowel as well as various combinations such as heart–lung, pancreas–kidney, liver–bowel, and heart–liver–kidney. Great progress also has been made in transplanting bone marrow for a wide range of diseases.

Success rates for transplantation, recorded in terms of graft survival and patient survival and also in terms of quality of life, vary from organ to organ. According to data from 1991, the 2-year survival rate for living-donor recipients of kidneys was 95.6 percent and for cadaveric kidney recipients was 90 percent; graft survival for the first group was 87 percent and for the second 72.8 percent. Of the best candidates for liver transplant, that is, those who were healthy enough to be working full-time when their transplant occurred, 85.7 percent survived for as long as 2 years; of the worst candidates, those in intensive care, 54.6 percent survived for as long as 2 years.

The best results for heart transplantation were found in recipients between the ages of 19 years and 44 years—80.5 percent survive for 2 years; the poorest results were for children up to age 5, of whom 64 percent survived as long as 2 years. The graft survival rate for pancreas recipients was 65.2 percent for 2 years, but these patients can be supported by exogenous insulin after graft failure, just as kidney graft failure can be countered by dialysis. Results were better for simultaneous kidney–pancreas transplants: 71.6 percent survived for 2 years. The graft survival rate for lung transplantation was 65.8 percent at 1 year, but patients are often retransplanted after graft failure. The heart–lung transplant survival rate, both for grafts and for patients, was 55 percent at 1 year.

Behind these simplified statistics lie many complications. Many recipients who reach the 2-year survival statistic live many years; others suffer late rejections or die prematurely from an underlying disease that required the transplant but was not cured by it. Quality of life may vary greatly for the survivors and varies according to type of transplant. Some recipients live an almost ordinary life, others are plagued by incessant disability. The age and gender of patients, the stage of their illnesses, and their ethnic origin often affect outcomes. The survival rate for black renal recipients, by 1991 data, was 66 percent—8.6 percent lower than the survival rate for whites; similar gaps exist for liver and heart recipients. Asian recipients of livers had poor outcomes.

Certain procedures, particularly the cluster transplants and visceral transplants, remain experimental, but the others have passed into the category of common and accepted medical practice. Between 1988 and 1991, the total number of organ transplants increased by 26 percent, from 12,784 to 16,053. Of these transplants, approximately 10,000 were kidney transplants, 3000 were liver transplants, 2000 were heart transplants, 500 were pancreas transplants, 400 were lung transplants, and 50 were heart–lung transplants (United Network for Organ Sharing 1993).

Thus, organ transplantation is well established. Its science will progress and, in all probability, will show greater prospects for success and will prompt greater boldness. In what sense does this medical and surgical accomplishment raise ethical problems more specific than the general question, What does one human being owe another? Are there special questions associated with the expansion of organ transplantation into a common and accepted medical practice? Are there special questions attendant on particular forms of transplantation? This chapter reviews these issues and the opinions of scholars about them: the intrinsic morality of transplantation, the determination of the death of the source of a cadaveric organ, the right of persons to donate their own organs, the selection of recipients for scarce organs, and the procurement and allocation of organs as a scarce social resource.

THE INTRINSIC MORALITY OF ORGAN TRANSPLANTATION

Is it morally legitimate to remove a vital organ from one person and place it in another's body? The answer seems obvious. Certainly it is moral to do so if the donor consents or if the source of the organ is one who has died. Certainly it is moral if the recipient needs the organ for continued life. However, on closer inspection, the "obvious" answers are not so obvious—each of them has given rise to much debate. Is it morally right for the donor to consent to the deliberate excision of an important bodily part? What does it mean to say that a person is dead, and, morally, what can be done to a dead body? Does a person in need of an organ have any moral claim on the organs of another? Whose moral claims take priority when there are more needy persons than there are available organs? The discussion of these questions and their reasonable resolution constitutes the ethics of organ transplantation.

The most fundamental moral question asks whether a person has the right to give up, for any purpose, an important bodily part. This is an ancient question, raised long before organ transplantation was possible: Do persons have the moral authority to mutilate their bodies, that is, to separate from themselves a part or organ that is a natural, constitutive part? Roman Catholicism and Judaism have long forbidden self-mutilation. A person is only the steward of his or her body; dominion over the body is God's purview. Mutilation is morally justified only if it will contribute to the well-being of the person whose body is mutilated. Thus, removal of a diseased limb to save one's life is permissible.

The advent of successful corneal transplant called for refinement of these traditional positions. In both faiths, the predominant opinion at present allows that the removal of an organ for immediate and genuine benefit of another person should not be considered a reprehensible self-mutilation—indeed, it is an act of charity. However, this position envisages that the removal of the organ will not cause serious detriment to the donor; certainly, it would not be tolerated if the removal of the organ precipitated the donor's certain death. Thus, donating one's heart while one was still living would be forbidden and condemned as suicide (Kelly 1956; Rosner 1979).

Although Roman Catholicism and Judaism condemn a donation that would be tantamount to suicide, could not an argument in support of such an act be constructed in secular ethics? Contemporary secular ethicists rarely argue against suicide. Further, would not a suicide that benefits another seem praiseworthy? In fact, several cardiac transplant centers have reported such offers. Arguments against such a practice would have to rely on the possibility of coercion and inducement that would undermine the presumption of free consent. Also, the reaction of the living recipient to being alive as the result of another's deliberate death might be devastating. Thus, donation of an organ that would directly lead to the death of the donor would seem ethically unacceptable.

Thus, the ethics of donation in the Roman Catholic and Jewish traditions seems sound. Persons are morally justified in giving up a bodily part for the benefit of another, but they cannot do so if that donation would directly lead to their own death or serious physical detriment. Thus, the donation of a kidney, of a cornea, of bone marrow, is morally acceptable. However, the problem is more complicated. The donor should make the donation responsibly, that is, with an understanding of what donation entails and with free consent (informed consent). From the earliest days of organ transplantation, it has been recognized that informed consent poses a particularly difficult ethical problem.

Because the body rejects tissue that its immunological system does not recognize, the most successful transplants are those between persons who are genetically related. Given this biological phenomenon, the social and psychological pressure to donate an organ to a close relative can be extreme, even to the point of coercion. An honest effort must be made to relieve the pressure that may come from a concerned family; however, it is difficult to relieve the internal compulsion that arises from a sense of duty to save one's relative. There is, of course, a difference between a sense of duty and actual duty.

Here a second ethical question, almost the opposite of the problem of mutilation, arises, Is there an ethical duty to risk one's own well-being to contribute to the well-being of another? Again, this ethical question antedates transplantation; the Catholic and Jewish traditions have long debated the problem in other contexts. Their answer is a qualified "yes"; such a duty does exist and its stringency depends on the degree of affinity to the one in need, on the seriousness of the need and of the risk that must be taken, and on the likelihood that the helping action will really help.

This sort of duty has generally been identified as an obligation in charity, rather than a duty in justice. Its force is less strict, that is, certain circumstances can be exempt from it and the recipient has no right to demand its fulfillment. Thus, donation of bone marrow, which poses little risk to the donor, imposes a greater, but not absolute, obligation on a potential donor. The higher likelihood of failure of this sort of therapy might justify a refusal to undergo even the lesser risk. On the other hand, the greater possibility that a renal transplant might succeed would place on the potential donor an obligation to undergo the greater risk of contributing a kidney.

To many people, the traditional approach to the morality of altruistic action seems more reasonable than a utilitarian approach in which one's moral obligation is dictated by the "greater good of the greater number." The latter approach seems to lead to the absurd conclusion that, since the two kidneys of one person could save the lives of two persons in need, the first person has a utilitarian duty to sacrifice both kidneys. Critics of utilitarianism point out that such a doctrine would oblige persons to make extreme sacrifices for the greater good; defenders of utilitarianism have countered that the existence of rules favoring one's own welfare and absolving one from continual and excessive sacrifice are sufficient to preserve the greater good.

Even if a qualified moral duty to donate can be established, such a duty has not been recognized by the law. The effort of a person in need of a bone marrow transplant to force his cousin, who was the most compatible donor, to contribute was rejected by the court. The court noted that, although it found the cousin's refusal to undergo the minor risks of bone-marrow aspiration morally reprehensible, the law's respect for the privacy of persons and their right over the integrity of their bodies could not be overcome by a duty of charity or supererogation (*McFall v. Shimp* 1979).

The free and informed consent of the donor is thus required, even if the donor has a moral duty, because a moral duty must be carried out—or rejected—by means of responsible decisions. In this respect, the use of minor children as donors for their siblings has posed a difficult problem. The first case that came to public notice involved a sibling who was retarded. The court approved the taking of the retarded brother's kidney only through the tortuous reasoning that the retarded child would himself be benefited by the continued life of his brother, to whom he was devoted. In so reasoning, the court upheld, though shakily, the principle that a person should not be put at risk unknowingly and unwillingly unless a benefit would accrue to the person himself (*Strunk v. Strunk* 1969).

In recent years, the practice of taking a kidney from a minor sibling has disappeared (fortunately, advances in immunosuppression have made the practice less necessary). At the same time, there seems to be little hesitation to take bone marrow from a minor, which is justified on the grounds that the risk is trivial. However, the invasion of the body of an unconsenting person is not justified by the smallness of the risk, but by the existence of a moral duty to benefit another. Some authors have argued that such a duty exists on the presumption that the child would consent if he or she were able to comprehend and choose. This is a controversial position (McCormick 1974; Ramsey 1976).

THE DETERMINATION OF DEATH

Organs can be removed from the body of a dead person and transplanted into the body of a living one. The procedure can be done for all major organs and must be done in cases in which the organ is essential for life; thus, hearts, livers, and lungs come from cadaver donors and kidneys and bone marrow can come from either living or cadaver donors. The removed organ must be viable, in the sense that it retains the biological properties that will enable it to function within the recipient. Thus, the body of the donor must still have some sort of vitality at the time of removal of the organ. At the same time, removal of the heart renders life impossible for the donor (unless another heart or artificial prosthesis is substituted).

Removal of a heart from a living human would appear to be homicide in the moral and legal understanding of that term. Yet removal of a heart from a cadaver in which the vital functions, particularly the perfusion of organs by oxygenated blood, have totally ceased provides an organ too damaged for transplantation. Thus, the first attempt to grapple with this problem, *A Definition of Irreversible Coma: Report of the Ad Hoc Committee of Harvard Medical School to Examine the Definition of Brain Death*, opened with the remark that their revision of the criteria for defining death was prompted by the belief that "obsolete criteria for definition of death can lead to controversy in obtaining organs for transplantation" (Ad Hoc Committee 1968).

Indeed, there was controversy; the medical ethics literature of the late 1960s and early 1970s is filled with it. During the several previous decades, it had become possible to maintain vital functions by mechanical support. At the same time, ability to diagnose extensive destruction of the brain had become sharper. Thus, the way out of the impasse appeared to be adoption of a new basis for determining death. The old basis had relied on clinical perception that heart and lungs had ceased to function because heart beat, pulse, and breathing had stopped. The new basis relied on the clinical perception, assisted by the technique of encephalography, that the activity of the brain had ceased. Thus, on the new basis, an individual might still have heart beat and respiration supported mechanically and, at the same time, be declared dead because no brain activity was detectable. From this point of view, partial death seemed possible—an individual was dead in the brain but was still living in the rest of the body. If medical practice adopted this approach and if the law could be brought to sanction it, vital organs could be removed from dead bodies.

This approach was filled with ambiguities. Yet, under pressure to clarify the legal status of cadaveric transplantation, states began to enact brain-death statutes to replace or supplement their "obsolete" cardiorespiratory statutes. Peculiar cases began to appear in the courts. Trauma services hesitated to cooperate with transplant services. Philosophers argued about the meaning of death. Medical practitioners were uncertain of the differences between total brain death and permanent coma or vegetative state. The media reflected the doctors' confusion. In 1978 the Congress of the United States created the President's Commission for the Study of Ethical Problems in Medicine and in Behavioral and Biomedical Research. The enabling legislation directed the Commission to study "the ethical and legal implications of the matter of defining death, including the advisability of developing a uniform definition of death" (Veatch 1976).

The Commission published its report, *Defining Death*, in July 1981. After an extensive review of the theological, philosophical, legal, and medical literature and wide consultation with experts and with the public, the Commission recommended that legal jurisdictions enact the following Uniform Determination of Death Act:

> An individual who has sustained either (1) irreversible cessation of circulatory and respiratory functions, or (2) irreversible cessation of all functions of the entire brain, including the brain stem, is dead. A determination of death must be made in accordance with accepted medical standards (President's Commission 1981, 2).

This formulation expressed the Commission's conclusion that death should be considered a unitary phenomenon that can be demonstrated either by the traditional grounds of irreversible cessation of heart and lung function or on the basis of irreversible loss of all functions of the entire brain. At this writing, 50 state legislatures have enacted the Commission's recommended Uniform Statute, either as new legislation, by amending earlier state statutes, or through case law. Thus, the ethical issue that plagued the first decade of organ transplantation has been resolved. In one state, New Jersey, the law contains an explicit exemption for persons whose religious beliefs are incompatible with the brain-oriented determination of death (New Jersey Advance Directives for Health Care and Declaration of Death Acts, November 1991).

Once the distinction between total brain death and persistent coma has been established in conceptual and clinical terms, the question can still be asked, Is it ethical to remove major organs from persons in persistent coma for purposes of transplantation? Presumably, if no ethical objection were raised to such a practice, legal authorization could be obtained by statute. In a widely noted article, "Harvesting the Dead," physician Willard Gaylin suggested that the proposed benefits would not surpass the costs in intangible effects on our sense of human dignity and respect; philosopher Hans Jonas vigorously dissented (Gaylin 1974; Jonas 1974). However, another philosopher, Rolston, argued against the "vivisection" of an irreversibly comatose person for purposes of transplantation. Rolston proposed that whatever is biologically vital has ethical value and that there is "an obligation to respect the body that is still fighting death" (Rolston 1982, 332).

The legal and ethical preference for the whole-brain criterion also eliminates the retrieval of organs from an anencephalic infant. At present, this supply of organs is generally considered beyond reach. Thus, the acceptance of the whole-brain criterion for determination of death had two effects—it legitimized the salvage of organs from the dead and, at the same time, restricted the supply of organs by rejecting salvage from irreversibly comatose persons. Thus, there is another ethical problem: the distribution of a scarce resource.

THE SUPPLY OF ORGANS

Human organs in their natural sites, the human body, are abundant, but they become a scarce resource for transplantation into another body. The first reason is that human tissue is suited peculiarly to the person in whom it originated—a person's immunological system powerfully rejects the insertion of foreign tissue. Other than the cornea of the eye and, to a lesser extent, bone, in which the vascular system that mediates the immune response is not involved, major organs are repudiated in a violent (often lethal) graft-versus-host or host-versus-graft disease by the body into which they are transplanted. Thus, organs are not simply interchangeable between human persons and, even less so, between humans and other species.

The first significant breach of the immunological barrier was the recognition that the immunological system is genetic. Identical twins share an identical immunological response and, thus, the organs of one twin are not rejected by the other twin. The first successful kidney transplant in 1954 transplanted a kidney from one identical twin to his brother. As the principles of immunology became clearer, immunological similarities less complete than those of identical twins provided an opening for transplantation. Similarities in tissue types are more frequent between blood relatives but can also be found among strangers. Thus, during the past three decades, the natural immunological limits of transplant have been widened.

In addition to the ability to match persons who are likely to be immunologically compatible, scientists discovered drugs that suppressed, to a great extent, the natural processes of rejection. A variety of these drugs, mostly steroids with varying efficacy, appeared in the 1960s, but in 1983, the Food and Drug Administration approved cyclosporine, a drug that rapidly proved safer and more effective than all others. Cyclosporine and a series of successors—tacrolimus (FK 506), gusperimus trihydrochloride, and mycophenolate mofetil—widened vastly the possibilities for organ transplantation. Although these drugs create a safer environment in the recipient's body for the new organ, they also have short- and long-term adverse effects that can be bothersome, serious, and sometimes lethal.

The second reason that organs are a scarce resource is that most major organs are essential to the life of the donor. The removal of the heart causes death; removal of the lung, liver, or pancreas causes death or severe disability. The human body, however, has two kidneys and one can be removed or cease to function without severe detriment. Thus, the kidney was the first accessible organ. Within the past decade, segments of liver and lung have been transplanted between living persons, and hearts have been moved from a person about to receive a heart–lung transplant to another in so-called domino operations. Nevertheless, despite this technological virtuosity, the ability to acquire organs from living persons remains limited.

Thus, the primary source of organs for transplantation is a dead body. As the process of death sets in, the organs of the body begin to deteriorate rapidly. Organs viable for transplantation must be retrieved quickly and, if possible, must be retrieved from a dead body whose vital functions are being sustained artificially. Such bodies are often of persons who die after a trauma that destroys their central nervous system but leaves other organs intact. To meet this situation death was redefined in the 1960s to allow brain-related clinical criteria to support a legal and medical determination of death.

Most organs for transplantation come from *cadavers*, persons judged dead on the basis of brain-related criteria. In 1991, 7727 kidneys came from cadaveric donors and 2262 came from living donors; only 22 partial livers contributed to 2951 liver transplants; in domino operations, four hearts from living donors went to 2127 heart recipients. In all, cadaveric donors contributed 13,761 organs and living donors contributed 2292 (United Network for Organ Sharing 1993). Dependence on cadaveric donors creates two significant problems, both of which are ethical problems. First, to what extent is consent necessary and how can it be attained from a cadaveric donor? Second, how can the supply of donors, both living and dead, be increased?

Although in the early days of transplantation, some organs were confiscated from cadavers by eager medical examiners, there has been general agreement that consent for cadaver donation is an appropriate and necessary social practice. Just as consent of relatives to autopsy is customary, so consent for use of a decedent's organs is suitable. The practice of willing one's corneas after death has been in vogue since the 1940s and seems to have set a precedent for the idea that a person could "will" or permit the use of other organs after his or her death.

In the 1960s, the idea that the donation of organs should be legally formalized led the National Conference of Commissioners on Uniform State Laws to draft the Uniform Anatomical Gift Act, which was adopted by all 50 states by 1970. The law enables competent adults to indicate their intention to donate the organs of their body at the time of death by signing a legally valid document. In the absence of such a document, specified family members may authorize the taking of organs unless the deceased had specifically denied the intent to donate (Uniform Anatomical Gift Act 1968). Many states made it simple to prepare such a document by allowing persons to signify their willingness to donate organs by a notation on their driver's licenses.

Despite these legal practices, a critical shortage in the supply of organs persists because not enough organs are donated and retrieved and because medical indications for organ transplantation have expanded. In 1991, 25,000 patients were on the waiting list for all types of solid organs—16,000 organs were available. Median waiting time for kidneys increased from 356 to 514 days between 1988 and 1992; waiting time for a heart increased from 108 to 198 days during that time, with 788 patients dying while they waited (United Network for Organ Sharing 1993).

In 1985, it was estimated that approximately 200,000 persons were declared dead each year on the basis of brain-related criteria, but organs were obtained from only about 2000 persons. Yet, the need at that time for hearts, lungs, and kidneys was estimated as 50,000 or more (Schwartz 1984). Since 1985, serious efforts have been made to improve donation and retrieval of organs technically by use of older donors, expanded use of nonrelated donors, and use of nonheartbeating donors. Yet the shortage worsens. What social arrangements can be made to ameliorate this situation? What ethical principles should govern the social arrangements?

The Anatomical Gift Act was built on a concept that modern ethics finds congenial, namely, the autonomy of individuals, which endows them the right to control disposition of their bodies, even after death. Similarly, common law has allowed persons to determine how their bodies will be disposed of, within certain limits, and has granted next-of-kin rights of disposal in the absence of the specific directives of the deceased. Antecedent donation of organs seems in accord with these accepted concepts. Because the Anatomical Gift Act does not force a person to donate an organ, persons who have moral objections to dissection or organ removal can decline donation.

There are contrary traditions about the disposition of the body. Several religious traditions, Jewish, Muslim, and Buddhist, have ancient prohibitions against dissection and it would appear that these prohibitions cannot be overridden by the choice of the decedent. It is interesting, however, how these religious traditions have responded to the novel situation of transplantation.

Jewish religious law explicitly prohibits mutilation of the dead body. Contemporary developments have refined that position and allowed it to be interpreted as permitting removal of an organ when the life of another can thereby be saved. Even then, care must be taken that contact with the dead not cause religious defilement (Rosner 1979; Tendler 1978). Islamic beliefs about resurrection require bodily integrity at the time of death. Buddhism also abhors mutilation of the body and transplantation has been viewed skeptically. Nevertheless, in most Islamic and Buddhist countries, donation after death has been permitted if the explicit consent of the donor has been obtained before death (Kimura 1995; Nakasone 1995; Prottas et al. 1995; Sachedina 1995; Stiller et al. 1995).

In Japan, however, a persistent public reluctance, particularly over the question of brain death, has prevented the medical profession from instituting heart, liver, and lung transplantation, but kidneys and corneas can legally be transplanted (Brannigan 1992).

Even if a person wills organs for transplantation, can an ethical case be made that organs should be removed and used for transplant without or against the explicit wishes of the family of the decedent? Does the cadaver, in some sense, belong to the state or to society? The severe shortage of organs and the significant benefit to recipients makes such a question plausible. Although transplanters and policy makers generally avoid so bold a proposal, its ethics are worth considering. One modern ethical theory, utilitarianism, provides a plausible argument that any use of the body of a decedent that could benefit society should be mandatory unless society's revulsion or discomfort at certain uses counterbalances the advantages.

Nevertheless, most ethicists have argued against routine salvaging of organs without personal or familial permission. Ramsey proposed that "the routine taking of organs would deprive individuals of the exercise of the virtue of generosity" (Ramsey 1970, 210). Veatch also states that, in a "society which values personal integrity and freedom, we must be able to control our bodies not only in our lifetime but within reasonable limits after that life is gone" (Veatch 1976, 268).

A philosopher, J. L. Muyskens, argues against both Ramsey and Veatch. Against Ramsey, he maintains that routine salvaging does not deprive persons of the opportunity to exercise the virtue of generosity because there are many ways to demonstrate that virtue. Against Veatch, he counters that salvaging does not undermine individual autonomy of the individual and collectivity because not all powers vested in the state threaten the autonomy of the individual. Thus, "with regard to organs such as kidneys—given the relatively good chances of successful transplantation—we (pragmatically) ought to be (hence, if acting rationally would be) willing to relinquish our right to be buried intact" (Muyskens 1978, 97).

This thesis implies the acceptance of the utilitarian principle: Actions are ethically right if they contribute to the greater good of the greater number. Such a principle points to such beneficial use of organs that otherwise would simply corrupt. Even then utilitarianism might recommend respect for individual choice on the basis that salvaging organs without permission might have some social disutility, such as undermining, in a progressive fashion, the inviolability of the human body before death. Also, it might offend the religious or moral feelings of many persons and lead to feelings of outrage and discrimination, which are also social disutilities. In addition, it would also be important to acknowledge, if not the absolute authority, at least the privacy and sensitivity of the family.

Some commentators have moved between the utilitarian view and the view requiring previous consent by proposing a presumed consent position. Arthur Caplan once suggested that organs might be salvaged without explicit consent (Caplan 1983). He proposed that unless a person or a family explicitly objected to removal of organs, it could be presumed that the person is willing to donate for the good of others. Ian Kennedy made the same suggestion in Great Britain (Kennedy 1979). In France, the law approves such an approach—cadaver organs can be taken unless the decedent has objected or the family objects (Raymond 1978). Taking the right to refuse seriously would require complex and perhaps impossible recordkeeping and coordination. Caplan subsequently modified his concept to "required request"— hospital personnel would be required by law to request permission of the family. Most states and the federal government have already enacted such legislation, but with little apparent effect on increasing the supply of organs; rates of compliance did not exceed 50 percent, probably because of continued reluctance of health-care providers to introduce this subject in the tragic circumstances of death (Caplan 1984, 1988).

However, the proposals to increase the supply of organs do not come to grips with the central ethical issue: Does the state, or some other party, have moral claim on a cadaver when the cadaver can be used for social benefit? The Task Force on Organ Transplantation, established in accord with the National Organ Transplant Act (Public Law 98-507) makes the bold statement that "each donated organ be considered a national resource to be used for the public good" (US DHHS 1986, 302). The Task Force uses the phrase "donated organ," which implies consent, but is it not plausible to argue that these "national resources" might be harvested without consent? It is not clear to what extent public good should prevail over private rights.

Even if thoughtful philosophical consideration of this issue leads to the conclusion that social authority over use of organs is ethical and, in general, supersedes the ethical value of individual or familial right to prohibit such use, there might be important policy reasons for not adopting this position. A policy that afforded certain legal protections to the refusal of individuals and families, as well as requiring the permission of next-of-kin, when available, might be preferable. It is important to have law devised to make organs available with ease, but also to have, at the same time, law that respects these limitations (Sadler and Sadler 1984).

It is persistently suggested that the supply of organs would be enhanced by establishing an open market in which organs are bought and sold for financial consideration. A market for blood and sperm has long existed: Why should major organs be treated differently? Almost from the beginning of the era of transplantation, the concept that an organ transferred from one person to another is a "gift of life" has been the dominant theme. The market in blood had been trenchantly criticized by the British scholar Richard Titmus in *The Gift Relationship* (Titmus 1971) in which he saw blood donation in a free, noncommercial system as a significant and necessary demonstration of altruism in an industrial society of strangers. This concept, together with the lifesaving drama of transplantation and the American predilection for voluntary assistance to others in need, built around transplantation a strong ethos of gift. The proposal that a market replace the ethos of gift, although rational to the economic mind, shocks the ethically sensitive. Sociologists Renee Fox and Judith Swazey, pioneers in the study of the social and ethical world of transplantation, have decried the "de-gifting" tendency that they see in increasingly commercial attitudes toward organ retrieval (Fox and Swazey 1992, 206).

Would a market for the buying and selling of organs increase the supply? This can only be answered by experience. From the earliest years of corneal and renal transplantation, indigent persons have on occasion offered to sell one of their "disposable" organs. In India, particularly, an open, thriving market for kidneys exists—2000 sales were reported in 1991. Most purchased organs probably flow into the developed world. In 1983, an American physician established a brokerage that offered to negotiate a price between sellers and buyers of organs. This idea was firmly repudiated by the transplantation community and led to the explicit prohibition of acquiring, receiving, or otherwise transferring "any human organ for valuable consideration for transplantation if the transfer affects interstate commerce" (1984 National Organ Transplantation Act, Public Law 98-507). Even after prohibition, several leading transplant centers in the United States were reported to have allowed wealthy patients from abroad to bring with them their paid "donor," who was passed off as an altruistic relative (Freedman 1985; Pittsburgh Press 1985).

Still, some commentators find no objections to a market in organs. Some wonder why the organ supply should operate any differently than the rest of American medicine, which is essentially a commercial industry (Blumstein and Sloan 1989). In one publication, a physician and a philosopher discuss the question. The philosopher saw no morally relevant difference between selling one's time and selling one's organ and noted that in the transplant situation, the donor is now the only one who does not profit financially. The physician agreed. He remarked that sale would be good for both provider and recipient and doubted that a slippery slope would start.

However, these views are in the minority, even in the sparse literature on the subject. The opponents reject the market in organs, on the grounds that a traffic in organs would be degrading and the profit motive would be likely to reduce care and caution in selection of suitable organs (Frier and Mavrodes 1980; Kennedy 1979). The market would destroy the gift-of-life motif that has powerful psychological and social repercussions that are of great value to the society and to interpersonal relationships (Fox and Swazey 1992). In the most extensive article to analyze the ethics of a market in organs, Perry (1980) reviews the arguments for and against the two options usually discussed, namely, the donation of organs and the harvesting of organs. He comes to the conclusion that a modified market would be tolerable. The market would allow reimbursement and incentives but not profit. A transplant surgeon subsequently proposed a similar concept of a "death benefit" paid to the family of a deceased donor (Peters 1991).

Weighty objections attend a policy of reimbursement. Desperate persons might be enticed to offer organs for sale, pre- or postmortem. There would be an opportunity of exploitation of the poor. An ethicist criticized the death benefit proposal as "ethically flawed—a policy that resorts to monetary inducements, that replaces altruism by selfish self-interest and that manipulates consent by monetary incentives, has too many ethical liabilities to be acceptable either as a policy or as an experiment" (Pellegrino 1991, 1306).

Organ exchange may belong in the category of "blocked exchanges" of which Michael Walzer speaks. Certain sorts of human exchange that might be accomplished with efficiency through a market system are not permitted by a society primarily because they are "desperate exchanges or trades of last resort . . . this is a restraint of market liberty for the sake of some communal conception of personal liberty, a reassertion . . . of the ban on slavery" (Walzer 1983, 102).

There are other objections. A market system would encourage the development of a class of middle men and entrepreneurs whose practices might be less than savory. They would be modern counterparts of the nineteenth century graverobbers. A market might also make it difficult to sustain the sort of quality control over organ accrual that is necessary for the best medical care. One philosopher (Caplan 1983) writes:

> Allocating lifesaving organs by the ability of those in need to pay what the market will bear is blatantly unfair to the poor. Nor can medicine morally allow itself to be used by those who would risk their own health out of greed, desperation or ignorance. To argue that the sale of organs is a business motivated by humanitarian concerns for the well being of those in need simply flies in the face of the fact that selling organs can only increase the cost for those who now receive them for free.

The supply of organs may be increased by means other than routine harvesting or marketing. Legislation and social arrangements could tip the balance in favor of donation. Arguments against a market in organs do not rule out certain arrangements that might involve monetary considerations. Tax deductions or reduction in hospital bills might increase the incentive to donate. The idea of organized giving to charity based on similar incentives was frowned on in the earlier years of this century by those accustomed to giving solely for the sake of charity, unmotivated by anything but generosity.

The critical shortage of organs has prompted unusual proposals, two of which raise interesting ethical questions. The first proposes that animal organs (xenografts) be used if they are anatomically and physiologically possible. In the first two decades of the transplantation era, 20 xenografts were performed between humans and primates, all unsuccessfully. In 1984 a surgeon transplanted the heart of a baboon into a newborn girl whose heart lacked a left ventricle (Altman 1984). The infant died several days later. This operation, unlike the earlier ones, was widely noted in the press and aroused much criticism, primarily because the scientific preparation for such a transplant was inadequate and thus offered the dimmest prospect for success. However, questions about the propriety of exchanging organs between species were raised.

Some objected on religious grounds, claiming that God puts an impassable barrier between animals and humans. The religious argument was not supported by the conclusions of a group of distinguished theologians who were asked by the President's Commission for the Study of Ethical Problems in Medicine to advise whether Christian theology or Jewish law contains any specific Divine prohibition against crossing species. The theologians concluded that there was no definitive prohibition (President's Commission 1982). In addition, the evolutionary process shows many examples of transfer of genetic material between species.

Another argument against xenografts came from the proponents of animal rights. They objected not only to the killing of animals for human purposes, but to the use of already endangered species, the most likely sources of usable organs. The animal rights arguments have a growing persuasiveness at the present time, but still run counter to strong values that favor benefiting humans even at the cost of animal life.

Although a moratorium prevailed on human–animal transplants between 1984 and 1992, a baboon liver and a porcine liver were transplanted into patients in Pittsburgh and in Los Angeles (both patients died, although the Pittsburgh patient survived 71 days). It is now known that the immunological response to animal grafts is qualitatively the same as the response between humans, although considerably more severe. Advances in immunosuppression are expected to make xenografts feasible soon. When this happens, the ethical arguments will surface, particularly the accusation of "speciesism," that is, humans have no presumptive claim on animal lives as a way to save their own (Caplan 1992).

A second proposal to alleviate the shortage of organs suggests that organs from anencephalic infants be used for transplantation into newborns and infants in need. *Anencephaly* is a genetic anomaly in which the higher portions of the brain and the skull remain undeveloped in the fetus; after birth, an anencephalic infant may live for a few hours or even a few days but will inevitably die. About 2000 anencephalic infants are born in the United States each year; it is estimated that approximately the same number of infants are in need of hearts, livers, and kidneys. However, the anencephalic infant, once born, is a living being protected by law. Although lacking higher brain portions, the anencephalic infant has a functioning brain stem and, thus, is not legally brain-dead. Salvaging viable organs would, it appears, constitute a direct act of killing the donor infant.

In the mid-1980s, several commentators proposed that the determination of death by brain criteria be modified to include the *brain absent*, those born without the major portion of their brains (Harrison and Meilander 1986). A debate ensued over the propriety of considering the anencephalic infant as a donor. Opponents countered that expansion of the criteria was clearly the first step that would lead to the use of many other brain-damaged but not brain-dead persons as donors (Fletcher et al. 1986; Churchill and Pinkus 1990). The Ethical and Judicial Council of the American Medical Association concluded in 1994 that the anencephalic infant could be considered as a potential organ donor and made a limited exception to the requirement of a dead donor "because of the fact that the infant has never experienced, and will never experience, consciousness" (American Medical Association 1994, 30).

One transplant center, acknowledging that anencephalic infants did not meet the legal definition of death, instituted an experimental protocol in which the infants were ventilated for 2 weeks and, if they met traditional cardiorespiratory death criteria, were to be used as donors. The experiment failed to produce a single donor and was discontinued (Peabody et al. 1989). There is at present little interest in this source of organs.

THE EXPERIMENTAL FRONTIER

Transplantation moves on a constantly advancing, and often faltering, frontier. Many forms of organ transplantation, although always a serious personal and medical event, have become standard and accepted medical practice. Yet, the science and techniques of organ transplantation continue to advance. As transplantation moves ahead, new ethical problems arise.

During the 1980s, considerable interest surrounded the possibility of neural transplantation for the treatment of Parkinson's disease, a degenerative neurological disease that usually strikes persons in their middle or late years. Among the possibilities, one was particularly intriguing, namely, transplantation of tissue taken from the brains and adrenal glands of aborted fetuses into the brains of persons afflicted with parkinsonism. This procedure was first performed in Mexico in 1988 (Madrozo 1988).

A similar interest focused on the use of fetal pancreatic tissue for transplantation into patients with insulin dependent diabetes, of whom there are nearly 1 million in the United States. Although attempts at pancreatic transplants have been made since 1921, with the discovery of insulin as a product of the pancreas in the late 1980s, a number of fetal tissue transplants were attempted. In general, fetal tissue seems appropriate for transplants because it has not yet developed the strong immunological properties that instigate rejection.

The utility of tissue from aborted fetuses immediately raised ethical questions. The federal government had imposed a moratorium on fetal research in 1974, but after the *Report on Research Involving the Human Fetus*, issued in 1975 by the National Commission for the Protection of Human Subjects of Biomedical and Behavioral Research, allowed research involving the human fetus only under the most restrictive conditions. However, the new question did not constitute research with the human fetus but with the use of the human fetus for research on another person, the patient who would be the recipient of its tissues. In 1987, a symposium on the ethics of fetal transplantation was held, at which the investigators and bioethicists reviewed the ethical and legal implications of this innovation (Mahowald 1988).

The next year, an NIH researcher submitted a proposal to transplant fetal tissue into a patient with Parkinson's disease. The Director of NIH was anxious about the legality and ethics of approving such a protocol and requested advice from the Assistant Secretary for Health and Human Services, who imposed a moratorium on funding for all research on fetal tissue transplantation and ordered the convocation of an advisory panel to answer 10 ethical questions. The principal question concerned the morality of using tissue that had been obtained from elective abortions—it could be charged that the mother who chose abortion abdicated the right to give consent regarding use of fetal tissue, that the possible beneficial uses of aborted tissue would attribute moral value to the abortion, and that the utility of the tissue might induce women to abort who would not otherwise do so.

The Human Fetal Tissue Transplant Research Panel concluded that it was possible and appropriate to distinguish between the morality of elective abortion and the morality of use of fetal tissue for transplant research. The panel found, although after considerable controversy and with some strong dissent by those who believed that use of fetal tissue necessarily involved complicity in abortion, that such research should be permitted as good public policy. The panel recommended that the moratorium be lifted (Fetal Tissue Panel 1988). This did not happen, however, until the Bush administration was replaced by the Clinton administration in January 1993. Several research protocols are now investigating the efficacy of fetal tissue transplantation (Greely et al. 1989; Vawter et al. 1990).

As transplantation surgical techniques become more sophisticated and as immunosuppression becomes more effective, bolder forms of transplantation are considered. Each bolder form must confront the ethical questions faced by all biomedical research: How is the risk to be compared with the benefit in the face of unknown results, and how is consent to be obtained? To what extent should one person assume risks to save another?

These questions were posed to the investigators and the participants who contemplated an innovative segmental liver transplant between a parent and a child. Because the liver regenerates itself, it is possible to remove a lobe for transplant. However, removal of a liver lobe is not an inconsequential procedure. Although similar procedures had been performed, the exact nature of the risk to the donor was unclear. In 1990, a group of Chicago investigators and ethical consultants explored the question with care and concluded that the benefits justified the risks and that the consent of parents to donate to their threatened child was free and uncoerced. Their thoughtful consideration, however, was not unanimously accepted by the transplantation community; some leaders questioned the comparable efficacy of liver transplant from live donors versus transplants from cadavers, while others questioned whether the consent of parents in these cases was truly uncoerced (Singer et al. 1989; Busatil 1991). As the practice of using live donors expands, these questions will be asked again and again.

Liver transplantation has also forced reconsideration of a question that faced the very earliest practitioners of renal dialysis and transplant: Should the lifestyle and behavior of a potential recipient be considered as a qualification for admission to treatment? The developers of renal dialysis, faced with an acute shortage of dialysis machines and organs, were forced to select patients whom they could treat—nonselection meant death. When that terrible choice had to be made, decision makers found themselves using selection criteria drawn from the basis of "worth to society."

The advance of liver transplantation has again raised that issue. Liver failure is often caused by end-stage cirrhosis, which is often produced by excessive use of alcohol. Should persons who have destroyed their livers by abuse be given transplants when livers are in short supply? Should they be retransplanted in the event of rejection or repeated liver failure? Patients with alcoholic cirrhosis reportedly have transplant survival rates equivalent to liver recipients with other diagnoses, and they apparently have good records of abstinence from alcohol after transplantation (Starzl et al. 1988). In 1991, Medicare coverage for liver transplantation caused by alcoholic cirrhosis was conditioned on a demonstrated period of abstinence.

Despite these facts, providers may feel discomfort at "wasting" an organ on someone whom they suspect will abuse the organ again. Social policy about provision of health services is now seriously questioning whether resources should be limited for persons who have caused their condition by abusive lifestyles (Moss and Siegler 1991). In a field that has learned to select patients on the grounds of efficacy, the reintroduction of debate about social worth and personal deserts is troubling.

The field of transplantation is particularly prone to incidents that are ethically perplexing, personally dramatic, often tragic, and highly attractive to the media. At almost regular intervals, a story appears of a child whose life can be saved only by transplanting a cluster of organs, of a child whose life can be saved only by a very expensive transplant for which insurance will not pay, of the President of the United States ordering a military plane to rush an organ to a dying patient. Among the most widely publicized of such events was the continuing drama, played out over several years, in which physicians attempted to replace the failing human heart with an artificial device.

The artificial heart, developed initially by the NIH in the 1960s and then by commercial bioengineering groups with heavy federal funding, is essentially a mechanical blood pump implanted in the chest and powered by an external pneumatic engine connected by tubes through the chest wall to the internal pump. Aware of the momentous ethical and social implications of this new technology, the National Heart, Lung, and Blood Institute commissioned two special panels to review the questions (National Institutes of Health 1973, 1985).

Surgeon William deVries implanted an artificial heart for the first time in patient Barney Clark in Salt Lake City, Utah, on December 2, 1982. Clark died 112 days later. During the next 3 years, five more patients were implanted; the longest survivor was William Shroeder who lived for 620 days and suffered one medical crisis after another. Despite years of testing the device in dogs, sheep, and calves, unanticipated physical and physiological problems plagued human patients. The course of each patient was followed closely by the media and persistent debates occurred about the usefulness of the artificial heart, which promised (and cost) so much, but delivered so little (Jonsen 1986; Preston 1985).

After the discouraging series of clinical failures, the National Heart, Lung, and Blood Institute decided to terminate support for artificial heart transplantation and concentrate on more limited heart support technology; however, pressure from several influential senators forced a reversal of this decision and research has continued (Shaw 1984; Fox and Swazey 1992; Culliton 1988; Hogness and Van Antwerp 1991).

Among the most painful decisions created by any medical technology that pushes ahead into unexplored areas are those involving the cost of the new intervention on the individuals who are its experimental subjects. Often, the medical costs of early experiments are covered by federal agencies and commercial developers. However, as the technologies move from the earliest stages of investigation into broader, but not yet generally accepted use, sources of funding diminish. Costs are increasingly imposed on the patients and on their insurers. Insurers frequently refuse to cover "investigational" procedures. Throughout the evolution of organ transplantation, this problem has faced individuals in need of forefront procedures. These persons must often appeal to the public for donations.

The most famous appeal was a nationally publicized campaign by Charles Fiske to obtain a liver and insurance coverage for his daughter Jamie who was dying of biliary atresia. Fiske appeared before the national meeting of the American Academy of Pediatrics to make his case. As a result, not only did Jamie receive her transplant, but Congress mobilized to provide funding for pediatric liver transplantation, another decision, like the 1972 decision to provide national health insurance for renal dialysis and transplantation, made organ by organ (Fox and Swazey 1992, 85–89).

SELECTION OF PATIENTS FOR A SCARCE RESOURCE

Organs for transplantation are, at present and for the foreseeable future, in short supply. Many persons who might benefit by organ transplantation will not be able to receive an organ. Thus, the ethics of selecting patients to receive a scarce resource arises. On what principle should available organs be distributed, so that a fair and equitable allocation is achieved? The question first arose in the late 1960s when chronic hemodialysis was introduced as a life-sustaining therapy for persons with end-stage renal disease. The few centers in which the skills and machinery existed for this procedure were forced to select a handful of patients from among thousands throughout the United States who were in need.

One center, Northwest Kidney Center in Seattle, devised a method to select patients by submitting the names of all medically suitable candidates to a lay board that was to choose the few fortunate recipients of this lifesaving therapy. The committee became known as the "God Committee" because it had the power to choose who would live and who would die. The choice often turned on the social worth or productivity of candidates.

Renal transplantation, the parallel therapy for end-stage kidney disease, also requires allocation of a scarce resource—available organs; heart transplantation faces the same situation. The problem of fair and equitable distribution of scarce medical resources has been widely discussed in the press and by scholars. Scholarly discussion has generally centered on two quite different approaches to the problem of allocation: One favors distribution of the scarce resources on the basis of the principle of social utility; the other favors egalitarian principles. The egalitarian approach leads its advocates to recommend a system of random selection as the only mechanism consonant with the dignity and equality of all candidates. The utilitarian approach requires explicit assessment of the qualifications of candidates, although this approach also allows random selection if there are two candidates equally in need and equally qualified.

The argument between the utilitarian and egalitarian approaches is carried on at two levels—on the level of the basic principle and on the level of practicality. At the level of basic principles, one confronts the perennial philosophical question of whether the foundation of moral judgment is social utility, namely, the achievement of the greater good for the greater number in a society, or the absolute moral claims or rights of each person to the human goals of life and liberty.

In one of the earliest philosophical analyses of this problem, Rescher asserts that "society 'invests' a scarce resource in one person as against another and is thus entitled to look to the probable prospective 'return' on its investment" (Rescher 1969). This statement endorses the principle of social utility. It is one way of measuring the value of individual lives in society as a whole. According to this view, much as one might respect the life of an individual, the value of that life is, in the last analysis, only one factor within the welfare of the society as a whole. Even if the most serious efforts are made to protect and enhance the value of individual lives, the design and limits of these efforts must be dictated by the needs of the general good.

On the level of principle, many philosophers offer criticisms of this position. In the debate about patient selection, Childress notes that "the individual's personal and transcendent dignity, which on the utilitarian approach would be submerged in his social role and function, can be protected and witnessed to by a recognition of his equal right to be saved" (Childress 1970). From this viewpoint, society's investment is not merely the resources poured into a medical device or procedure, nor is its return the measurable usefulness and productivity of certain social rules and functions. Rather, its investment is the incalculable and multiple contribution that a society makes to the very existence of each individual; its return is the very life of individuals, saved and fostered by multiple social interventions.

When applied to the distribution of lifesaving resources, the analogy of investment is plausible but inadequate. Its plausibility comes from the fact that significant resources of knowledge, time, money, and materials are brought to bear on the development of certain medical interventions. Even when these resources do not come from the government, they draw, in a collective and cumulative way, from the store of human potential available to any society. Their devotion to one purpose subtracts them from other purposes. This holds true in public and private sectors and in various spheres, such as education, arts, recreation, and commerce. Presumably, the bending of efforts to certain tasks has some purpose, some goal. Some potential value is sought, some good is to be created. Those who make these efforts often do so in the hope that their children, their fellow citizens, and others unknown to them will benefit. Thus, the plausibility of the investment analogy lies in the recognition that out of significant efforts, significant goods should come.

The analogy, however, is inadequate because it does not help in discovering what good, how much good, and to whom the good should flow. At best, in the debate about lifesaving medical resources, it suggests that the good should be health. If the resources are antibiotics, health is freedom from infection; when the resources replace the heart, health is a revitalized cardiovascular system. But, from the utilitarian perspective, the good envisioned by the investment theory is not health in the abstract, nor even health as a personal attribute of individuals. The good is more likely to be health insofar as health contributes to social productivity. The healthy person is the employed person or the active person contributing to, and not subtracting from, the welfare of society. Overall welfare is always what the utilitarian principle envisions. This apparently laudable goal is fraught with ethical perils.

Ethical perils appear when authors turn to practical levels. Persons favoring the egalitarian approach are highly critical of any effort to assess the qualifications of individuals, but admit that society does evaluate persons in many ways and is frequently biased. In the provision of a lifesaving resource, evaluation approaches the impossible. In the words of Paul Freund:

> The more nearly total is the estimate to be made of an individual, and the more nearly the consequences determine life or death, the more unfit the judgment becomes for human reckoning. . . . Randomness as a moral principle deserves serious study (1969, xvii).

Authors critical of the utilitarian approach note the impossibility of weighing the multiplicity of valuable human qualities by the same scale— is the shrewd politician who maintains social peace through intricate compromises more valuable than the insightful novelist whose sharp criticism makes society uncomfortable? Critics call attention to the fallibility of predictions about future contributions by persons whose goals and attributes may change in a society where new needs are always emerging. They cite instances in which obviously irrelevant personal characteristics tipped the balance—for example, favoring a church-going Scout leader to a respectable person without strong civic or religious interests.

On the basis of these arguments, advocates of the egalitarian approach conclude that any system of selection that requires evaluation of personal qualifications will be flawed by fallibility, bias, ignorance, and capriciousness and, thus, be unfair in its working and results. Egalitarians recommend various systems of random selection, such as lottery or first come, first served. They see these systems as more consonant with fundamental human equality and as less open to the flaws of an evaluation system. It is possible, however, for an egalitarian to favor certain sorts of criteria, such as age, provided the criteria can be shown to be relevant to the selection and can be fairly applied.

Advocates of social utility do not generally discuss the weakness of assessment of personal characteristics. One author merely comments "the fact that the standard (of social contribution) is difficult to apply is certainly no reason for not attempting to apply it" (Rescher 1969, 619). Another admits that techniques of assessment are "imperfect, but that they succeed better than random chance in maximizing social value of the selected candidates . . . errors are regrettable but . . . more such errors would have occurred had we used any other allocative technique" (Basson 1979, 327). These authors frequently note that the type of assessment repudiated by egalitarians is intrinsic to evaluating any medical need and medical success. An appropriate diagnosis and prognosis rest not only on physiological information, but on many psychological and social features of a particular patient. The chances for successful treatment often depend on intellectual and emotional capability for understanding and following a regimen and on the network of support on which a patient can draw. As advocates of the maxim that where society as a whole makes an investment, society has the right to maximum return, they count return in terms of productive lives saved, persons restored to self-support, and a life of active contribution to society. Thus, the distribution of a scarce resource in which social investment has been made or by which society may gain or lose in significant ways mandates careful discrimination between persons to ascertain those for whom use will be "highest and best."

Advocates of the egalitarian approach do not deny these assertions but tend to see medical suitability as consisting of more objective data and, if psychological and social evaluations are involved, they recommend that "the attempt to establish fine degrees of prospective response to treatment should be avoided" (Childress 1970, 622).

The concept of a return on social investment does not address another crucial question: Who should determine what counts as a suitable return on the investment? If, as egalitarians assert, society invests in the development of means of health care, presumably, society should determine the level of return. Since society is constituted of individuals who explicitly or implicitly contribute to that investment out of their income and efforts by foregoing other sorts of benefits, it is plausible to suppose that they expect to enjoy that return for themselves or for their children. At least, it is plausible to suppose that persons expect to have a chance equal to others to be beneficiaries of the investment. This line of argument affirms a strong imperative of fair and equal distribution and appears to turn the argument of social investment on its head:

All persons in the present and all future persons should be given an equal chance.

Occasionally, it has been suggested that persons who are responsible for their own illness should not be the beneficiaries of scarce resources. Indeed, insurers and employers are beginning to make decisions about premiums and employment on the basis of judgment about personal responsibility for health; for example, smokers are considered high risk. However, this claim, which has some ethical plausibility at face value, is countered by arguments that the relationship between voluntary actions and any specific illness is generally statistical. Causes of any illness are complex and interrelated. In most conditions—certainly for those for which cardiac transplant is contemplated—it is factually impossible to blame any specific individual. Further, even if a casual connection could be established, the behavior in question might not be voluntary in the sense of being relevant for ascribing responsibility. Thus, the suggestion that persons should be excluded from health care because they have brought about their condition has carried little weight in the ethical literature (President's Commission 1983).

Those favoring egalitarian principles often propose a system of random selection of patients. The lottery is defended as most suitable to human dignity, least open to bias, most palliative of anxiety about "qualifying," and most likely to be chosen, if society were offered a referendum on various selection systems. In principle, the lottery seems, to many commentators, the only "fair" system. However, the lottery has also been criticized. Far from seeing a human lottery as appropriate to human dignity, some authors have been repelled by the idea. The jurisprudent Edmund Cahn considers "the stakes too high for gambling and the responsibilities too deep for destiny" (Cahn 1955, 71). Joseph Fletcher calls a lottery "literally irresponsible, a rejection of the burden, refusal to be rational" (Fletcher 1969, unpublished lecture). Even Katz and Capron, who ultimately favor a lottery, are critical:

> The Lottery is more blind than fair, for an evenhanded approach is desirable only insofar as it deals with like classes of individuals (1976, 193).

Other authors note the practical problem of a lottery. It requires a preexisting group from which lots can be drawn, a situation that is unrealistic because patients appear serially with a need for help; the patients' conditions can also change during the waiting time. One author stressed the fact that lotteries can be rigged and, in matters of such import, are likely to be (Harris 1975; Willard 1980). Some authors question the contention of those favoring lotteries that random selection would alleviate anxiety. Several authors distinguish between "natural" types of random selection such as first come, first served, and artificial random selection, such as lotteries. The queue for natural random selection, some note, is more in accord with the realities of illness and traditions of health care, but the queue can be "jumped"

(Fried 1974; Willard 1980). All systems of random selection make it possible for certain socially disreputable or dangerous persons to receive the gift of life, a prospect that critics of the lottery find unpalatable, but proponents consider the price of fairness.

ALLOCATION OF SCARCE RESOURCES

Jamie Fiske's father sought coverage for her expensive transplant from his private insurer and, in so doing, called attention to the overall problem of coverage for transplantation. Although the End Stage Renal Disease Act of 1972 provided Medicaid funding for renal transplantation, it has always done so in a restricted way. It covers the costs of surgery and immediate care but provides only 1 year of funding for the expensive and necessary immuno-suppressive drugs. Reluctance to spend more arises, it appears, from the fear of politicians and bureaucrats that a comprehensive policy of funding organ transplantation is a fiscal slippery slope. Yet, public pressure has gradually forced expansion of funding, organ by organ. In 1986, the Health Care Financing Administration agreed to reimburse heart transplantation. Many states and most insurers now pay for transplantations that attain the status of common and accepted medical practice and are, on occasion, pushed to support even the more investigational.

Despite help from federal programs, the significant cost of transplantation places a heavy burden on those who pay for health-care services. Organ transplantation is a visible target for budget makers and policy makers. In 1983 Massachusetts established a task force, under the chairmanship of ethicist–lawyer George Annas, to study the problem of state funding of organ transplantation (Annas 1984). The judicious conclusions of the task force were ignored by subsequent pressures to expand the availability and funding of transplantation in Massachusetts. In Oregon, a concerted effort to inaugurate a health-care system reform that would lead to universal coverage of all residents of that state began in the late 1980s. At first the reform focused on the costs of organ transplantation covered by Medicaid. Noting that the money expended on organ transplantation for an anticipated 34 patients was enough to expand basic medical care to several thousand indigent women and their children, the Oregon state legislature eliminated all funding for organ transplantation except for kidney and cornea transplants. This trade-off represented what an economist would recognize as a rational allocation of "opportunity costs" (Daniels 1989).

Within months of the decision, the media publicized the plea of a young mother for a bone marrow transplant for her son who was dying from leukemia, which forced reconsideration of the policy. Oregon then began a serious effort to create a priority list for health-care services, in which efficacy in saving and extending life of good quality, rather than costs, was the criterion for provision of any service. In the list, now in use in the Oregon

Medicaid program, major organ transplants are covered services if significant benefit can be demonstrated, a category that includes both extension and quality of life (Garland 1991; Hadorn 1991; Welch and Larson 1988).

Again and again, organ transplants appear in discussions of the high cost of medical services. In 1988, Mary Ann Baily, a health-care economist, noted how difficult it is to determine precisely the costs of transplantation. Figures are reported in different ways—full costs, such as those for follow-up care, are often not included, individual cases vary widely because of differences in the patient's course, and true costs are often obscured by accounting conventions. Nevertheless, using the approximate estimates (1988) of $25,000 to $50,000 for a 1-year survivor of kidney transplant, $95,000 to $148,000 for heart transplants, and $130,000 to $320,000 for liver transplants, Bailey offers some cost estimates. For 2000 heart transplants (the number actually performed in 1990) the cost would be $249 to $354 million. The estimated need, however, is 75,000 recipients annually, reduced by donor availability to 16,000. For 5000 liver transplants, the cost would be $738 million to $1,688 billion (2520 liver transplants were performed in 1990). For 10,000 kidney transplants, the cost would be in the range of $9.88 million. The total cost, at the high estimate of need for heart, liver, and kidney transplants would be $13 billion to $19 billion; at the low-estimate need, the cost would be $3.3 billion to $4.4 billion (Baily 1988).

These are large numbers. Even compared with a nationwide health-care expenditure of $80 billion in 1991, they are significant. The $2.2 million cost of Oregon's estimated 34 transplants seemed a significant saving to the Oregon legislature. The crucial issue is that transplantation may be highly valuable to individual recipients, but it benefits only a small number of persons within any population. Mary Ann Bailey estimated that 10,000 annual kidney recipients constitute 0.0044 percent of the U.S. population; 2000 heart recipients represent 0.0007 percent of the U.S. population (Bailey 1988, 203). Thus, significant health-care resources are allocated to a tiny segment of the population.

The debates of the 1990s over health-care reform have forced the public and policy makers to consider how health-care resources in general are to be distributed within the population. What sorts of services should be available to what classes of persons and at what cost to whom? This is sometimes called the problem of *macroallocation*, as distinguished from *microallocation*, which is the selection of particular persons as recipients of a service. In the United States we have traditionally allowed the market to distribute health-care services—people buy the services they need through direct payment or insurance—and we have supplemented the market with public funding of services for those unable to buy what they need.

The advent of organ transplantation put the issue in a new light. The ability to save specific lives, in a highly visible way, by expensive transplantation raised the question of whether any individual should be allowed to die because he or she could not afford the high costs of transplantation. In

1972, almost without hesitation, Congress approved the End Stage Renal Disease Amendments to the Social Security Act. The amendments provided broad financial support to all persons in need of kidney transplantation and dialysis. In its first phase, the program appeared modest—11,000 patients were cared for at a cost of $280 million—but the program rapidly assumed major proportions. Today, it serves approximately 50,000 patients at a cost of more than $1 billion.

In addition, the United Network for Organ Sharing (UNOS) was established in the 1980s. UNOS is a private, nonprofit corporation with a contract with the federal government to operate a registry of transplant recipients and a system of organ procurement and distribution. The system, set up in accord with the National Organ Transplantation Act of 1984 (Public Law 98-507), attempts to effect an efficient and equitable access to transplantation for all who are medically suitable. In this system, all patients are entered in a single, coordinated waiting list for all organs, and each patient is given priority in terms of length of time on the list, histocompatibility, urgency, and so forth.

Thus, the original ethical crisis faced by doctors and advisory committees forced to choose patients one-by-one for life or for death has dissipated. Although some have criticized the UNOS system for lapses in equity and for inefficiencies, it has done much to relieve the inequities of access that faced earlier transplantation resources (Caplan 1992).

The spontaneous altruism of the 1972 Congressional decision to fund the End Stage Renal Disease Amendments has, in the eyes of some, become a social burden, not only because the considerable costs serve relatively few persons, but because the funding raises the question Should not this be afforded to all who need any organ transplant? In the years since the enactment of the End Stage Renal Disease Amendments, the costs of medical care and the proportion of the gross national product devoted to its financing have become a major public concern (Rettig 1980).

In 1978 Congress asked the President's Commission on the Study of Ethical Problems in Medicine and Biomedical and Behavioral Research to study the question of access to health care from an ethical viewpoint. The Commission's report, *Securing Access to Health Care*, was an extended analysis of the problem of justice in health care. Many scholars in philosophy, economics, social policy, science, and health sciences contributed to its formulation. The report concluded that "society has an ethical obligation to ensure equitable access to an adequate level of health care without the imposition of excessive burdens" (President's Commission 1983, 4).

Adequate is defined as the level of care that enables individuals to achieve sufficient opportunity, information, and evidence of interpersonal concern to facilitate a reasonably full and satisfying life. Recognizing that the concept of adequacy is indefinite, the Commission refrained from attempting to specify what adequate care should include. Instead, the Commission suggested characteristics of adequacy that deserve attention in any discussion of an equitable health-care policy. These characteristics are the relationship between various forms of care and the health-care needs of an individual and the relationship between the benefits of care and its costs, including diversions of resources from other socially desirable endeavors. The Commission concluded:

> Consequently, the level of care deemed adequate should reflect a reasoned judgment not only about impact of the condition on the welfare and opportunity of the individual but also about the efficacy and the costs of the care itself in relation to other conditions and the efficacy and cost of the care that is available for them . . . and the cost of each proposed option in terms of foregone opportunities to apply the same resources to social goals other than that of ensuring access [to health care] (1983, 36–37).

The "reasoned judgment" is made by drawing on criteria such as professional expertise, average current use of health resources, and lists of services deemed necessary. The Commission also recognized the extreme complexity of the problem posed by the principle of ensuring equity of access and recommended a variety of means to resolve the problem: better data on health-care needs, analysis of health-care needs and the costs and efficacy of forms of care, education of the medical profession and of the public, and various financial strategies to limit and distribute costs.

Some philosophers reject the concept of rights in their approach to health care. The rejection arises from awareness that accepting the notion of rights would require dedicating unlimited resources to the health-care benefits of individuals. Claiming such a right would rule out establishment of priorities for various sorts of good derived from health care as well as priorities for those benefits compared with priorities for different sorts of good regarding other aspects of social needs. Thus, these philosophers repudiate the proposal that any particular health-care intervention, such as cardiac transplantation or artificial heart implantation, must be provided as a matter of right to every individual needing such an intervention, regardless of whether it is lifesaving (Green 1983; McCullough 1981).

However, the lifesaving nature of organ transplantation seems to obstruct all efforts at rational philosophical or economic analysis that might lead to a restrictive policy. The Oregon rationing system that excluded all major organ transplants except kidneys was wrecked on the rock of a mother's plea for her dying child. The revision of the Oregon rationing system acknowledged that the rule of rescue, a strong psychological and social imperative to save those threatened by death, must have a place even within a limited system (Hadorn 1991; Jonsen 1986).

The attempt to apply the President's Commission's principle of adequacy seems to lead to a paradox. Organ transplants are potentially lifesaving. Persons who need organ transplants are threatened with death, regardless of ethnic origin, social class, or economic status. In the face of this great equalizer, it seems unfair that only those who can afford the technology should benefit from it. Thus, to rectify this unfairness, we seem obliged to make the lifesaver available to all. In so doing, we add a charge to the publicly supported medical budget, which may have the effect of pushing other services—services that deserve to be among those judged adequate—to the fringes, or out of existence. This solution may be an unfair solution to a problem of unfairness.

The other horn of the paradox is that we demand that a technology not jeopardize access by all persons to an adequate level of care. We intuitively believe that health-care services such as prenatal care, access to physicians for early diagnosis or reassurance, treatment of reversible disorders that without care would be lethal or crippling, and palliation of ravages of chronic disease must all be supplied at the "adequate" level. We envision that an expensive new technology made available to all, that is, supported by public funds, may jeopardize or restrict many useful and necessary services. But the only place that could happen, with any probability—one might say certainty—is within the segment of health care that is supported by public funds. Medicare is a real budget. It has a dollar limit, fund balances, and a bottom line. Within such a budget, funds can be reduced, eliminated, or moved from one line to another.

On the other hand, the so-called health-care budget of the United States is a fictitious or metaphorical one. Its bottom line is a sum added up from a diversity of sources over which no budget officer has any control. The addition of a large expense to a real budget implies that, unless new money is added, the budget will be stressed and to balance the budget less visible, less dramatic, less necessary items may be threatened (Jonsen 1986). The addition of expenses to the metaphorical budget does not necessarily lead to the consequences that befall a real budget.

In the last analysis, the principle of equitable access is noble. It is probably the best statement of the principle of justice in health care that our present wisdom can generate. But the ability to carry the principle into practice eludes us, given our current health-care budget system. An expensive technology should not be financed by the same tax dollars that finance presently available health care if it appears that new technology will derogate from currently available services. Yet, the new technology will be on the market and will be purchasable by persons who desire it (unless there were a way to prohibit its purchase). Thus, some will acquire the embargoed device, and others will not, although the need may be the same. Is this outcome unfair or merely unfortunate (Engelhardt 1984)? A Federal Task Force on Organ Transplantation struggled with this question and tended to see the situation as unfair. The task force concluded that, for purposes of public policy, major organ transplantation should be financed by government funds. However, governmental agencies who must pay the bill may be inclined to see the situation as unfortunate (US DHHS Task Force 1986).

CONCLUSION

The paradox over expensive but lifesaving therapies is only one of the moral ambiguities that permeate the field of transplantation. Some moral issues are settled: the intrinsic morality of transplantation, the right of persons to donate organs, the principles of fair access and distribution. However, many questions remain. Does a family have the moral right to countermand a donation? Probably not. May organs be taken from those not dead but in permanent coma? Possibly, but serious doubts remain. Does the state have the right to take cadaver organs without consent? Probably not, but the question remains open. Can a society prohibit or limit lifesaving transplantations to some in the name of fairness? Probably, but not without serious doubts. These questions represent the profound ambiguity of the question with which we opened this chapter—What does one human being owe another?

This pervasive ambiguity impresses the most sensitive observers and participants in the world of transplantation. After several *cluster* operations—transplantations en bloc of liver, pancreas, stomach, and intestines—were reported in 1989, the doyen of U.S. transplant surgeons, Francis Moore, expressed his dismay. Although he admired the courage of the families, the enterprise of the surgeons, and expressed wonder about the progress of a field Moore had pioneered, he noted, nevertheless:

> We often read in the medical literature that some patient was so desperately ill that almost anything was welcomed by the patient, the family and the physicians. This sort of hyperbolic "desperate remedies" pressure . . . should be looked on with skepticism. There must be some likelihood of success before the desperate remedy becomes more than a desperate search for an opportunity to try a new procedure awaiting trial (1989, 1483).

In almost every case, organ transplant constitutes a desperate remedy. Certainly, in those areas in which outcomes for survival and for quality of life are good, the rescue is reasonable, worthwhile, and often cost effective (renal transplant can save years of dialysis costs; heart transplant often costs as much or less than long hospitalization before inevitable death). Yet, in many situations, the possibility of rescue is more remote and is attended with great suffering and eventual disappointment. This is the endemic state of the world of organ transplantation.

The ambiguity of transplantation has frustrated two scholars who for many years chronicled with sympathy and sensitivity its growth, its successes and failures, and the courage of physicians and patients. In 1992, they announced that they were "leaving the field." Among their concerns, Fox and Swazey noted that the ethos of the leaders of transplantation includes not only "a classic American frontier outlook: heroic, pioneering, adventurous, optimistic, determined . . . ," but also "a bellicose, 'death is the enemy' perspective; a rescue-oriented and often zealous determination to maintain life at any cost; and a relentless, hubris-ridden refusal to accept limits." They were also convinced that, "if society is to engage in such endeavors, we have a moral obligation to ensure equitable access to organ replacement" (Fox and Swazey 1992, 201). Their discouragement reflects one side of the ambiguity that splits the field of organ transplantation.

A contrasting view comes from a group of ethicists and physicians who are impressed with the ethical achievement of the field of transplantation: "no part of the health care system has done more to resolve questions of justice than transplantation" (Benjamin et al. 1994, 860). They note the seriousness with which transplanters and policy makers have taken the responsibility for setting up a fair allocation system and repudiating market and commercial schemes that would distort fair allocation. They praise physicians for sticking by the rules for allocation, which are designed to maximize the chance of successful outcomes and to minimize organ wastage. Benjamin and associates see an integrity and equity in the ways in which physicians serve the two masters—their own patients and the population of future patients—and they consider this a model for reform of the general system.

> References to justice and equal access have become part of the everyday vocabulary of those involved with transplantation. We think this change may soon become equally pervasive in the health care system as a whole . . . experience with organ transplantation may teach us that some of the thorniest difficulties associated with rationalizing medical care are within our power to resolve (1994, 860).

The alternative pessimistic and optimistic views of organ transplantation manifest the ambiguity of this extraordinary realm of modern medicine, an ambiguity that appears in its daily practices and decisions, in its ethical disputes, and in the policies that the profession and the public fashion to procure organs, to allocate them fairly, and to manage the crisis that pits personal desperation against public welfare.

DISCUSSION QUESTIONS

1. What criteria should be used for selecting the recipients for scarce organs? How would such factors as medical need, probability of success, lifestyle, and ability to pay fit into a selection scheme?

2. Should organs be bought and sold on the open market? What would be the economic, social, and medical implications of such a policy?

3. Should organ transplantation be included in the commonly understood notion of "adequate" or "minimal" health care?

4. What are the advantages and disadvantages of the following policies: harvesting organs from cadavers? routine inquiry? presumed consent?

Who would be most harmed and who would most benefit? Are fundamental moral rights jeopardized by such policies?

5. Should organs procured from U.S. citizens be used for noncitizens (e.g., nonimmigrant aliens, citizens of other countries who come here to be transplanted, etc.)?

REFERENCES

Books and Articles

Altman, L. K. "Learning from Baby Fae." *New York Times*, Nov. 18, 1984, 1, 30.

Ad Hoc Committee of the Harvard Medical School to Examine the Definition of Brain Death. "A Definition of Irreversible Coma." *JAMA* 205 (1968): 337–340.

Annas, G. *Report of the Massachusetts Task Force on Organ Transplantation*. Boston: Boston University School of Public Health, 1994.

American Medical Association Council on Ethical and Judicial Affairs. *Code of Medical Ethics: Current Opinions with Annotations*. Chicago: American Medical Association, 1994.

Baily, M. A. "Economic Issues in Organ Substitution Technology." In D. Mathieu, Ed., *Organ Substitution Technology. Ethical, Legal, and Public Policy Issues*. Boulder, CO: Westview Press, 1988: 198–210.

Basson, M. "Choosing among Candidates for a Scarce Medical Resource." *J Med Philos* 4 (1979): 313–334.

Benjamin, M., Cohen, C., Grochowski, E., for the Ethics and Social Impact Committee. "What Transplantation Can Teach Us about Health-Care Reform." *N Engl J Med* 330 (1994): 858–860.

Blumstein, J. F., Sloan, F. A. Eds. *Organ Transplantation Policy. Issues and Prospects*. Durham: Duke University Press, 1989.

Brannigan, M. "A Chronicle of Organ Transplant Progress in Japan." *Transpl Int* 5 (1992): 180–186.

Busatil, R. W. "Living-Related Liver Donation: CON." *Transpl Proc* 23 (1991): 43–45.

Cahn, E. *The Moral Decision: Right and Wrong in the Light of American Law*. Bloomington: Indiana University Press, 1955.

Caplan, A. *If I Were a Rich Man, Could I Buy a Pancreas?* Bloomington: Indiana University Press, 1992.

———. "Organ Transplants: The Costs of Success." *Hastings Cent Rep* 13(6) (1983): 23–32.

———. "Ethical and Policy Issues in the Procurement of Cadaver Organs for Transplantation." *N Engl J Med* 311 (1984): 981–984.

Childress, J. "Who Shall Live When All Cannot Live?" *Soundings* 53 (1970): 339–355.

Churchill, L., Pinkus, R. The Use of Anencephalic Organs: Historical and Ethical Dimensions. *Milbank* 68(2) (1990): 147–169.

Culliton, B. "Politics of the Heart." *Science* 241 (1988): 283.

Department of Health and Human Services. Reports of the Task Force on Organ Transplantation: Issues and Recommendations. Washington, DC: Department of Health and Human Services, 1986.

Daniels, N. "Justice and the Dissemination of 'Big-Ticket' Technologies." In D. Mathieu, Ed., *Organ Substitution Technology. Ethical, Legal, and Public Policy Issues.* Boulder, CO: Westview Press, 1988: 211–218.

Engelhardt, H. T. "Allocating Scarce Medical Resources and the Availability of Organ Transplantation: Some Moral Presuppositions." *N Engl J Med* 311 (1984): 66–71.

Fetal Tissue Panel. *Report of the Human Fetal Tissue Transplantation Research Panel.* Bethesda, MD: National Institutes of Health, 1988.

Fletcher, J., Robertson, J., Harrison, M. "Primates and Anencephalics as Sources for Pediatric Organ Transplants." *Fetal Ther* 1 (1986): 150–164.

Fox, R., Swazey, J. *Spare Parts: Organ Replacement in American Society.* Oxford and New York: Oxford University Press.

Freedman, B. "The Ethical Continuity of Transplantation." *Transpl Proc* 17 (1985): 17–23.

Fried, C. *Medical Experimentation.* New York: Elsevier, 1974.

Frier, D., Mavrodes, G. "The Morality of Selling Human Organs." In M. Basson, Ed., *Ethics, Humanism, and Medicine.* New York: Alan R. Liss, 1980.

Freund, P. "Introduction to the Ethical Aspects of Experimentation with Human Subjects." *Daedalus* 98 (1969): vii–xiv.

Garland, M. "Justice, Politics and Community: Expanding Access and Rationing Health Services in Oregon." *Law, Med Health Care* 19 (1991): 1–23.

Gaylin, W. "Harvesting the Dead." *Harpers* 249 (1974): 23–30.

Greely, H. T., Hamm, T., Johnson, R., et al. "The Ethical Use of Human Fetal Tissue in Medicine." *N Engl J Med* 320 (1989): 1093–1096.

Green, R. "The Priority of Health Care." *J Med Philos* 8 (1983): 373–380.

Hadorn, D. C. "Setting Health-Care Priorities in Oregon. Cost-Effectiveness Meets the Rule of Rescue." *N Engl J Med* 265 (1991): 2218–2285.

Harris, J. "The Survival Lottery." *Philosophy* 50 (1975): 81–87.

Harrison, M., Meilaender, G. "The Anencephalic Newborn as Organ Donor." *Hastings Cent Rep* 16, no. 2 (1986): 21–23.

Hoffmaster, B. "Freedom to Choose and Freedom to Lose." *Transpl Proc* 17 (1985): 24–32.

Hogness, J. R., Van Antwerp, M., Eds. *The Artificial Heart. Prototypes, Policies and Patients.* Washington DC: National Academy of Sciences, 1991.

Jonas, H. *Against the Stream: Comments on the Definition and Redefinition of Death. Philosophical Essays.* Englewood Cliffs, NJ: Prentice Hall, 1974.

Jonsen A. "Bentham in a Box: Technology Assessment and Health-Care Allocation." *Law, Med Health Care* 14 (1986): 172–174.

———. "The Artificial Heart's Threat to Others." *Hastings Cent Rep* 16 (1986): 9–11.

Katz, J., Capron, A. *Catastrophic Diseases. Who Decides What?* New York: Russell Sage Foundation, 1975.

Kelly, G. "The Morality of Mutilation: Toward a Revision of the Treatise." *Theolog Stud* 17 (1956): 332–344.

Kennedy, I. "The Donation and Transportation of Kidneys: Should the Law Be Changed?" *J Med Ethics* 5 (1979): 13–21.

Kimura, Rihito. "Medical Ethics, History of 'Subsection' Contemp. Japan." In W. T. Reich, Ed., *Encyclopedia of Bioethics*, Revised Ed. New York: Simon & Schuster/ Macmillan, 1995: 1496–1505.

Lombardo, P. "Consent and Donations from the Dead." *Hastings Cent Rep* 11, no. 6 (1981): 9–11.

Madrozo, I., León, V., Torres, C., et al. "Transplantation of Fetal Substantia Negra and Adrenal Medulla to the Caudate Nucleus in Two Patients with Parkinson's Disease" (Letter). *N Engl J Med* 318 (1988): 51.

Mahowald, M. "Neural Fetal Tissue Transplantation: Scientific, Legal and Ethical Aspects." *Clin Res* 36(3) (1988): 187–188.

Mathieu, D., Ed. *Organ Substitution Technology. Ethical, Legal and Public Policy Issues.* Boulder, CO: Westview Press, 1988.

McCormick, R. "Proxy Consent in the Experimental Situation." *Perspect Biol Med* 18 (1974): 756–769.

McCullough, L. B. "Justice and Health Care: Historical Perspectives and Precedents." In E. E. Shelp, Ed., *Justice and Health Care.* Boston: Reidel, 1981: 51–71.

Menzel, P. *Medical Costs, Moral Choices.* New Haven: Yale University Press, 1982.

Moore, F. D. 1989. "The Desperate Case: CARE (Costs, Applicability, Research, Ethics)." *JAMA* 261 (1989): 384–386.

Moss, A., Siegler, M. "Should Alcoholics Compete Equally for Liver Transplantation?" *JAMA* 206 (1991): 384–386.

Muyskens, J. L. "An Alternative Policy for Obtaining Cadaver Organs." *Philos Pub Aff* 8 (1978): 88–99.

Nakasone, Ronald Y. "Buddhism." In W. T. Reich, Ed., *Encyclopedia of Bioethics.* New York: Free Press, 1978: 312–317.

National Institutes of Health. *The Totally Implantable Artificial Heart: Economic, Ethical, Legal, Medical, Psychiatric and Social Implications.* Bethesda, MD: National Institutes of Health, 1973.

———. *Working Group on Mechanical Circulatory Support: Artificial Heart and Assist Devices: Directions, Needs, Costs, Societal and Ethical Issues.* Bethesda, MD: National Institutes of Health and Human Services Publication No. 85-2723, 1985.

Outka, G. "Social Justice and Equal Access to Health Care." *J Relig Ethics* 2 (1974): 11–32.

Peabody, J., Emery, J., Ashwal, S. "Experience with Anencephalic Infants as Prospective Organ Donors." *N Engl J Med* 321 (1989): 344–350.

Pellegrino, E. D. "Families' Self-Interest and the Cadaver's Organs: What Price Consent?" *JAMA* 265 (1991): 1305–1306.

Perry, C. "Human Organs and the Open Market." *Ethics* 91 (1980): 63–71.

Peters, Thomas G. "Life or Death: The Issue of Payment in Cadaveric Organ Donation (commentary)." *JAMA* 265 (1991): 1302–1305.

Pittsburgh Press. "The Challenge of a Miracle: Selling the Gift." November 3–8, 1985.

President's Commission for Study of Ethical Problems in Medicine and Biomedical and Behavioral Research. *Defining Death.* Washington, DC: Government Printing Office, 1981.

———. *Securing Access to Health Care.* Washington, DC: Government Printing Office, 1983.

Preston, T. A. "Who Benefits from the Artificial Heart?" *Hastings Cent Rep* 15 (1985): 5–7.

Prottas, Jeffrey, Childress, James F., Ubel, Peter A., Mahowald, Mary B. "Organ and Tissue Procurement." In W. T. Reich, Ed., *Encyclopedia of Bioethics.* New York: Free Press, 1978: 1852–1871.

Ramsey, P. *Patient as Person.* New Haven: Yale University Press, 1970.

———. "The Enforcement of Morals: Non-Therapeutic Research on Children." *Hastings Cent Rep* 6 (1976): 21–30.

Raymond, A. "France, The Automatic Transplant." *Washington Post,* August 16, 1978.

Report of the Massachusetts Task Force on Organ Transplantation. *Law, Med Health Care* 13, no. 1 (1985): 8–27.

Rescher, N. "Allocation of Exotic Lifesaving Medical Therapy." *Ethics* 79 (1969): 173–186.

Rettig, R.A. "The Politics of Health Cost Containment: End-Stage Renal Disease." *Bull NY Acad Med* 56 (1980): 115–137.

Rolston, H. "The Irreversibly Comatose: Respect for the Subhuman in Human Life." *J Med Philos* 7 (1982): 337.

Rosner, F. "Organ Transplantation in Jewish Law." In F. Rosner and J. D. Bleich, Eds., *Jewish Bioethics.* New York: Sanhedrin Press, 1979.

Sachedina, Abdulaziz. "Islam." In W. T. Reich, Ed., *Encyclopedia of Bioethics,* Revised ed. New York: Simon & Schuster/Macmillan, 1995: 1289–1297.

Sadler, A. M., Sadler, B. "Organ Donation: Is Voluntarism Still Valid?" *Hastings Cent Rep* 14, no. 5 (1984): 6–9.

Schwartz, H. S. "Bioethical and Legal Considerations in Increasing the Supply of Transplantable Organs: From UAGA to 'Baby Fae.'" *Am J Law Med* 10 (1984): 397–438.

Shaw, M., Ed. *After Barney Clark. Reflections on the Utah Artificial Heart Experience.* Austin: University of Texas, 1984.

Singer, P. A., Siegler, M., Whitington, P. F., et al. "Ethics of Live Transplantation with Liver Donors." *N Engl J Med* 321 (1989): 620–622.

Starzl, T., Van Thiel, D., Tzakis, A., et al. "Orthotopic Liver Transplantation for Alcoholic Cirrhosis." *JAMA* 260(217) (1988): 2542–2544.

Stiller, Calvin R., Fox, Renee C., Swazey, Judith P, Caplan, Arthur L. "Organ and Tissue Transplants." In W. T. Reich, Ed., *Encyclopedia of Bioethics.* New York: Free Press, 1978: 1871–1894.

Tendler, M. D. "Cessation of Brain Function. Ethical Implications in Terminal Care and Organ Transplant." *Ann NY Acad Sci* 315 (1978): 394.

Titmus, Richard. *The Gift Relationship: From Human Blood to Social Policy*. London: George Allen and Unwin, 1971.

United Network for Organ Sharing. *Annual Report of U.S. Scientific Registry of Transplant Recipients and Organ Procurement and Transplant Network. Transplant Data: 1988–1991*. Bethesda: Division of Organ Transplantation, Health Resources and Services Administration, Department of Health and Human Services, 1993.

Vawter, D. E., Kearney, W., Gervais, G., et al. *The Use of Human Fetal Tissue: Scientific, Ethical and Policy Concerns*. Minneapolis: Center for Biomedical Ethics, University of Minnesota, 1990.

Veatch, R. M. "The Whole Brain Oriented Concept of Death: An Outmoded Philosophical Formulation." *J Thanatol* 3 (1975): 13.

———. *Death, Dying and the Biological Revolution*. New Haven: Yale University Press, 1976.

———. "What Is a 'Just' Health-Care Delivery?" In R. H. Veatch, Ed., *Ethics and Health Policy*. Cambridge: Ballinger, 1976: 127–153.

Walzer, M. *Spheres of Justice*. New York: Basic Books, 1983.

Welch, H. G., Larson, E. B. "Dealing with Limited Resources: The Oregon Decision to Curtail Funding for Organ Transplantation." *N Engl J Med* 319 (1988): 171–173.

Willard, D. "Scarce Medical Resources and the Right to Refuse Selection by Artificial Chance." *J Med Philos* 5 (1980): 225–229.

Wolstenholme, G. E. W., O'Connor, M. *Law and Ethics of Transplantation*. London: Churchill, 1969.

Statutes and Cases

End Stage Renal Disease Amendments, 1972.

McFall v. Shimp. No. 78-17711. (Allegheny County, PA), July 26, 1978.

National Organ Transplantation Act, 1984.

New Jersey Advance Directives for Health Care and Declaration of Death Acts, 1991.

Strunk v. Strunk. 445 S.W.2d. 145 (Kentucky), 1969.

Uniform Anatomical Gift Act, 1968.

Uniform Determination of Death Act, 1981.

Moral Problems
in Psychiatry

The Role of Value Judgments
in Psychiatric Practice

LORETTA M. KOPELMAN

SUMMARY

More critical attention should be given to the role of value judgments in psychiatry because such evaluations influence how we make decisions about people's capacities to understand, reason, choose, or act. This chapter focuses on how both moral and nonmoral value judgments shape the practice of psychiatry and directly affect how people are viewed and treated. Value judgments about fairness, promoting people's well-being, encouraging their self-determination, promoting social utility, and duties of beneficence are among the most important of these assessments.

Value judgments also affect court decisions about who will be convicted of crimes, involuntarily committed to hospitals, treated without consent, allowed to raise their children, or be regarded as mentally ill. When people disagree about these matters, their controversies may represent value disagreements rather than scientific disputes. Included herein are discussions about the Americans with Disabilities Act, the President's Commission analysis of competency, liberty-limiting principles (e.g., weak paternalism and the Harm Principle), confidentiality, competency, the moral basis of diagnosis, involuntary commitment, and research guidelines.

Note: This chapter is dedicated to my father, the late Frank M. Criden, M.D., a psychiatrist.

Societies reveal a good deal about themselves by how they treat people with mental illness. Cultures show their scientific views, but they also display their values. The role of science is well recognized in assessments about people's mental health, illness, or diagnosis. Yet value judgments also have an essential role to play in these judgments. For example, they affect how psychiatrists envision their duties to patients, including their goals in making diagnoses, maintaining confidentiality, assessing competency, and in judging who merits liberty and who should be involuntarily committed to a hospital. Value judgments also help determine consent and research regulations, and influence how to mark thresholds between the healthy and ill, or between the able and disabled. They also influence court verdicts about who will be convicted of crimes, involuntarily committed to hospitals, treated without consent, allowed to raise their children, regarded as mentally ill, or given compensation for mental disabilities. When people disagree about these matters, their controversies may represent value disagreements rather than scientific disputes. In this chapter I argue that more critical attention should be given to the role of such value claims in understanding psychiatric practice. Value judgments about promoting people's well-being, obligations of fostering self-determination, enhancing beneficence (the duty to do good or prevent harm), and social utility are among the most important of the judgments affecting psychiatric practice, and they should receive special attention.

MORAL AND NONMORAL VALUE JUDGMENTS

The founders of modern psychiatry helped change how the public envisioned mental illness because they reclassified mental illness from moral to nonmoral categories of badness. This revolutionary accomplishment also altered how people with mental disability were treated. Leaders such as Benjamin Rush and Sigmund Freud taught that if people's behavior resulted from mental illness, they need not be held responsible for their behavior and that compassionate care, not blame, was the proper response to their behavior.[1] In 1812 Rush wrote, "For many centuries they have been treated like criminals, or shunned like beasts of prey; or if visited, it has only been for the purposes of inhumane curiosity and amusement. . . . Happily, these times of cruelty to this class of our fellow creatures and insensibility to their sufferings are now passing away" (1979, 243). This reclassification, however, does not eliminate moral notions from psychiatric practice or policies. Both moral and nonmoral values have important roles to play in psychiatric practice and policy.

A *value judgment* expresses a positive or negative assessment about someone's or something's worth, importance, significance, ability, or merit

---

[1]See collected works of Rush (1979) and Freud (1959).

to us in some way. *Nonmoral value judgments* assess the goodness or badness of things (not people) and the actions that are useful to obtaining those things we consider valuable or to avoiding those we dislike. For example, part of what "illness" means is that it is bad, but the badness is nonmoral. Illnesses make us feel terrible and interfere with what we want to do. One cannot consistently speak of a "good" illness unless the illness allows one to avoid something worse (like an exam). Cowpox, a mild viral illness, was considered good and sought when it was the best available protection from smallpox. Diagnosing someone as ill is evaluative, therefore, because it means that people have been judged to have something bad or wrong with them. Since they are not responsible for their sickness, the badness is not moral. They fail, not morally but through disability, to meet certain health norms or ideals considered good, desirable, or worthwhile.

Moral judgments express whether people's actions are right or wrong, whether people have duties or obligations, and what motives or character traits we consider good, bad, blameworthy, or virtuous (Frankena 1973). Moral judgments have helped define professional goals and principles since ancient times by clarifying the duties and the virtues of good physicians.[2] The physician's duty of beneficence to patients is of particular importance in these codes and covenants, and is expressed in concerns about the relief of suffering; the restoration of health; and the diagnosis, treatment, and prevention of illness. Duties of beneficence are even part of what we mean by "therapy" and "therapist." To be a *therapist*, one must provide therapy; and, to count as a *therapy*, it must be intended to help the patient. Virtuous physicians are also supposed to protect public health, promote personal health, prevent illness and disabilities, maintain confidentiality, and improve their knowledge and skills.[3]

Both moral and nonmoral value judgments, then, have important roles to play in psychiatric practice. The reclassification of mental illness from moral to nonmoral badness, however, represented a major step in the humane treatment of psychiatric patients. Mental illnesses came to be seen as fundamentally similar to physical illness and not the result of sin. This led to a similar posture between the study, diagnosis, treatment, and prevention of physical and mental illnesses. To understand the role of values in psychiatric practice, moral and scientific judgments should also be distinguished.

---

[2]The terms *ethical* and *moral* are used interchangeably here.

[3]Like other dynamic traditions, there are differences of opinion about how to benefit people through medicine and fulfill stated goals and virtues (MacIntyre 1981). Moreover, like other fast-moving fields in science and medicine, practices considered good a short time ago may be discredited today. Because moral guidelines have been a part of medical practice for so long, they have affected the law. Consequently, there are often similarities in the moral, professional, and legal duties to provide proper therapy.

DISTINGUISHING MORAL AND SCIENTIFIC JUDGMENTS

To consider how to distinguish the role of scientific and moral judgment in medical practice, consider Case 10.1.

CASE 10.1

Peter has applied to medical school. He has a straight A average, excellent letters of recommendation, outstanding test scores, and praise from his interviewers. Dr. R, a physician serving on the admissions committee, knows that Peter has been seen for many years by a psychiatrist for a serious psychotic disorder and has been hospitalized more than once for this. Peter functions poorly when he has to deal with people. He has succeeded academically because his work has been confined to learning material from books and working in the library. On the basis of what is known about this condition, Dr. R concludes the stress of medical training would be very bad for Peter and that in the unlikely event he finished, he would be an unfit physician. If Dr. R says nothing, Peter will be admitted and another candidate will be denied admission. What ought Dr. R to do?

Dr. R contemplates four options: (1) tell the committee what he knows about Peter; (2) tell the Dean of Admissions privately; (3) tell the committee that he knows something about Peter that he cannot share but that makes Peter an entirely unsuitable candidate for admission; or (4) say nothing. Suppose, too, that because of the competitive nature of the admissions process and the esteem in which the committee holds Dr. R, he knows the first three options would result in Peter not being admitted to medical school. Dr. R cannot recommend that the committee ask Peter about his medical and psychiatric history because that would be illegal for the committee to do (Americans with Disabilities Act, 1990; U.S. Rehabilitation Act 1973). Each of the above options has undoubtedly been taken at some time by admissions committee members, but what *has been* done does not settle the moral question of what *ought to be* done. Dr. R wants to select and act on a morally justifiable opinion, not merely state a personal, social, or institutional preference.

To put forth a judgment as moral, one must be willing to defend it in a certain way. Philosophers often call this defense *practical reasoning* or advancing a moral justification. This justification is a goal toward which we strive when we claim to be making a moral judgment. Because this goal is so demanding, none can say with certainty that it has been achieved. The goals in a moral justification are to be clear, to use all relevant information, and to give cogent reasons for one's views. Advancing a moral also requires consistency or a willingness to apply the reasons universally and impartially; it presupposes that one is not being egoistic, but will apply the reasons to all, even oneself. Furthermore, one must always assess one's reasons critically in relation to other relevant, albeit fallible, considerations such as legal, social, and religious traditions or other stable views about how we should act or what we should be. Although fallible, these traditions hold the preserved wisdom about how to understand and rank values. It also includes a willingness to be sensitive to moral conflicts and problems, to beliefs about what is compassionate, and to the feelings, preferences, and rights of others.

If we assume Dr. R has sufficient information, then Dr. R's problem is more moral than scientific because, unless the conflict is solved in another way (e.g., Peter might volunteer the information to the committee), Dr. R has to decide how to rank certain important values. Dr. R might decide to honor Peter's privacy and confidences by saying nothing. Alternatively, Dr. R might decide the duty to act on the information is greater than preserving confidentiality as a way to select the best candidates for medical training, or to protect people, including Peter, from harm. The way we rank values is sometimes affected by our roles. Arguably, Dr. R has a greater duty to be silent if he is Peter's psychiatrist. Furthermore, if Dr. R shares his knowledge about Peter, will he help to undermine the important practice of respecting privacy and medical confidentiality? If Dr. R does not tell, is he responsible if Peter becomes much sicker in medical school or harms others? Is he unfair if by his silence he denies a more suitable candidate a place in the class? To reach a morally justifiable conclusion, Dr. R must presume he knows about Peter's illness and its consequence well enough to predict how Peter will respond to medical school, as well as how to rank important values. It is the *method* of reasoning, not just the arrived at opinion, that makes a judgment worthy of being considered a moral judgment. Similarly, it is the method of reasoning that makes someone's claim worthy of being called scientific.

Psychiatry, like any other branch of Western medicine, not only employs many values but is also committed to the scientific method. It is a matter of debate how moral judgments differ from factual or scientific claims or how methods of reasoning in ethics and science differ. This issue need not be resolved, however, to distinguish between moral and scientific judgments. *Scientific judgments* are based on data collected or appraised in relation to hypotheses or theories for the purpose of predicting future events and consequences. The purpose of gathering data and building scientific theories is to describe, explain, predict, or control events. Such claims serve in medicine as the empirical basis for the activities of diagnosis, prognosis, prevention, or treatment of illness. Scientific judgments are necessary, but not sufficient for the practice of psychiatry, because psychiatry also includes values, duties, goods, goals, and virtues as an internal part of this tradition. Dr. R would not be justified in expressing his opinion about Peter's prognosis as a psychiatric opinion unless he could justify it in ways the scientific community considered credible. For example, if reliable studies show that 90 percent of those with Peter's condition become acutely ill with the kind of stress experienced in medical school, Dr. R could predict problems for Peter with a high degree of certainty.

Scientific claims, including psychiatric opinions, must generally be testable or falsifiable. Certain schools of psychiatry are held to be unscientific because their theories cannot be used to derive testable hypotheses. Philosophers Karl Popper (1962) and William P. Alston (1967), for example, argued that certain psychoanalytic theories are not scientific because they cannot be confirmed or refuted. If this is correct, whatever utility such theories may have, insofar as they do not derive testable hypotheses, they are not scientific. For example, suppose one study found that 90 percent of the people with Peter's condition became seriously incapacited in stressful situations, but another study with similar subjects and methods found that only 5 percent had this result. Investigators would not be satisfied with these different findings and would try to give some account of the different results. In science it is usually assumed that similar situations result in similar findings and consequences—this is called the assumption of the uniformity of nature. Diversity of views and opinions in science generally creates a problem to be solved by investigators, although some debates, such as those on the level of quantum theory or cosmology, may be difficult to resolve. In science, great emphasis is placed on systematic power, elegance, and simplicity in resolving disagreements when two accounts square with what is known.

Although there are many controversies in the sciences, it is generally assumed that disputes can be resolved by better methodologies, studies, data, hypotheses, or theories. In contrast, there may be a diversity of views in the moral life that cannot be resolved by these means. This does not mean that rational discourse is any less important in morality than it is in science or that science is value-free or theory-neutral. Rather, it means that reasoned differences of opinion in moral life can occur; and they may result from differences in the balance given to conflicting goods, rights, duties, goals, principles, virtues, or values. When more than one ranking of them can be justified, different reasoned views should be tolerated. Thus, even when we do not agree in our moral judgments we can sometimes recognize that alternative views have merit. Moral differences, however, can often be resolved by gaining more relevant information, by clarifying the language we use, by examining the worthiness of our reasoning, by looking at the consequences or implications of our reasoning, or by identifying the nature and ranking of the importance of principles proposed as justifiable and worthy. For example, to decide what to do for Peter in Case 10.1, Dr. R might want to have more information about how legal and moral commentators understand the duty to maintain or override confidentiality.[4]

Thus, attaching the title "moral," "scientific," or "psychiatric" to one's judgment means that one believes a certain method of reasoning has been used properly, and the assertion is not just a matter of preference, mores, traditions, aesthetics, or social approval. If one calls one's claim a moral judgment, this means a moral justification can be given; and if one calls one's view a psychiatric opinion, this means that a scientific justification can also be given. Moral and scientific reasoning share many goals. They both require one to be clear in stating the problem, to collect relevant and unbiased information, to reevaluate opinions in light of new information, to defend opinions with reasons, and to be consistent. A dissimilarity between moral and scientific reasoning is that different views in science are almost always seen as a problem to be solved. Although moral problems are often solved by better data, studies, methods, or theories, sometimes reasonable and informed people of good will may rank important values differently. Insofar as they do, it may be proper to be tolerant of different views. It is possible, therefore, to disagree in both morals and science while acknowledging that alternative choices are rational.

THE MORAL BASIS OF PSYCHIATRIC DIAGNOSIS

There are at least five important but different views about the role of value and scientific judgments in the diagnosis of mental disease or illness. The views are distinguishable in terms of whether or how advocates believe a value judgment can be subject to rational confirmation or rejection.

Subjective Opinion

One view is that judgments about mental disease or illness are merely a matter of subjective opinion that cannot be given a rational defense. This view fully acknowledges that values cannot be eliminated from psychiatric

---

[4]Ethics is a field of philosophy especially concerned with conflicts of important values, rights, principles, duties, goals, or ends, where reasonable and informed people of good will can reasonably disagree. Interest in moral conflicts and forced ranking of values can bias the problems studied by philosophers. Although most moral problems are resolvable in a fairly straightforward manner, philosophers tend to be especially interested in conflicts of important values, rights, duties, principles, ends, or goals that are hard to resolve, regardless of whether they are rare. For example, studies show that persons with mental illness are, as a group, probably little or no more dangerous than the general public (Zembaty 1982). Nevertheless, theoretical discussions often focus on the rare cases in which a person may be a danger to self or others to test the fair limits of liberty or the power of the state to intervene, constrain, or coerce citizens. Furthermore, many reasonable people are more interested in resolving or avoiding the head-to-head conflicts that force such rankings.

diagnoses but denies that the judgments are subject to rational confirmation or rejection. This view, for example, would state that we have no way to evaluate, confirm, or reject the judgment of a minister who in 1860 decided his wife was mentally ill and committed her to an institution for no other reason than that she disagreed with him (Szasz 1970). Or consider Case 10.2.

CASE 10.2

Mrs. Q seeks counseling from Dr. B. Mr. Q is a visiting professor from a country Dr. B believes to favor the subjugation of women's interests to men's. Mrs. Q, as a result of living in this country while her husband went to graduate school, wants to learn to achieve more personal independence. Her husband forbids this, regarding such views as symptoms of mental illness. Dr. B believes Mrs. Q is not mentally ill but understandably angry about the way her husband says she must live her life. Is she mentally ill or is her health just a matter of subjective opinion?

It certainly matters to Mrs. Q whether she is viewed as healthy or mentally ill. Yet, if diagnoses are just a matter of subjective opinion, then diagnosing cannot be done well or badly or for good or bad purposes. Moreover, according to this view, there can be no scientific basis or moral justification for determining whether people have mental illness. This view is incompatible with viewing psychiatric practice as scientific or as a profession.

The Medical or Physiological Model

Another view, associated with the work of psychiatrist Thomas Szasz, holds that psychiatric diagnoses are defensible only where there is a known bodily disease causing the symptoms. Otherwise, "mental" illness is a metaphor to describe or control behavior we do not like (Szasz 1961, 1970); physical illnesses are real and mental illnesses without a demonstrated pathophysiology are social fictions. If this view is correct, it is wrong to diagnose people like Peter in Case 10.1 as having an illness unless we know his condition to be a physical disease.

There are serious problems with this view. First, the so-called medical model fails as a general account of maladies, even if we limit ourselves to physical disease or illnesses. When people have had unexplained but similar symptoms, such as those of asthma, multiple sclerosis, and schizophrenia, physicians diagnose the conditions as diseases before knowing their physical causes. Thinking of illness or disease as a pathophysiological process began with the nineteenth-century pathologist Rudolf Virchow. Virchow expanded but did not invent the concepts of illness and disease.[5] The older notion of illness or disease was understood in terms of the patterns in people's complaints, sufferings, and disfunctions. Virchow's insight, although of great importance in initiating the age of scientific medicine, cannot be the single basic notion of disease. To seek and identify a process or function as pathological presupposes we first identify a pattern in people's complaints, suffering, or dysfunction. It may take many decades to learn about the underlying pathology of diseases and how they are affected by environmental, social, and genetic factors. A pattern of illness related to people's suffering, complaints, or dysfunction is often sufficient to say something is an illness or disease even before satisfactory explanations of its cause are found.

In addition, it seems inappropriate to sharply distinguish mental and physical diseases or illnesses because they seem interrelated. For example, depression can bring on physical illness, and physical illness can cause depression. Psychiatric practice has traditionally focused on ailments in which suffering involves impairment of a person's ability to understand, reason, choose, or act. Sometimes physical lesions or processes are found to explain these impairments.

Psychiatrists are unwilling to say they are interested in mental as opposed to physical illness (American Psychiatric Association, *DSM-IV*, 1994; see glossary on mental disorder). They have always been interested in diseases of the brain such as Alzheimer's disease in which underlying physical pathologies are clear. Moreover, some ailments once regarded as purely mental conditions, such as certain forms of manic depressive illness and schizophrenia, are now seen as having physical causes, but they are still treated in psychiatric practice.

A final objection to the view that a rational defense of psychiatric diagnoses requires proof that the diseases or illnesses are physical disorders is that there are inherent problems within the reductionist or materialistic approach that this view presupposes. One assumption made by reductionists and materialists is that the human point of view can be eliminated from scientific inquiry so that it is possible to arrive at a purely material account. Yet this is problematic because one needs a perspective to make judgments that material things are the same or different. These accounts also presuppose that some laws can explain human behavior and illness and do so without exception. Yet no successful example of this has ever been produced and critics suggest there are good reasons for supposing these materialistic or reductionist programs cannot succeed (Margolis 1966; MacIntyre 1981; Chisholm 1956).

The Statistical Frequency Model

A third view is that judgments about psychiatric diagnosis are subject to rational confirmation or rejection only when they are purged of values. Some claim that the statistical frequency model can result in value-free testing

---

[5]For a discussion of the relation of concepts of illness and disease, see Fulford 1989.

and judgments (Mercer 1973). According to this view, distribution of a trait (e.g., fearfulness) is determined on a basis of a standardized test; traits judged two or more deviations from the mean are considered abnormally low or abnormally high.

Although such methods have been extremely important in removing bias and partiality in making diagnoses and determining the prevalence and incidence of mental illness, this method does not eliminate values (Kopelman 1984; Macklin 1972, 1973). Researchers must make certain choices and they may do so well or badly, or for good or bad purposes. Values are introduced in the selection of norms judged appropriate for the purpose of the test, in the selection of the test instrument itself, in the uses to which the test is put, in the selection of a significance level, and in the interpretation of the results. For example, thumb-sucking has a different meaning among preschool and premedical college students. In interpreting this behavior, then, it is important (a value) to distinguish groups by age. Researchers also employ values in deciding when there is enough of a difference between groups to end a study and conclude the variance was not due to chance alone. Just as a teacher selects what to test and what grade is passing, so an investigator decides what to test and when differences between study arms are significant. This may be done well or badly, fairly or not. Thus, despite defenders' beliefs, values are introduced in many ways by this statistical frequency method.

Ethical or Cultural Relativism

A fourth view is that diagnoses about mental illness are value laden, but that the values are based entirely on what is approved or disapproved in one's culture. According to this view, no rational basis exists for establishing that one set of cultural values is right and the other wrong. This is the extreme version of *ethical cultural relativism* and has the consequence that there can be no judgments about how patients ought to be treated having intercultural authority. The profession of psychiatry, however, is an international and intercultural activity that sets moral duties for psychiatrists and evaluative standards for diagnosis, treatments, and research. If the extreme version of ethical relativism is true, the judgments of international psychiatric organizations have no genuine intercultural moral authority and merely reflect the particular cultural views of individual members. Consider Case 10.3, which is based on Block (1981) and Reich (1981).

CASE 10.3

In the 1970s and 1980s, international psychiatric organizations criticized psychiatrists in the Soviet Union for misdiagnosing people who exhibited no signs of serious illness, and for detaining and treating people as mentally ill for political reasons. Psychiatric diagnosis was employed, critics charged, as a weapon by the Soviets to silence dissidents advocating human rights or nationalism for republics within the Soviet Union. It was also used to repress persons seeking to emigrate, who had religious convictions, or who caused other embarrassment to the Soviet government. The Soviet psychiatrists defending these practices argued that the criticisms were unfounded. They said the people were sick because they were maladjusted, nonconformist, and abnormal within their society and that this was demonstrated by their deviant and inappropriate social behavior. Soviet psychiatrists are taught to view such behavior as mental illness. Diagnoses and practices, they argued, are framed by society's own norms and values. These patients were seen as sick people and should be detained and treated in Soviet society, even if they might not be in other societies. Can diagnoses ever have moral or professional authority from one culture to another?

This version of ethical relativism claims to give an account of duties, rightness, wrongness, goodness, and badness in terms of *cultural* approval and disapproval. Thus, to work, defenders must tell us how to differentiate or identify cultures so we can find out what is good or bad, or right or wrong. Or to put the point another way, how do we count cultures? Is the international community of psychiatrists itself a culture? If not, why not? If it is, people from different parts of the world can share cultural norms; consequently, their value judgments have moral authority, and ethical relativism is false.

In short, ethical relativism is not a helpful theory if we cannot distinguish people's cultures well enough to decide what is good or bad, or right or wrong. Nor is it useful if defenders fail to distinguish between cultures but merely observe that each of us belongs to many cultures, or that cultures overlap and have many similarities with others and differences within. Although these observations seem true, they defeat ethical relativism. That is, if cultures cannot be clearly distinguished, or if it is extremely difficult to mark a particular culture, it is equally difficult to say what is approved or disapproved within a particular culture.[6] Consider that the first criticisms of the Soviets' practices came from psychiatrists *within* the Soviet Union, who openly challenged what they viewed as a political misuse of psychiatry. Social deviance is not mental illness and to hold it is, they said, violates international psychiatric values. These groups condemned the national control of professions for political purposes. Their criticisms were taken up by members of international psychiatric organizations who believed psychiatric organizations should control psychiatric diagnoses and practices, not psychiatrists in the service of a political agenda. Of course, people from different

---

[6]For a fuller discussion of the problems with ethical relativism, see Kopelman (1994b).

cultures sometimes *do* act differently and have distinct norms, but the point at issue is whether cross-cultural value judgments with moral or other authority is *ever* possible. Making value judgments that have moral authority in different cultures, then, is an important part of the psychiatric profession, and consequently incompatible with this extreme version of ethical relativism.

Meaning and Use

A fifth view, and the one that seems correct to me, is that psychiatric diagnoses are inherently evaluative, but we have to consider how the diagnoses are used to determine their meaning and reasonableness. Some ways to use diagnoses are psychiatrically respectable and some are not. For example, to say "He behaves like a psychopath" could express a sound psychiatric judgment, or be a way to express fear, humor, hate, or prejudice. When used as a psychiatric judgment, the authority for accuracy belongs to the international psychiatric profession and should be grounded in scientific descriptions, explanation, or prediction of events. Similarly, if someone is described as having anorexia nervosa, we would expect to see a thin person who has an eating disorder. But diagnosing disease or illness also conveys an evaluation about that condition: It is bad to have anorexia nervosa or any other disease.

We need to examine, then, the justification for saying some condition is bad as well as the scientific grounds for asserting that the condition causes disfunction or disability. Our views on both counts may change. For example, Benjamin Rush, the leading psychiatrist of eighteenth-century America, held that sexual promiscuity was a deplorable and pathetic disease of the mind and caused physical illnesses such as "pulmonary consumption, dyspepsia, dimness of sight, vertigo, epilepsy, hypochondriasis, loss of memory, monologue, fatuity and death" (Rush 1979 (reprint), 347). These views were undercut by impartial studies and more attention to the values used in making such judgment. More recently, psychologist Carol Gilligan and others have argued that so-called scientific information often has a gender bias about normal behavior (Gilligan et al. 1988).[7]

Complexity in the meaning and use of psychiatric terms also stems from choices about how to draw the line between health and illness. Like physicians in other branches of medicine, psychiatrists treat a broad range of illnesses and problems. They range from mild disturbances that would correct themselves in time to chronic debilitating conditions (such as schizophrenia), and to life-threatening disorders from which people can recover (such as anorexia nervosa and severe depression). Some psychiatric patients are

---

[7]Freud's views about the psychological dynamics of women and their so-called penis envy were limited by his cultural beliefs.

competent people seeking counseling for the problems of living that thwart them: how to cope when they feel trapped by a job, marriage, or school; how to respond to an abusive person in their life; what to do when they feel very sad. Psychiatrists also see patients who are extremely impaired, even suicidal or violent. Some are unable to act as they wish, and cannot, for example, leave their homes without experiencing great anxiety. Others cannot be responsible for their actions because they have a picture of reality distorted by hallucinations, delusions, or irrational misconceptions. Psychiatrists seek to diagnose, study, prevent, and treat this broad range of maladies, and, as in other branches of medicine, they do so with varying degrees of success.

Which of these conditions should be regarded as "mental illnesses"? Psychiatrist Will Gaylin (1982) argues that milder disorders have increasingly received psychiatric labels; inhibitions, episodes of aberrant behavior, the absence of normal behavior, and anger have been pulled into the web of psychiatric diagnoses. To add to the confusion, some rich countries and generous third-party payers were willing to recognize milder conditions as mental illnesses. The various assessments of where to draw the line between health and illness, however, do not seem fundamentally different from other areas of medicine, and, in part, seem to be social and economic choices. For example, at some point, neurological discharges are excessive enough to merit a diagnosis of epilepsy, and overweight is excessive enough to be called obesity. Thus, our choices about where to draw the line between health and disease, especially for milder conditions, in part, seem to be socially determined. Although this is true of both physical and mental maladies, prejudices exist for people with psychiatric diagnoses—assigning labels based on mild conditions may cause more harm than good.

To help address the problems of subjectivity, prejudice, and cultural differences, international psychiatric organizations try to reserve *mental disorder* for very serious, well-defined conditions. They also press for standard, worldwide acceptance of psychiatric nosology, in which both the scientific and evaluative elements have been justified. These restrictions have moral and scientific purposes. Morally, they minimize the harm done to people through inappropriate labeling and the stigmatization of others as a result of mistakes, inconsistency, or politics. They also serve the purposes of science because consistent classification is needed to study and test theories about disorders. On these grounds, both national and world psychiatric organizations condemned the Soviet psychiatrists for misusing psychiatric diagnosis and giving inappropriate therapy. The American Psychiatric Association (*DSM-IV* 1994), for example, states that mental illnesses are not to be locally defined and that social deviance, however disagreeable, is not in itself a basis for ascribing mental illness. Mental disorders, they hold, are not different in kind from physical diseases, and diagnoses should be based on their associations with specific conditions that are painful, disabling, and nonmorally bad.

DUTIES IN DIAGNOSES

There are three interrelated duties for those given the authority to diagnose others. As we shall see, these obligations sometimes conflict (Kopelman 1984).

One reason for giving a diagnosis to someone is for *accuracy or integrity of observation and descriptions*. If a man believes his thoughts are being controlled by satellites, he should be described as delusional. Accurate, individual descriptions of people's illnesses or problems are the first step to understanding, explaining, and treating illnesses, and thus fulfilling scientific goals and goals in medicine. Soviet physicians were condemned by psychiatric organizations on scientific as well as moral grounds for deliberately using diagnoses inaccurately for political purposes.

Some have charged that psychiatrists are more willing to recognize abuses due to inaccuracy of diagnoses in the Soviet Union than in their own countries (Szasz 1970; Reich 1981). Warren Reich charges that what the Soviets did was different in degree, but not in kind, from what we sometimes see in the United States. Psychiatrists have used diagnosis of mental illness to help people "circumvent the law, get abortions, or to help them evade the military draft. Psychiatrists often saw little danger from such humanitarian deeds, and responded to the requests willingly. But the danger was there, and we only need look to Russia during the Soviet regime to appreciate its extreme potential" (Reich 1981, 84). It is not obvious that the actions merely differed in degree but not in kind. One relevant difference is that the patients in the Soviet Union were diagnosed against their will so that others could restrict their freedom for political purposes; the Western patients Reich describes sought the diagnoses to gain or evade certain constraints. Reich, however, makes a good point that deliberate misdiagnosis is a kind of lie.

A more widespread abuse of accuracy in psychiatric diagnoses is the *redescription* of people in psychiatric terms to control them or to disvalue them or their reasoning. People are sometimes called "depressed," "paranoid," or "psychotic" because others do not like their views. In Case 10.4, an accurate diagnosis by a psychiatrist helped someone about to be mistakenly described as incompetent and treated over her objections.

CASE 10.4

Mrs. J is 57 years old and has just learned she has a cancerous, rapidly growing brain tumor. She is already blind and knows that people with her condition usually die within six months; none have survived one year. She knows she will become increasingly disabled both mentally and physically. She refuses any procedure that would prolong her life and says she wants to commit suicide. Her physician seeks a psychiatric consultation. A psychiatrist judges her competent, finding that her choice is neither impaired nor the product of mental illness. The nurses and her physician, however, persist in thinking her decision shows she is depressed and should therefore be declared incompetent. Should clinicians decide that people are incompetent based on the content of their decisions?

Second, another important reason that professionals have for diagnosing a person as mentally ill is to *benefit the person* by signaling he or she has important and unique needs. This purpose is closely associated with moral duties of beneficence to people, duties of great importance in the medical profession. Diagnosis may help people by gaining them access to aid, programs, research protocols, third-party payments, or by excusing them from blame. Moreover, descriptions of the number of people who are mentally ill can help them collectively by showing that we need more funds for facilities, treatment, or research. If benefit to the person is given as a reason for diagnosing others by those with special authority to do so in our society, however, people have a right to expect that there are good grounds to hold that the diagnosis will produce more good than harm for them. In balancing likely benefits and harms, one should consider not only the efficacy of treatments, but their side effects and psychosocial dangers (such as risks of prejudice, loss of esteem, misconceptions about mental illness, and the "spread" effect—the tendency to view disabled persons as more handicapped than they are).

Third, professionals sometimes have duties to provide accurate diagnoses *to benefit society.* An accurate diagnosis may be more useful to people who want someone committed or declared incompetent, or to third-party payers, employers, researchers, and the courts than to the person getting the diagnosis. Someone's diagnosis, for example, may reveal that a person is a threat to others and must be detained involuntarily. Accurate diagnoses can also benefit society by allowing us to conduct good research about a condition to help future patients. Or, it may be socially useful to gain information about the incidence and prevalence of diseases so a society can decide how best to allocate resources fairly.

These three reasons for accurate diagnosis represent important values of scientific integrity, beneficence, and utility. Unfortunately, they can conflict. For example, the diagnosis of a patient as mentally ill might be accurate and socially useful, but not be of benefit to the person, as when the diagnosis results in the loss of guardianship or control of property. Because different and potentially conflicting moral responsibilities arise in ascribing diagnoses, it is important to distinguish and justify which are being used. We will now consider other important values shaping psychiatric practice, beginning with the duty to maintain confidentiality.

DUTIES REGARDING CONFIDENTIALITY

When Freud began to see psychiatric patients in his office, he scheduled them so they would never meet. Thus, almost from the beginning of modern psychiatry, extraordinary precautions were taken to ensure patients' privacy and confidentiality. One reason for maintaining confidentiality is therapists' duty to help patients and protect their well-being. Assurances of confidentiality encourage patients to disclose sensitive information that may be crucial for good health-care decisions, yet could harm them if generally known. For example, a surgeon may wish to discuss with his psychiatrist that he has delusions of grandeur, a stockbroker that she may be manic depressive, or a college president that he has an irrational dislike for certain groups of people. Another reason for maintaining confidentiality is that people generally have a right to control information about themselves and can be especially harmed if certain psychiatric information about them is released. Thus, confidentiality is important because of duties of beneficence, rights of self-determination, fairness, and its social utility.

The duty to maintain confidentiality, however, is not absolute. Although there is a presumption in favor of confidentiality, this can be overruled if there is a greater value at stake. Exceptions to confidentiality include the duty to protect an identifiable person or persons (as in child abuse), and the duty to protect the patient (as in protecting a very depressed and suicidal person). In some cases, confidentiality is overridden by a duty to protect unidentified third parties or the general community (for example, patients with dementia should not have driver's licenses because they pose a serious risk of harm to others in the community). The least controversial of the exceptions to the duty to honor confidentiality are situations in which there is a clear, immediate, and grave threat of harm to some identifiable person(s); for example, see Case 10.5.

CASE 10.5

Dr. T is a psychiatrist counseling Mr. and Mrs. N. They tell Dr. T that they keep their three-year-old child locked in the attic for long periods of time as punishment. Should Dr. T tell authorities about this, even if Dr. T is uncertain whether the information is true?

Dr. T is legally and morally obligated to report suspected child abuse to the authorities for investigation because protecting the child from clear, immediate, and grave threats of harm is more important than maintaining patients' confidentiality.

To override the duty of confidentiality, one ought to consider both the severity of the harm and the probability of its occurrence. Disclosures are usually justified when they prevent serious and predictable harms to others.

The more uncertainty that exists about the probability and magnitude of the harm predicted or the benefit to be gained, the more controversy there is about whether to break confidentiality. Reasonable and informed people of good will may sometimes disagree about whether the probability and magnitude of the harm to be avoided or the benefit to be gained justifies exceptions, or about the nature or extent of the duty to respect people's rights of privacy and confidentiality. These value disputes affect not only moral discussions, but legal and psychiatric disputes about when to override confidentiality.

Great controversy, for example, was generated by the decision in the precedent-setting case *Tarasoff v. Regents of the University of California* (1976) as described in Case 10.6.

CASE 10.6

A patient, Prosenjit Poddar, confided to Dr. Moore, a psychologist, that he intended to kill his former girlfriend, Tatiana Tarasoff. Dr. Moore believed him and notified his superior and the police. No action was taken to warn the woman, whom Poddar eventually killed. The California Supreme Court ruled in favor of the family who sued claiming that the psychiatrist and psychologist had a duty to warn her. "When a therapist determines, or pursuant to the standards of his profession should determine, that his patient presents a serious danger of violence to another, he incurs an obligation to use reasonable care to protect the intended victim against such danger" such as warning the intended victim, notifying the police or "Whatever other steps are reasonably necessary under the circumstances" (1976, 204). Did they have a duty to warn her?

This is a controversial precedent because the standard used is difficult to apply. Many patients during therapy express great hostility, even saying they will kill others. Clinicians cannot always predict which of the very few among the many who say such things really mean it. Psychiatrists have argued that they are being required to deliver psychiatric opinions about who is a genuine threat when there is insufficient data to make such predictions. They charge that forcing them to report too widely, for example, for fear of litigation, would undermine the important practice of confidentiality as well as the patient–therapist relation. The debate in law and medicine over the Tarasoff ruling continues. Another important class of exceptions to the duty to honor medical confidences concerns the person who poses a risk of harm to self, as in Case 10.7.

CASE 10.7

Mr. D is taken to his internist, Dr. S, who learns Mr. D has become thin and withdrawn since the death of his son two months earlier. Mr. D blames himself for his son's death. Assurances that he is in no way to blame cannot touch his unshakable belief. He thinks he is worthless, talks openly about how he could go about killing himself, but forbids his physician to say or do anything to stop him. He believes himself unworthy of treatment or hospitalization. Mr. D's physician does not regard his desire to die to be rational and he views Mr. D as depressed and suicidal. Dr. S seeks hospitalization and treatment for Mr. D over his objections because the condition is treatable and he needs to be protected from harming himself. Is Dr. S justified in overriding Mr. D's confidentiality and in seeking psychiatric hospitalization and treatment for Mr. D over Mr. D's objections?

The more the evidence for the psychiatric opinion that the probability or magnitude of harm is great, that the condition is reversible, or that the person is impaired, the more the justification for regarding the situation as an exemption to medical confidentiality. Mr. D's condition is probably reversible, and there is evidence that great harm can come to Mr. D because of his impaired reasoning. Dr. S's decision seems justified for suicide prevention. Suicide is a means some people use to escape pain (Hume 1965; Heyd and Block 1981). Both Mr. D in Case 10.7 and Mrs. J in Case 10.4 sincerely wanted to commit suicide. There is no evidence, however, that Mrs. J's decision, unlike Mr. D's, is the product of mental illness, or that her condition is reversible. These decisions, then, sometimes turn on whether the person is competent, and competency determinations use many values requiring careful justification.

JUDGING COMPETENCY

Competency decisions made in courts reveal some central social values because they involve balancing the rights of the individual to steer his or her own course through life with the power of the state to control people.[8] (Competency and capacity evaluations are sometimes differentiated in that the former is taken to be a legal notion, and the latter is not; but they are not differentiated here.) Consider the controversy in Case 10.8.

CASE 10.8

Joyce Brown was a high school graduate, who had been a secretary for ten years. In her mid-thirties (1983), she lost her job for absenteeism after she began to use drugs. Evicted from her apartment, she

---

[8]Portions of this section were adopted from Kopelman (1990); portions of the section on "Discrimination" from Kopelman (1996); and portions of the section on "Research" from Kopelman (1994a, 1995).

began to live on the streets of New York. She came to the attention of the national press at age 40 when Mayor Edward Koch who, as the winter months approached, instructed New York City personnel to pick up the homeless, against their will if necessary. Many of the homeless who avoid shelters in the cold weather suffer from psychiatric illnesses, and city officials believed that they needed to be protected from their own impaired judgments. Joyce Brown was committed to Bellevue Hospital against her will and was diagnosed as having a paranoid schizophrenic disorder. She had slept over hot air grates, eaten poorly, cursed do-gooders, relieved herself in the streets, abused African American men, sung loudly in public, and ripped up money people tried to give her (Hornblower 1987). Her family was unhappy about her life on the streets. Believing she could be helped, they wanted her committed and treated.

The American Civil Liberties Union defended Ms. Brown, arguing that she was competent and ought not to have been forcibly treated or committed. The judge was confronted by seven psychiatrists, four representing The City of New York who said she was incompetent, and three from the defense who said she was competent. Found to be articulate, calm, and persuasive in the court and on national television (possibly because her lawyers made sure she took her medication), she was declared competent. Was Joyce Brown competent enough to live as she wished or were her preferences the product of her illness?

Joyce Brown's trial was about whether she was competent, but it was also about what kind of society we have and how to rank conflicting values. Placing rights of self-determination higher than duties of protection, some argued she was competent. Others claimed she needed to be protected and treated so she could become well enough to direct her life more autonomously. How should we understand and justify value judgments used in competency decisions?

Charles Culver and Bernard Gert (1982) identified the core meaning of competency as the ability to do a certain task well enough for a certain purpose. To determine if someone is competent or capable, then, we have first to determine: *competent for what?* For example, a student shows competency in college algebra by passing appropriate tests. To say someone is competent (or not) means that the person did certain things that reveal what the person can do. This has led authors to regard competency as a threshold concept that is task-specific (Brock 1989; Faden and Beauchamp 1986). Someone can be competent in one thing (algebra) but not in another (basketball). Someone who cannot jump or shoot baskets is not a competent basketball player. In assessing competency in algebra or basketball, it is fairly easy to identify the appropriate tasks, criteria, tests, and thresholds. Other assessments may be more complex, but the same three features are present. Judgment that someone is competent or has the ability to do a task involves assessments:

1. Someone tries to do a task associated with some ability.
2. The association of the task and the ability is defensible.
3. A justifiable threshold exists to separate those who can and cannot perform the task.

Values arise at each of the three stages. They arise in assessing who tries to do a task, in judging if a task is associated with an ability, and in defending the threshold. In some cases, however, it is not as easy as it was for basketball to identify the tasks, criteria, tests, or thresholds used to assess competency. In the case of legal competency, the notion is so complex that we simply pick an age for which the presumption is that persons over the age of majority are competent and those under that age are not. One can rebut these presumptions by showing that in certain cases an adult can be incompetent and a child competent (Brock 1989).[9]

In competency determinations for medical decisions (a special case of assessing competency generally) these assessments concern: (1) looking at people's actions to assess their ability to reason and deliberate about treatments and their consequences; (2) defending association of these actions with certain important goals and values, typically whether the person is prepared to make decisions that reflect his or her established values and goals (this condition captures whether people are acting characteristically or "like themselves"); (3) defending some threshold to separate competent from incompetent decision makers.[10]

The President's Commission for the Study of Ethical Problems in Medicine (1982) identified the moral values that professionals should use in decisions about a patient's decision-making capacity:

> Thus, a conclusion about a patient's decision-making capacity necessarily reflects a balancing of two important, sometimes competing objectives: to enhance a patient's well-being and to respect the person as a self-determining individual. . . . In the view of the Commission, any determination of the capacity to decide on a course of treatment must relate to the individual abilities of a patient, the requirements of the task at hand, and the consequences likely to flow from the decision. Decision-making capacity requires, to greater or lesser degree: (1) possession of a set of values and goals; (2) the ability to communicate and to understand information; and (3) the ability to reason and to deliberate about one's choices (President's Commission 1982, 57).

---

[9]If the tasks are unspecified, the competency or capacity judgment is elliptical. That is, it leaves open exactly what is entailed by making and defending such a judgment.

[10]The assessments change depending on the values used in the assessments. For example, doctors might use a lower standard of judging competency when there is not too much at stake and a higher standard of judging competency when the risk is very high.

The Commission considered and rejected competency determinations made solely on the basis of one's status (such as age), or on the nature or outcome of the choice alone (such as Mrs. J's decision to forgo lifesaving treatments in Case 10.4). The Commission recommended that in assessing a patient's capacity one should relate the specific tasks to an individual's circumstance as well as to the consequences of performing that task. This is called a functional approach because people's competency is judged by what they do, and because they may be competent to make some decisions for themselves for some purposes but not for others. The President's Commission proposal is useful because it identifies the important moral values that are at the heart of competency or capacity judgments, namely, the duty to consider and balance respect for people's self-determination with protecting them. People with serious mental illness may, though legally incompetent, be capable of representing their own interests to some degree.

Sometimes people disagree about what abilities, thresholds, or tests are relevant to assess competency. In Case 10.9, Miss O is competent by some standards but not by others.

CASE 10.9

Miss O is 21 and has been seeing Dr. Z as a psychiatric outpatient. Miss O has anorexia nervosa and weighs 70 pounds. Dr. Z believes if Miss O does not enter the hospital she will soon die. Dr. Z explains to Miss O that her prognosis is poor even if she enters the hospital, but that there is a 20 percent chance she can recover if she is hospitalized and cooperates. Miss O is cheerful, intelligent, and accurately discusses the risks and benefits of hospitalization, but she refuses to enter the hospital. Is Miss O competent?

The position favored by the President's Commission (1982), by philosophers Buchanan and Brock (1989), and Kopelman (1990), and by many psychiatrists (Appelbaum et al. 1982; Roth et al. 1977) is to balance the standard of competency with the ratio of the risk of harm to risk of benefit. If the treatment or intervention has a low or uncertain likelihood of helping the person, a lower test of competency is acceptable. In the case of Miss O, it is uncertain whether she will recover even with treatment. With such uncertainty, some would refuse to override what appears to be a rational decision. Others would favor involuntary treatment of Miss O even in the face of such uncertainty and argue that her attitude is a manifestation of her illness. In contrast, forcing treatment on Mrs. J (Case 10.4) who has a terminal illness clearly has a low or uncertain benefit. Furthermore, her judgment is not a feature of her illness and she is competent by a high standard. Thus, it is wrong to interfere. If treatment is likely to help, a higher standard of competency for refusal is used. Treatment is likely to help Mr. D in Case 10.7, and he seems very sick. Thus, it is wrong not to interfere.

A danger exists for this policy, however; people may reintroduce unjustified paternalism by adjusting the level of competency simply by whether they like the choice. For example, one could set a high standard for Miss O and for Joyce Brown and thereby declare them incompetent just because they want them hospitalized for their own good. But good intentions do not solve the original controversy of whether it is justifiable to set the threshold so high. Thus, although a functional approach seems reasonable in clarifying the nature of the problems and in calling for flexibility, this approach cannot itself indicate what values, norms, or standards to adopt. Depending on how it is used, the functional approach can introduce flexibility or permit arbitrary verdicts.

To summarize, value judgments are necessarily used in determining whether people lack capacity or competency to do certain things. The judgments should be grounded, however, in reliable information about which tasks, criteria, tests, and thresholds are reliable predictors of future performance. Values are internally related to these assessments about competency because these judgments mean people do, or do not, meet established norms. The norms or values may be nonmoral, as when we judge that someone is demented or lacks the intelligence to accomplish a certain task, or the values may reflect moral or social values, as in deciding that someone is too abusive to raise a child.

In addition to having values as part of the meaning of competency assessments, values are also introduced by the obligations and duties of those authorized to make decisions. Some duties involve moral and professional duties such as how to choose criteria, thresholds, and tests and to be accurate and seek the best available data. Many conflicts about determination of competency or capacity reflect underlying moral disputes among professionals about how to understand duties to respect people's choices and protect their well-being. People can be helped by being judged incompetent. This assessment can make special programs or funds available to them, or show the inappropriateness of certain reactions, such as frustration, anger, or blame. Moreover, descriptions of the plights of incompetent people in general can help them. Many homeless people, for example, have incapacitating psychiatric illnesses and need more attention. Mayor Koch claimed he was concerned about all New York City's homeless people when he focused attention on Joyce Brown (Case 10.8).

As we saw, when benefit to persons is given as a reason for the competency evaluations, there should be some evidence the assessment is likely to produce more good than harm. One would want to consider, for example, evidence that Ms. Brown cannot find food or shelter, or proof that the involuntary hospitalization and forced therapy would really benefit her. Joyce Brown's family and physicians focused upon her vulnerability, personality changes, and the possible benefits of therapy. Ms. Brown and her lawyers focused on her capacity to survive on the streets and her preference for freedom. Facing so much disagreement, Judge Lippman decided that Joyce Brown, who was not malnourished, incoherent, or suicidal, was competent. The dispute, in part, was over the proper limitations of protecting others despite their objections.

The case below also reflects how disagreements about competency or capacity can reflect underlying moral disputes about how to understand the limits of duties of beneficence (Case 10.10).

CASE 10.10

Mr. W, age 44, has been incapacitated by schizophrenia for many years and has been hospitalized repeatedly. He is somewhat less incapacitated than usual, but he and others expect this is temporary. He has repeatedly said such things as "My suffering is constant and greater than anything you can imagine, far worse than the pain of my heart attack last year." He plans to kill himself because he now has the capacity to do so and wants to depart his horrible existence. He sees his life as a terrible burden to himself, his family, and his community. Most of the psychiatric staff who have known him over the years believe they would feel exactly as Mr. W does if they were in Mr. W's place. Should he be hospitalized for suicide prevention?

Is Mr. W, who is severely impaired, competent to make this decision? Are others able to understand his anguish? The decision about whether a person is competent to make a certain decision or do certain things is important in determining whether it is morally permissible to interfere.

BALANCING PATERNALISM WITH FREEDOM

When people become mentally ill, they may suffer a loss of freedom from a diminished capacity to understand, choose, or act. There is no conflict between the need to protect people and to honor their self-determination when sick people agree to appropriate treatments or hospitalization. The difficulties arise when we have to choose between respecting someone's refusal of treatment or hospitalization and trying to protect them. In the end, we may enlarge someone's liberty by forcing them to undergo a certain treatment or hospitalization (Feinberg 1978). Self-determined persons act authentically when they deliberately select their beliefs and values and have the liberty to act upon their life plans (Dworkin 1976). When people are very ill, they are "not themselves" and cannot protect their own interests. In short, they are not choosing autonomously and others may have to help them.

Since ancient times, physicians have acknowledged that they have duties of beneficence to patients, and some charge that this promotes unwarranted paternalism. It would be unjustly paternalistic if the duty meant that all one has to do is to decide sincerely what one believes is in the patient's best interest, and then to do it (Veatch 1981). In that case, it would not matter what the standard of care was, what patients thought, or what the laws required. Believing that one is acting in the best interest of another shows sincerity of purpose. This is important because going against one's conscience may never be correct. One's conscience, however, may be informed or not, prejudiced or not, empathetic or not, or partial or not. Thus, doing what is best, or what one thinks is best, is not sufficient to justify actions. The moral rule to protect patients and act in the patient's best interest, however, does not entail unwarranted paternalism where it is understood as a test of conscience of the virtuous practitioner. The clinician asks, "Am I doing my best to help and not harm my patient?" Nor does it lead to unjustified paternalism where it is understood as one of many duties to patients that must be balanced. Disrespect to others can take many forms, not only unwarranted paternalism, but indifference or abandonment of people who make irrational or impaired choices.

The development and use of new technologies generate additional questions about the limits of justified paternalism. First, competent adults may resent having to get permission from psychiatrists to use mind-altering drugs they believe will enhance their lives. In some cases, drugs make people feel better and even seem to enhance people's performance.[11] Why should society decide that such drugs will be controlled substances for competent people until we learn more about the drugs? Second, the worse the mental illness, the more reasonable it may be to consider using risky, invasive, uncertain, or irreversible therapies. At the same time, the worse the mental illness, the less patients are probably able to assess competently for themselves the risks and benefits of treatments and the harder for others to claim clear moral authority for making decisions for patients.

Moral disputes about how to justify paternalism or limit the liberty of people who may be mentally ill usually center on the following questions: What standard should we use to decide to limit someone's liberty on the basis of mental illness? Who should make decisions for people who are incompetent? How should decisions be made for someone who is incompetent? In exploring answers to these questions, most agree that we need to find solutions that fairly promote people's well-being and their opportunities to become self-fulfilled persons. The difficulties arise when we disagree about how to balance protection with respect for self-determinism.

---

[11]See, for example, psychiatrist Peter Kramer's *Listening to Prozac* (1993).

LIBERTY-LIMITING PRINCIPLES

Several important standards have been offered to serve as a basis for limiting the liberty of others; the three most frequently discussed are reviewed here.

Strong Paternalism

Strong paternalism is a liberty-limiting principle stating that people can interfere with the freedom of another if they decide it is for the person's own good. Strong paternalism is controversial because someone's decision about what is good for another person may be wrong. Thus, it offers insufficient respect for people's self-determination, especially for competent persons' abilities to make decisions for themselves. People find it intrinsically valuable to plan their own lives and live as they wish. In addition, there is utility or instrumental value in living as one wishes because people generally are the best judges of what is best for themselves. In deciding for oneself, moreover, people develop their potential as autonomous persons, may gain respect from others, and do not feel thwarted (Mill 1859). Case 10.11, the case of Dax Cowart, is most frequently discussed in this regard.

CASE 10.11

In the film *Please Let Me Die* (1974) a patient, Dax Cowart, is interviewed ten months after being burned over 65 percent of his body. Blind, disfigured, and without use of his fingers, he has consistently insisted on his right to refuse medical treatment, including extremely painful procedures that will result in a quality of life he finds unacceptable. He would die quickly without treatment but also talks of committing suicide. Two psychiatrists find him competent and hold that his decision is not the product of mental illness. He cannot get the court hearing he wants and is treated despite his objections. His refusals have been unwavering for ten months but are discounted as incompetent, childish, manipulative, or insincere. Ten years later, Cowart uses similar reasoning to defend the right of competent patients to make decisions for themselves (Cowart 1984). Cowart is now a lawyer working to help patients gain their rights. Is Cowart's later success in life a vindication of the decision to treat him despite his objections?

With the best intentions, people may be entirely wrong about what harms or benefits others. They may be mistaken on the basis of factual or evaluative considerations. For example, the doctors were incorrect in predicting Cowart would regain some vision, use his hands, be able to dress himself, or attend to his personal needs. They were also wrong in supposing that they knew best which values really were most important to him. Patients now have some protection from the paternalistic enthusiasms of others because of relatively recent laws and social policies that have resulted from past abuses. What we sincerely believe is best for people may in fact harm them. Thus, this version of strong paternalism is rarely defended today.

Some form of protection, however, seems justified when people cannot make decisions for themselves, suffer incapacitating mental illness, show involuntary self-destructive behavior, or make choices so inappropriate to their own established life goals that we doubt their autonomy. Interference seems justified in the presence of people's nonautonomistic, self-destructive behavior or when they resort to acts that are irrational, unreasonable, and uncharacteristic. The next two standards are widely defended as grounds for limiting people's liberty.

The Harm Principle

John Stuart Mill offered an important standard for deciding when it is justifiable to interfere with the liberty of others. The standard has come to be called the *Harm Principle*. Its name comes from Mill's view that competent adults should not be restrained or compelled against their will except to prevent harm to others (Mill, 1859). If Dr. T in Case 10.5 reports Mr. and Mrs. N as a way to protect their three-year-old child from abuse, Dr. T uses the Harm Principle. The physician in Case 10.7 could also have used the Harm Principle to have depressed and suicidal Mr. D committed involuntarily to a hospital for treatment. Mill argued that incompetent people, like Mr. D, were exempt from the Harm Principle, and paternalism for them was justified. He also argued that children and retarded persons were exempt because they need more protection.

The Harm Principle, when justified, is probably the most widely accepted and least controversial principle for limiting the liberty of others. Yet it is controversial in several ways that directly relate to how to understand or rank values. First, we may disagree about whether the harm is sufficient in magnitude and probability to justify the restriction of another's freedom. For example, some may deny Mr. D is really incompetent and a threat to himself. Second, we can disagree about what to do with genuinely borderline cases. When, for example, is the threat of harm to children by parents serious enough to justify denying them custody of their children? Third, as in Case 10.6 describing the Tarasoff ruling, we can disagree about the duties of people, such as lawyers or psychiatrists, who learn, in the course of providing service, that their clients plan to harm or have harmed others. Psychiatrists hear many threats they should discount. In some cases, however, it seems clear that people pose a risk of harm to others and should be restrained (see Case 10.12).

CASE 10.12

A two-year-old boy, John, has been admitted to the hospital with multiple fractures, cuts, and bruises. His father, Mr. U, claims he has been sent from the future to destroy John, who will be the next Hitler if he is allowed to live. Mr. U says he must also destroy all John's friends because they will be the next Gestapo leaders.

Weak Paternalism

Critics of the Harm Principle argue that it offers insufficient protection to certain people. Sometimes we do not know whether persons who are about to harm themselves are competent or understand what they are doing. In such cases, it seems appropriate, perhaps even a moral duty, to interfere to determine whether the person is competent. For example, a seemingly competent person may want to fly from a 15-story window. If we believe we ought to interfere because the action seems so self-destructive and bizarre, then we must modify the Harm Principle. *Weak paternalism*, a position associated with the work of philosopher Joel Feinberg (Feinberg 1971), is such a modification. Feinberg permits interference with "self regarding harmful conduct only when it is substantially nonvoluntary or when temporary intervention is necessary to establish whether it is voluntary or not" (Feinberg 1971, 113). Weak paternalism would permit interference with the liberty of others as a way to determine whether they are competent or capable of making a rational choice (Feinberg 1971, 1978; VanDeVeer 1986).

Weak paternalism allows people to show a parent-like interest in someone who is possibly incapacitated. Yet it, too, can generate controversy. For example, does weak paternalism permit hospitalization of Joyce Brown who lives in the street, Miss O who has anorexia nervosa, or the suicidal and depressed Mr. D? A weak paternalist would permit interference with the liberty of others as a way to determine whether they are competent or capable of making a rational choice. Thus, the weak paternalist might recommend hospitalization to evaluate the competency of Joyce Brown, Miss O, or Mr. D. If the person is found competent and capable, however, the weak paternalist favors noninterference with the person's liberty as long as the person does not harm others.

Defenders of the Harm Principle and weak paternalism agree that interference with the liberty of adults requires a heavy burden of proof to show they are incapacitated, incompetent, or a threat to themselves or others. It requires proving that the probability and magnitude of the harm merits the interference. In addition, it necessitates showing that the means to interfere are effective and the least restrictive means available. If the reason given is to prevent harm or to benefit the person, moreover, there must be adequate evidence that, on balance, the interference will actually prevent harm or will benefit the person. If the reason for limiting someone's liberty appeals to social utility, there must be adequate evidence that, on balance, the inter-ference will prevent harm to others or will benefit society. These two views differ in that weak paternalism extends more protection to people who are impaired by such things as illness, ignorance, drugs, or fear.

DECIDING FOR INCOMPETENT PEOPLE

If adults are judged not mentally competent, who should make decisions for them? Several means exist to reach decisions, and the circumstances deter-mine which means ought to be used.

The Legal Guardian

When adults are declared legally incompetent, someone gets authority to make health-care or other decisions for them. This person is appointed by the courts and is often a family member who, presumably, is the most knowledgeable and interested in the well-being of the person. Family members are often ap-pointed guardians, moreover, because they usually bear the consequences of the choices; clearly certain choices and consequences suit certain families better than others. In addition, a family member can represent the values and stan-dards shared within the family and help make health-care choices that would probably suit the incompetent patient (Buchanan and Brock 1989).

Guardians maintain this authority as long as they promote the well-being and opportunities of those under their care, and prevent, remove, or minimize harms to them. Moral disputes about when to challenge guard-ians' authority to make health-care decisions often center on the point at which harms or dangers to incompetent people warrant interference with guardians' authority and what restrictions on their choices are needed to secure the person's well-being. Guardians who abuse, neglect, or exploit their wards may lose custody temporarily or permanently. Physical, sexual, or emotional abuse constitute grounds for loss of parental authority. In addi-tion, guardians who make imprudent or neglectful decisions may lose cus-tody temporarily or permanently.

Shared Decision Making

Ideally, important health-care choices should represent a consensus of the patient and the doctors, nurses, and, when appropriate, a family or guardian. Together they should find the option best suited to the person (President's Commission 1982). Even if the person is legally incompetent, he or she may have a point of view that should prevail, or at least should be acknowledged as important, in shaping the final decision. A person with Alzheimer's disease may have little short-term memory, but be able to use knowledge gained long ago to reason and make choices. To honor the value of self-determination while protecting incompetent persons, the persons themselves should participate in health-care decisions as much as possible when they can understand and reason about their options and life plans.

The Incompetent Person's Assent

Even when informed consent in a legal sense cannot be obtained, patients should, when possible, be encouraged to make or participate in their own treatment choices. For example, Culver and Gert (1982) concede that patients with a major depression have difficulty making decisions, yet believe that it is in their best interest to try to choose between the different therapies available. It promotes cooperation and involvement. Physicians should give their expert advice and discuss the risks and benefits of various treatments but promote patient choice.

Often it is important, then, to include people who are legally incompetent in decisions about their health care. This is intrinsically valuable because it helps them feel some responsibility and control. It can also be useful to them by enhancing their self-esteem, their decision-making abilities, their sense of control over their lives, and give them assurance that others respect them as persons. In addition, they may have a point of view that should be considered, or they may want to understand and participate in the decisions about their health care. For example, consider patients under the care of the esteemed eighteenth-century physician Benjamin Rush. He tried "therapies" of copious bleeding and purging for mental illnesses; he strapped people to "tranquilizing" chairs, and spun them in gyrating chairs to treat them for the congestion of blood in the brain which he believed to be the cause of mental illness. Even relatively incapacitated people might have reasonably objected to these means.

In seeking assent, one must be candid, and this in itself can have value. A lack of candor can cause people additional suffering by making them feel isolated from discussions, decisions, and support. Truthfulness generally has good consequences by promoting cooperation and enhancing trust in the credibility of caretakers. Some other reasons for being truthful with people are: (1) most people are offended if they are not told the truth, (2) trust is destroyed when we are not truthful, (3) allegations that people cannot bear to hear the truth are generally not borne out by observation, (4) deceiving and lying undermine the practice of truth telling, (5) most people are bad liars and others see through the deceptions, and (6) people often find out the truth from other sources.

What should be done, however, if the intended intervention is in the patient's best interest, and people are candid, but the incompetent person does not want it? For example, Mrs. Yetter, a mentally incapacitated woman, consistently refused needed surgery for suspected cancer (*In re Yetter* 1973). The court agreed with her physicians and family that the surgery was in her best interest and that her reasons for refusal were delusional. Yet the court ruled that her steadfast refusal and fear of death during surgery, not the delusions, were her primary reason for refusing surgery; it honored her right to refuse surgery even though judging it was in her best interest to have it. Thus, determining that something is in someone's best interest is not sufficient to impose it, even on someone who is unquestionably mentally ill. Her family and physicians were probably frustrated by her steadfast refusal. But they let the courts decide what to do rather than forcing surgery or abandoning her to her decision.

STANDARDS FOR DECISION MAKING

There are four important standards for making health-care decisions in psychiatric and other medical practice for patients.

Self-Determination

The first standard, that of self-determination, applies primarily to competent and informed adults, who should generally be free to make their own choices about their well-being and opportunities as long as they do not harm or violate the rights of others. For competent psychiatric patients, this is the appropriate standard.

Advance Directives

Adults and others may leave advance directives about their health-care choices in case they become incompetent. People who realize that they have Alzheimer's disease, for example, may leave an advance directive that they want no medical treatment to prolong their lives. There is a consensus that a moral and legal duty exists to follow advance directives drafted by competent people.

Substituted Judgment

A third standard, that of substituted judgment, applies to someone who was once competent enough to express preferences. Using this standard, people select the option that they believe the person would have chosen were he or she able. Families often know their relatives well enough to make the choices the relatives would have made. They may know, for example, that their relative had strong views opposing electric-convulsive therapy (ECT) and, using substituted judgment, reject it for him or her. A problem with this standard, however, is that it is more difficult to apply as we move farther from expressed views of the once competent person. It is sometimes difficult to determine whose preferences are operative when no advance directives have been left.

Best-Interest Standard

The best-interest standard applies to those who lack the ability or authority to make decisions for themselves and have left no advance directives. It maintains that decision makers should try to identify the person's immediate or long-term interests and then determine whether the benefits of an intervention or procedure outweigh its burdens. Such paternalism is justified for incompetent people. It does not mean decisions makers seek what is absolutely best, because that may be impossible (the best doctor cannot treat everyone), but the best among the available options. The best-interest standard permits complex judgments about what, on balance, is likely to be best for the individual, given the available options (Buchanan and Brock 1989).

INVOLUNTARY COMMITMENT

Basic social, moral, and legal questions are raised in determining the basis for involuntary civil commitment to a mental hospital. The laws a society adopts show how a society balances rights of self-determination and duties to protect people. Jurisdictional statutes differ, but they generally permit involuntary psychiatric commitment only when there is good reason to believe that people are a danger to themselves or others, or are very seriously disturbed and too sick to provide themselves with the basic necessities of life (Holder 1985). An array of restrictions to involuntary commitments resulted from well-documented abuses. For example, people were horrified to learn about patients undergoing crude psychosurgery in the 1940s. It was sometimes done without patient consent and on people hospitalized involuntarily. They were irreversibly harmed (Macklin 1982). Until recently, in every area of medicine, invasive and powerful procedures were used "for people's own good" without their consent and without what today we would consider adequate criteria or testing. The appeals to strong paternalism seemed justified when psychoactive drugs caused near miraculous changes in psychiatry in the 1950s. They were widely used before much was known about their harmful side effects, such as tardive dyskinsea (a loss of motor control). It became apparent that better testing and consent were needed. Some seek to cure the abuses of the past by abolishing or severely restricting the practice of involuntary civil commitment. This has left many psychiatrists troubled that the cure is worse than the disease and that patients will be harmed by making it difficult to protect them or making it very easy for them to get discharges when they need longer hospital stays (McGarry and Chodoff 1981).

A very important case was *O'Connor v. Donaldson*, decided by the United States Supreme Court in 1975. In this divided decision, the court ruled that "a non-dangerous individual who is capable of surviving safely in freedom by himself or with the help of willing or responsible family or friends cannot constitutionally be confined. A finding of 'mental illness' alone cannot justify a state's locking up a person against his will and keeping him indefinitely in simple custodial confinement" (1975, 287). The court decided that J. G. O'Connor, the superintendent of the institution, acted malevolently to violate Kenneth Donaldson's constitutional right to freedom (Case 10.13).

CASE 10.13

Kenneth Donaldson, after making a political comment, was knocked unconscious by fellow workers in 1943. A judge, at the request of Donaldson's parents, committed him to a mental institution for treatment. He was given an 11-week treatment of ECT and released. In 1956, at the request of his father, Donaldson was arrested, jailed, and subsequently diagnosed as paranoid schizophrenic. Two physicians interviewed him very briefly, and a judge informed him he would be sent to the Florida State Hospital. He stayed there 15 years, during which time Donaldson asked for a hearing and petitioned various courts. When his case was finally reviewed in 1971, Donaldson was regarded as no longer incompetent and was released. He sued for having been committed without treatment. The jury found that two physicians acted in bad faith by being guided by what Donaldson's parents wanted, rather than by what would have been in Donaldson's best interest.

Courts have ruled that people in mental institutions must get appropriate treatment and be housed in proper facilities. Psychiatrists, who may be sued when these conditions are not provided, complain that they are unfairly blamed when the real cause is inadequate funding and facilities (McGarry and Chodoff 1981). In some cases, psychiatrists and mental health facilities are caught in a squeeze between the courts that order proper treatment and housing and state legislatures that allocate insufficient funds for this purpose. Those seeking to save money may team up with activists who want to protect patients' civil liberties. Large numbers of patients have been discharged from mental institutions because the institutions were crowded or did not provide treatment, or because it was argued that the patients, like Donaldson, were capable of "making it on their own," especially with the help of friends. But many of these patients, like Joyce Brown in Case 10.8, became "street people." Some psychiatrists charge that activists, in their enthusiasm for defending civil liberties or saving money, have forgotten that there also exists a duty of beneficence to protect people who need help and who cannot take care of themselves (McGarry and Chodoff 1981).

Some have argued, however, that involuntary civil commitment in any circumstance is wrong (Szasz 1963). One reason given for this view is that laws have been abused. People who were no threat to self or others were committed for long periods of time. A second reason offered is that the interests of justice would be better served if the criminal justice system were used to deal with dangerous people; if people are dangerous and violent, they should be tried and put in prison. Or, according to psychiatrist Thomas Szasz, with whom these views are closely associated, they should be put in a prison hospital where medical and psychiatric treatment could be provided along with incarceration. A third reason that Szasz and others argue that those considered mentally ill ought not receive special treatment is that they claim mental illness is a fiction (Szasz 1963).

Each reason given for doing away with involuntary civil commitment is problematic. A difficulty with the first reason is that all laws can be abused, but this does not mean we should abolish all laws that have been abused. Therefore, citing outrageous violations does not settle the issue of whether there should be such laws. What proponents for this view need to show is that such laws are always inappropriate, the way laws fostering racial segregation or sexual discrimination are always inappropriate. It does not seem obvious, however, that the interests of justice would be better served by forbidding involuntary commitment or forced treatments. Should Mr. D (Case 10.7), who is depressed over his son's death, be left to live as he wishes and likely commit suicide, or should there be a legal means (with many safeguards) to treat him for what is probably a reversible condition?

The second reason also has problems. If people are put in prison for doing bad things, why should they have to get psychiatric treatment? If Mr. U, who beats up his son (Case 10.12) is bad, it is appropriate to punish him for what he has done, but not subject him to psychiatric treatment without his consent. But if he is sick, and for that reason could not help what he did, then why is it appropriate to punish him by putting him in prison? Most psychiatrists believe Szasz's proposal to use the criminal justice system in place of civil commitment procedures would be far more detrimental to people who are mentally ill than the possible abuses that could result from the misuse of the involuntary civil commitment procedures (McGarry and Chodoff 1981).

A third reason Szasz and others oppose involuntary civil commitment is that they deny the reality of mental illness. Szasz argues that if we know of an underlying physical cause to explain someone's bizarre behavior, such as a brain tumor, we can treat him as sick; but we cannot treat him as sick if no underlying physical cause can be found. We have discussed difficulties with this view earlier. Those, like Szasz, who oppose involuntary civil commitment and forced treatment often protest on grounds of civil liberties and argue that informed consent is needed. They argue that involuntary commitment for treatment is neither fair nor compassionate. But other psychiatrists typically counter that the alternative frequently proposed, using the criminal justice system or leaving people untreated unless they give informed consent, is far less fair or compassionate.

INFORMED CONSENT

A moral, legal, and medical consensus now exists that competent adults' free and informed choices must be followed in devising treatment plans or enrolling them as research subjects (Brock 1987; Buchanan and Brock 1989; Faden et al. 1986). Ideally, patients share decision making with physicians as part of an ongoing process in which doctors clarify options and make recommendations. With few exceptions, competent adults' actual choices among these options must be followed even if doctors and nurses find them imprudent. Philosopher Tom Beauchamp and others write,

> Legal, philosophical, regulatory, medical, and physiological literature have generally tried to define or analyze informed consent in terms of its "elements." The following elements have been identified as fundamental to the concept: (1) Disclosure, (2) Comprehension, (3) Voluntariness, (4) Competence, (5) Consent. Thus, one gives an informed consent to an intervention if and only if one receives a thorough disclosure about it, one comprehends the disclosure, one acts voluntarily, one is competent to act, and one consents to the intervention. (1991, 159S)

When dealing with persons with major psychiatric illness, however, informed consent can be a problem because the very skills needed for proper consent are impaired (attending, comprehending, understanding, reasoning, competent choosing, or acting).

It is generally agreed that it is wrong to violate the consensus on informed consent, and thus presumptively wrong not to gain informed consent. This posture does not mean that breaching it is actually wrong, but that there is a burden of proof on those who waive or modify consent standards to justify their action. Overcoming the presumptive duty to gain informed consent may be accomplished by demonstrating that the treatment constitutes a well-established exception to the duty to gain consent. Incompetence is one of the well-established exceptions.[12] Hence the presumptive duty to gain informed consent from patients may be overcome if the person is incompetent.

The policy on informed consent acknowledges three important values: fostering people's well-being, encouraging their self-determination, and promoting social utility. These values generally do not conflict, but

---

[12]Faden and Beauchamp enumerate the exceptions: "The public health emergency, the medical emergency, the incompetent patient, the therapeutic privilege and the patient waiver. All but one of these exceptions, the controversial therapeutic privilege, are commonly taken as both morally and legally valid, and thus as being consistent with—or placing valid limits on—the duty to respect individual autonomy" (1986, 35).

psychiatric patients are sometimes so incapacitated that their preferences are the product of their diseases or illnesses. For example, a suicidal patient may welcome hazardous or painful procedures, but the "choice" may be the nonvoluntary result of illness.

Gaining some form of agreement or assent, however, when people cannot give genuinely informed consent for therapy or research helps to honor the person's wishes and generally is useful in promoting the person's cooperation in a therapeutic program. However, some procedures are so irreversible and invasive that they create special doubts about whether anyone should be able to give consent for incompetent people. For example, surgeons will not agree to do psychosurgery without consent from patients, and some physicians are unwilling to do it even with patients' consent when procedures are very risky or permanently alter personality (see Case 10.14).

CASE 10.14

A judge has contacted a surgical group at the request of two prison inmates. The surgeons discuss whether they should do as the judge and inmates propose. One inmate with pedophilia, convicted of sexual abuse of children, seeks castration. The other inmate is extremely violent and seeks psychosurgery. Both hope to shorten their incarceration. The surgeons who are contacted refuse because they hold that no one can give meaningful consent. Anyone mentally disturbed enough to need the surgery doesn't have the capacity to give it; no third party should be allowed to give consent in these circumstances. Are the surgeons correct?

There is much controversy about what constitutes proper consent as the risk increases. As discussed in the section on competency, a variable standard relating to risk may be useful in determining when to seek consent from someone who may not be competent (Dworkin 1975). That is, the higher the risk, the more one needs informed consent from someone who is competent.

A very controversial research study sought to compare the effects of drug therapy and psychosurgery on criminal sexual psychopaths. The court ruled in *Kaimowitz v. Department of Mental Health for the State of Michigan* (1973) that "Psychosurgery should never be undertaken upon involuntarily committed populations, when there is a high-risk, low-benefit ratio as demonstrated in this case. This is because of the impossibility of obtaining truly informed consent from such populations." The court refused to permit a willing subject to participate. The court's ruling in *Kaimowitz* has been praised for limiting psychosurgery. It has also been criticized for making it appear that a person is incompetent simply because the environment is potentially coercive (Appelbaum 1982; Murphy 1979).

RESEARCH

Medical progress requires medical research, but how should investigations be conducted to learn about mental illnesses? Treatments were not systematically tested until the middle of the twentieth century, so many treatments became standards of care without careful evaluation of their safety and efficacy. Certain widely used drugs are just now being fully evaluated. Some drug testing is conducted with doctors and patients knowing the drug and dosage being given to the patient. In contrast to these *open label studies*, there are *double-blind, placebo-controlled* studies in which certain drugs are tested against a placebo; neither doctors nor patients know who is getting a drug and who is not. To be ethical, it must be uncertain which group(s) will benefit most.

Those giving consent for research must understand the potential risks or benefits of the study. One difficulty is that the sicker the patients, the harder it is to obtain informed consent from them. To compound the difficulty, the most powerful or invasive drugs or procedures often have side effects and are generally justifiable for the sickest patients, but those persons are least able to give consent for themselves. The sickest individuals, moreover, are usually already receiving treatment and may misperceive the research as an extension of their therapy.

Thus, psychiatrists bear a heavy responsibility when conducting research with psychiatric patients. Investigators should put the well-being of patients ahead of getting good study results. There was severe criticism of a decade-long study begun in 1983 at the University of California at Los Angeles for sacrificing patients' best interest to gain knowledge. Investigators systematically tested what happened when 50 patients under treatment for early stages of schizophrenia had their medications withdrawn for one year. The medication had serious side effects and the investigators theorized the patients might be better off without it. Twenty-three of the 50 patients in the study suffered relapses, several severe. The families said investigators led them to think their psychotic relatives would receive outstanding treatment in addition to being enrolled in the research. Some patients said that they suffered for months with delusions, hallucinations, and feelings of paranoia and that pleas by them and their families about their sufferings went unheeded. One young man committed suicide after repeated attempts to get help from those conducting the study. Another man dropped out of college, threatened his family, and suffered severe hallucinations for months. The study was criticized as unethical for not providing proper standards of care, not responding when patients' regressed, and for failing to carefully monitor patients. The researchers tried to defend their actions. "All of the patients signed 'informed consent' documents stating that their condition might 'improve, worsen or remain unchanged'" (Hilts 1994). This consent document, however, satisfied no standard about what to reveal concerning potential harms or benefits. The study was also criticized by the Federal Office of Protection from Research Risks (*New York Times*, 1994).

This study failed to honor a therapist's moral duties to provide proper care for patients. The desire to gain new knowledge, however important, is secondary to a therapist's primary duty. Moreover, the investigators did not obtain genuine informed consent. Obtaining a signed consent form, which in this case seemed to be largely a meaningless ritual, did not relieve investigators of moral and professional duties to act in the best interest of patients and subjects. In any case, informed consent is not sufficient to conduct research.

Many people who are mentally ill are competent to consent or refuse to participate in research, but many are vulnerable. Potential research subjects are called vulnerable if they either lack capacity to give informed consent or are likely to be coerced or manipulated to participate. Those severely impaired by mental illness or retardation are typically regarded as vulnerable because they lack capacity to give informed consent. Many people who are severely mentally disabled live in institutions, and institutionalized people are additionally vulnerable to coercion or manipulation. Because the informed participation of these vulnerable subjects is problematic, enrolling them in research protocols often requires special justification and safeguards that investigators must follow.

Vulnerability to Coercion and Manipulation

There has been consensus about how to protect the rights and welfare of competent adults who are vulnerable to coercion or manipulation. First, since the right to consent is grounded in its utility and the right of self-determination, institutional review boards (IRBs) or research ethics committees (RECs) should ascertain that consent is voluntary and the risks of research are not unfairly distributed to vulnerable groups (U.S. Protection of Human Subjects Regulation 1991). Second, where it is difficult to supervise consent adequately, vulnerable groups should receive special regulatory protection. For example, institutions for the criminally insane are settings that are inherently coercive, so U.S. regulations permit only a limited range of studies (U.S. Protection of Human Subjects Regulation 1991). Studies with more than a minimal risk or studies that do not hold out benefit to prisoners require demonstrated utility, special safeguards, approval of experts, and authorization from the Secretary of the Department of Health and Human Services.

A third area of agreement about protecting vulnerable subjects from coercion concerns the importance of avoiding unjustified paternalism. There is less consensus, however, on how to do this. Someone who is mentally ill may want to participate in research and may resent restrictions saying he cannot. If the person seeks punishing experiences, however, his or her "agreement" to participate in a study may be the voice of illness. When vulnerable people are legally competent, moral and legal disagreements abound concerning what specific restrictions on their choices are fair, promote their well-being, and respect their self-determination because their choices might be manipulated or coerced. Too little protection risks their exploitation; too much protection risks unjustified paternalism. Before limiting the liberty of people, we should consider whether they want such protection, whether the probability and magnitude of harm warrant restricting their freedom, and whether the restrictions are the least invasive to secure their well-being.

Vulnerability Because of Incapacity to Consent

As with competent people, the ethical basis for research policy for persons lacking capacity to give informed consent concerns promoting their self-determination, fair treatment, and well-being. Different policies balance these primary values differently and offer different authority principles (stating who decides) and guidance principles (substantive directions about how decisions should be made).

In the United States, guidelines for research on persons institutionalized as mentally infirm were proposed for those who have impairments such as, or similar to, mental illness, senility, psychosis, mental retardation, or emotional disturbances (U.S. Department of Health, Education, and Welfare 1978). To try to balance the social utility of research with respect and protection of the person, the guidelines stipulate that the greater the risk, the more rigorous and elaborate the protection of subjects' welfare and the informed consent requirements. In general, no research that presents more than a minimal risk is permitted on subjects who cannot give meaningful consent unless there is evidence that the intervention holds out the prospect of direct benefit to the subjects (such as therapy). A *minimal risk* is understood to be the kind of risk encountered in daily life or in a routine physical examination and includes consideration of physical and psychosocial risks. This definition is problematic because some daily risks are not minimal, and highly sensitive information can come to light in routine office visits (Kopelman 1995).

According to the proposed federal guidelines, the consent of the mentally infirm person must be sought. None who refuse may be enrolled in any study that does not hold out direct benefit unless there is authorization from the courts. A guardian may consent for nontherapeutic studies only if the person cannot give consent, the risk is minimal, and the person does not object. For example, nontherapeutic studies might be epidemiological surveys of the infectious diseases in an institution; questionnaires about patients' preferences; or assessments of people's physical strength while they were patients in mental institutions.

Vulnerable subjects need the protection of good peer review committees and research guidelines. Excessive restrictions, however, also have dangers. They can thwart the advance of knowledge needed to improve medical care. When potential subjects are capable of giving legal consent but are vulnerable to pressure, agreement should be monitored to see whether it is coerced or manipulated. When potential subjects are not capable of giving consent, IRBs and RECs need to consider evaluative issues of utility, fairness, and protection to see whether others can give consent on their behalf.

DISCRIMINATION

People with mental illnesses and disabilities face prejudice, stigmatization, and unjustified discrimination based, in part, on mistaken beliefs that they are responsible for their conditions or behavior (Kopelman 1988). In an attempt to address this problem, the United States passed the Americans with Disabilities Act (ADA) (1990) to protect disabled persons' access to goods, services, and benefits and to promote equal opportunity. The ADA is designed to shield people with both physical and mental disabilities from discrimination in "employment, housing, public accommodations, communications, recreation, institutionalization, health services, voting and access to public services" (Americans with Disabilities Act 1990). Arguably, however, even this widely heralded and bold law reveals a limited commitment to protect people with mental disabilities (Kopelman 1996). To obtain the ADA's protection a person must be disabled, must be otherwise qualified, and accommodations for the disability must be of a certain sort. We shall review each of these three necessary conditions for protection.

Disability

To receive protection, the person must be disabled as defined by the law. Three groups of people are protected from discrimination. First, the ADA protects people with "a physical or mental impairment that substantially limits one or more major life activity." A *major life activity* is defined as "functions such as caring for one's self, performing manual tasks, walking, seeing, hearing, speaking, breathing, learning and working." Second, it protects those with a record of such impairments, for example, recovered alcoholics. Third, it protects people perceived as disabled by others, such as those with HIV infection (Americans with Disabilities Act 1990).

The ADA places specific restrictions on those who qualify. It excludes people with "(1) transvestism, transsexualism, pedophilia, exhibitionism, voyeurism, gender identity disorders not resulting from physical impairments, or other sexual behavior disorders; (2) compulsive gambling, kleptomania, or pyromania; (3) psychoactive substance-use disorders resulting from current illegal use of drugs" (Americans with Disabilities Act 1990). Thus, the ADA does not protect someone who is addicted to cocaine; it also excludes homosexuals and bisexuals from seeking protection under this law.

Otherwise Qualified

To gain protection the person must also be otherwise qualified to receive the benefits, goods, or services or to perform the essential functions of the job, with or without accommodations. This requirement may mean that the disabled person is qualified once certain accommodations have been made. For example, suppose a man who is well-qualified to work as a computer programmer is so obsessive–compulsive that he has difficulty dealing with the noise in a busy office. A reasonable accommodation might be that the man receive a secluded place to work. The ADA is clear, however, that the principle of reasonable accommodation has limitations. People are not qualified for protection under the ADA if they cannot perform the essential functions of the job or if they pose a risk to themselves or others. For example, someone with a psychotic disorder who believes that aliens are about to invade the world would pose too great a risk to others to be an air traffic controller.

Readily Achievable or Reasonable Accommodations

According to ADA, the changes needed to accommodate the disabled person must be reasonable in that they are not likely to produce an undue burden for employers or state or local governments (Title I and II) and must be readily achievable ways for private entities to provide access to goods and services without altering their fundamental nature (Title III). For this category, the ADA has several parts with somewhat different standards. Title I applies to employment; Title II to public services of the state and local government and to institutions receiving government funds, such as hospitals; and Title III to private entities offering public services, such as restaurants, bars, and doctors' offices. Title I and II use a higher standard for accommodation (no undue burden) than does Title III (readily achievable) (Department of Justice 1993). The ADA states that Title I and II accommodations must be no undue hardship to the covering agency in terms of financial resources, time, and energy. More accommodations are expected of large, affluent organizations than of small companies, and the ADA exempts companies employing fewer than 15 persons. No employer or agency, however, is expected to alter the essential functions of the position or be put at financial hardship to accommodate someone. Examples of accommodation that would most likely be "no undue burden" to the covering agency for an office worker or hospital employee might include flexible scheduling, unpaid leave for short-term psychiatric treatments or dialysis appointments, a private place to work to alleviate stress, reassignment of jobs, restructuring of jobs by switching nonessential assignments, individual assistance, architectural alterations, or allowing an employee to work at home. Some commentators argue that most accommodations for otherwise qualified disabled persons in the workplace will not be costly and that their impact may be further mitigated by available tax credits (Collins 1992).

There is a question concerning the sincerity of the ADA's commitment to those with mental disabilities, however. The ADA boldly promises to protect those with mental as well as physical disabilities. Yet, those who have mental disabilities and seek the ADA's protection may find themselves in a bind. For example, suppose they seek employment. On one hand, they must show they are otherwise qualified for the position including, usually, that they can perform in a work setting and get along well with people. On the other hand, they must also show they are disabled as defined by the ADA. According to some commentators (Symons 1992), this means they must show a permanent, nontransitory, mental impairment so severe that it substantially limits one or more major life functions. People who become extremely agitated and hallucinate in times of stress, for example, may meet such a requirement. In having a severe enough disability to qualify for the ADA's protection, however, they are for that very reason likely to be viewed as unable to perform the essential functions of a job. People who become agitated and hallucinate in times of stress are not otherwise qualified for most jobs. Thus, by fulfilling one necessary condition for the ADA's protection (disabled) they are likely to fail another (otherwise qualified). In contrast, people whose mental impairments are not so severe that they substantially limit one or more major life functions may find that they fulfill one necessary condition (otherwise qualified) but fail to fulfill another (not sufficiently disabled). Hence, the ADA seems to have a "Catch-22" for those with mental disabilities.

A second problem is that the ADA bases some exclusions on social mores. As discussed earlier, certain groups are explicitly excluded from ADA's protection not because of the severity of the condition but because of its nature. In another kind of society, an otherwise qualified compulsive gambler or transvestite whose accommodations required no undue burden to the covering agency would receive protection from discrimination. Those who worked to pass the ADA candidly admit that without these concessions they would not have secured passage through Congress. Members of Congress apparently believed their constituents would not support protection for those who had sexual or social aberrations. In many cases, people with conditions such as pedophilia, pyromania, and the others named are not otherwise qualified to hold certain jobs; so, arguably, omissions based on their diagnoses signal that society does not want to protect them from discrimination. Many of these exclusions, then, appear to be more an expression of prevailing social attitudes than the results of a principled choice.

The ADA appeals to many important values including equality of opportunity, beneficence, efficiency, social utility, and certain social mores. These values can conflict and we will not know the meaning and implications of the ADA's promise of protection and equal opportunity for mentally disabled persons until we have a better idea about how to understand or rank these values when they conflict. Until we as a society clarify how to resolve such disputes, the ADA is ambiguous and a central moral and social question is unresolved: How can we demonstrate commitment to the rights and welfare of those with severe disabilities while placing fair limits on their claims? Unfortunately, despite great strides in some areas, discrimination still remains a difficult problem for people with mental illnesses and mental diagnoses.

To conclude, value judgments shape the practice of psychiatry and directly affect how people are viewed and treated. Scientific information is, of course, also an important component of psychiatric practice. Our focus, however, is on the role of moral and nonmoral values in psychiatric practice and policies. We have seen that value judgments affect how the line is drawn between mental illness and health; how decisions are made about competency, responsibility, and blame; and how it is decided which people should be regarded as incapacitated in their capacity to understand, reason, choose, or act. Policies about when confidentiality must be maintained and when it should be overridden also contain value choices, as do regulations about when involuntary treatment and commitment are permissible. Disputes about value judgments may underlie disagreements about the moral basis of diagnoses and whether psychiatric diagnoses have a rational, intercultural, and sound basis. When people disagree about how to assign blame and responsibility, justify involuntary commitment, assign diagnoses, remove guardianship, permit surrogate consent, allocate resources, and make other decisions that are a part of psychiatric practice, their disputes may represent value disagreements rather than scientific quarrels. When unexamined or unjustifiable values are seeded into policy and decisions, the result may be a harvest of bias, injustice, and prejudice. More critical attention should be given to the meaning and justifications of value judgments that affect psychiatry's technical terms, theories, diagnoses, treatments, and research.

DISCUSSION QUESTIONS

1. What was revolutionary and important about the reclassification of mental illness from moral to nonmoral categories of badness?

2. How can moral judgments be distinguished from scientific or psychiatric judgments?

3. Which of the following views about psychiatric diagnosis are compatible with the current practice of psychiatry, and why: Psychiatric diagnoses are (1) subjective views; (2) myths, unless there is a known bodily disease causing the symptoms; (3) views subject to rational confirmation only when they are value-free; (4) views relative to the values of someone's culture and fully determined by cultural norms.

4. Discuss three kinds of duties for giving someone a psychiatric diagnosis and give an example when they may come into conflict. Why do the international societies try to restrict psychiatric diagnoses to conditions that are severe and insist that social deviance is not a basis for psychiatric diagnosis?

5. Why is confidentiality especially important in the practice of psychiatry and under what circumstances can it be overridden?

6. In what way must values be integrated into all competency judgments? How are they integrated into policies about a patient's decision-making capacity?

7. What characterizes the following liberty-limiting principles and which seems most justifiable for people with mild mental disorders, and why: strong paternalism, the Harm Principle, weak paternalism?

8. What is the ideal of shared decision making for health care? In deciding how decisions should be made for incompetent people, four standards have been offered. What are they, and when is it appropriate to use them?

9. Why does the controversy over involuntary treatment and commitment raise fundamental questions about what kind of society we are?

10. What are the elements of informed consent and why do they raise special difficulties with people who have serious mental illness?

11. Why are psychiatric patients in institutions often vulnerable subjects? Distinguish between subjects who are vulnerable due to coercion and manipulation and those who are vulnerable because they lack capacity to give consent.

12. Why has there been more discrimination and stigmatization for those suffering from mental illnesses than others? How does the Americans with Disabilities Act try to shield people with both physical and mental disabilities from discrimination? How would you assess the ADA's policy?

REFERENCES

Books and Articles

Alston, W. P. "Logical Status of Psychoanalytic Theories." In Paul Edwards, Ed., *The Encyclopedia of Philosophy*, Vol. 6. New York: The Free Press, 1967: 512–516.

American Psychiatric Association. *Diagnostic and Statistical Manual of Mental Disorders*, 4th ed. Washington, DC: American Psychiatric Association, 1994.

Appelbaum, P. S., Roth, L. H. "Competency to Consent to Research: A Psychiatric Overview." *Arch Gen Psychiatry* 39(8) (1982): 951–958.

Beauchamp, T. L., Cook, R. R., Fayerweather, W. E., et al. "Ethical Guidelines for Epidemiologists." *J Clin Epidemiol* 44(Suppl. 1) (1991): 151S–169S.

Block, S. "The Political Misuse of Psychiatry in the Soviet Union." In S. Block and P. Chodoff, Eds., *Psychiatric Ethics*. Oxford: Oxford University Press, 1981: 321–341.

Brazelon, D. "Psychiatry and the Adversary Process." In J. M. Humber and R. F. Almeder, Eds., *Biomedical Ethics and the Law*, 2nd ed. New York: Plenum Press, 1974: 185–193.

Brock, D. "Children's Competence for Health Care Decisionmaking." In L. Kopelman and J. Moskop, Eds., *Children and Health Care: Moral and Social Issues*. Dordrecht, Holland: D. Reidel, 1989.

Buchanan, A., Brock, D. W. *Deciding for Others: The Ethics of Surrogate Decisionmaking*. New York: Cambridge University Press, 1989.

Chisholm, R. "Sentences About Believing." *Proc Aristot Soc* 56 (1956): 125–148.

Collins, M. C. "Introduction to the ADA and Employment: How It Really Affects People with Disabilities." *Gonzaga L Rev* 28(2) (1992): 209–218.

Culver, C. M., Gert, B. *Philosophy in Medicine: Conceptual and Ethical Issues in Medicine and Psychiatry*. New York: Oxford University Press, 1982.

Dax's Case: Concern for Dying (film). New York: 1984.

Dworkin, G. "Can Convicts Consent to Castration?" *Hastings Cent Rep* 5(5) (1975): 18–19.

———. "Autonomy and Behavior Control." *Hastings Cent Rep* 6(1) (1976): 23–28.

Faden, R. R., Beauchamp, T. L. *History and Theory of Informed Consent*. New York: Oxford University Press, 1986.

Feinberg, J. "Legal Paternalism." *Can J Philos* 1 (1971): 105–124.

———. "Freedom and Behavior Control." In W. T. Reich, Ed., *Encyclopedia of Bioethics*, Vol. 1. New York: The Free Press, 1978: 93–101.

Frankena, W. K. "Value and Valuation." *The Encyclopedia of Philosophy*, 2nd ed., Vol. 8. New York: The Free Press, 1967: 229–232.

———. *Introductory Readings in Ethics*, 2nd ed. Engelwood Cliffs, NJ: Prentice Hall, 1974.

Freud, S. *Collected Papers*. Vols. 1–5. New York: Basic Books, 1959.

Fulford, K. W. M. *Moral Theory and Medical Practice*. Cambridge, UK: Press Syndicate of the University of Cambridge, 1989.

Gaylin, W. "In Matters Mental or Emotional, What's Normal?" In T. A. Mappes and J. S. Zembaty, Eds., *Social Ethics*, 2nd ed. New York: McGraw-Hill 1982: 269–271.

Gilligan, C., Ward, J. V., Taylor, J. M., Eds. (with Bardige, B.). "Remapping the Moral Domain: New Images of Self in Relationship." In *Mapping the Moral Domain*. Cambridge: Harvard University Press, 1988: 4–19.

Heyd, D., Block, S. "The Ethics of Suicide." In S. Block and P. Chodoff, Eds., *Psychiatric Ethics*. Oxford: Oxford University Press, 1981: 185–202.

Hilts, P. J. "Agency Faults a U.C.L.A. Study for Suffering of Mental Patients." *New York Times*, March 10, 1994: A1, A11.

Holder, A. R. *Legal Issues in Pediatrics and Adolescent Medicine*, 2nd ed. New Haven: Yale University Press, 1985.

Hornblower, M. "Down and Out—But Determined." *Time*, November 23, 1987: 29.

Hume, D. "Of Suicide." In A. MacIntyre, Ed., *Hume's Ethical Writings.* New York: Macmillan, 1965: 297–306.

Kopelman, L. M. "Respect in Retardation: Issues of Valuing and Labeling." In L. M. Kopelman and J. C. Moskop, Eds., *Ethics and Retardation.* Dordrecht, Holland: D. Reidel, 1984: 65–86.

———. "The Punishment Concept of Disease." In C. Pierce and D. VanDeVeer, Eds., *AIDS: Ethics and Public Policy.* Belmont, CA: Wadsworth, 1988: 49–55.

———. "On the Evaluative Nature of Competency and Capacity Judgments." *Int J Law Psychiatry* 13:4 (1990): 309–329.

———. "How AIDS Activists Are Changing Research." In John F. Monagle and David C. Thomasma, Eds., *Health Care Ethics: Critical Issues.* Gaithersburg, MD: Aspen, 1994a: 199–209.

———. "Female Circumcision/Genital Mutilation and Ethical Relativism." *Second Opinion,* 20(2) (1994b): 55–71.

———. "Research Policy/II. Risk and Vulnerable Groups." In W. T. Reich, Ed., *Encyclopedia of Bioethics,* Revised ed. New York: Simon & Schuster/Macmillan, 1995: 2291–2296.

———. "Ethical Assumptions and Ambiguities of the Americans with Disabilities Act." *J Med Philos* 21 (1996): 187–208.

Kramer, Peter D. *Listening to Prozac.* New York: Viking Press, 1993.

MacIntyre, A. *After Virtue: A Study in Moral Theory.* Notre Dame, IN: University of Notre Dame Press, 1981.

Macklin R. "Mental Health and Mental Illness." *Philos Sci* 39 (1972): 341–365.

———. "The Medical Model in Psychoanalysis and Psychotherapy." *Comprehensive Psychiatry* 14 (1973): 49–69.

———. *Man, Mind and Morality: The Ethics of Behavior Control.* Engelwood Cliffs, NJ: Prentice Hall, 1982.

Margolis, J. *Psychotherapy and Morality: A Study of Two Concepts.* New York: Random House, 1966.

McGarry, L., Chodoff, P. "The Ethics of Involuntary Hospitalization." In S. Block and P. Chodoff, Eds., *Psychiatric Ethics.* Oxford: Oxford University Press, 1981: 203–219.

Mercer, J. *Labeling the Mentally Retarded.* Berkeley: University of California Press, 1973.

Mill, J. S. *On Liberty* (1859). London: Penguin Books, 1974 (reprint).

Murphy, J. G. "Therapy and the Problem of Autonomous Consent." *Int J Law Psychiatry* 2(4) (1979): 415–430.

"Medical Ethics in the Dock" (Editorial). *New York Times,* March 14, 1994.

Please Let Me Die. Department of Psychiatry, Galveston: University of Texas, 1974.

Popper, K. R. "Science, Conjectures and Refutations." In K. R. Popper, *Conjectures and Refutations: The Growth of Scientific Knowledge.* New York: Harper & Row, 1962.

President's Commission for the Study of Ethical Problems in Medicine and Biomedical Behavioral Research. *Making Health Care Decisions,* Vol. 1. Washington, DC: Government Printing Office, 1982.

Reich, W. T. "Psychiatric Diagnosis as an Ethical Problem." In S. Block and P. Chodoff, Eds., *Psychiatric Ethics*. Oxford: Oxford University Press, 1981: 61–88.

Roth, L. H., Meisel, A., Lidz, C. "Tests of Competency to Consent to Treatment." *Am J Psychiatry* 134(3) 1977: 279–284.

Rush, B. *Medical Inquiries and Observations Upon Disease of the Mind* (1812). Birmingham: The Classics of Medicine Library, 1979 (reprint).

Symons, A. L. "The Three-Step Test for Determining When Compliance with the Americans with Disabilities Act Is Required." *Gonzaga L Rev* 28(2) (1992): 235–264.

Szasz, T. *The Myth of Mental Illness*. New York: Hoeber–Harper, 1961.

———. *Law, Liberty and Psychiatry: An Inquiry into the Social Uses of Mental Health Practices*. New York: Macmillan, 1963.

———. *Ideology and Insanity: Essays on the Psychiatric Dehumanization of Man*. New York: Anchor Books, 1970.

U.S. Department of Health, Education, and Welfare, National Commission for the Protection of Human Subjects of Biomedical and Behavioral Research. *Research Involving Those Institutionalized as Mentally Infirm: Report and Recommendations*. Publ. (05)78-0006 and Publ. (05)78-0007 (App.). Washington, DC: Government Printing Office, 1978.

VanDeVeer, D. *Paternalism Intervention: The Moral Bounds of Benevolence*. Princeton: Princeton University Press, 1986.

Veatch, R. *A Theory of Medical Ethics*. New York: Basic Books, 1981.

Zembaty, J. S. "Introduction: Mental Illness and Individual Liberty." In T. A. Mappes and J. S. Zebaty, Eds., *Social Ethics*, 2nd ed. New York: McGraw-Hill, 1982: 263–268.

Cases, Acts, and Regulations

U.S. Department of Justice. "Nondiscrimination on the Basis of Disability in State and Local Government Services." Order No. 1512-91. *Compliance Handbook* §504, App. III.D. See 28 *CFR* 35.150.

Americans with Disabilities Act, 42 USC §12101–12213 (Suppl II), 1990.

Kaimowitz v. Department of Mental Health for the State of Michigan, Civil Action No. 73-19434-AW. Wayne Co. Cir. Ct., July 10, 1973.

O'Connor v. Donaldson, 422 U.S. 563, 95 S.Ct. 2486, Vol. 45 L.Ed. 2d 396, 1975.

Tarasoff v. Regents of the University of California, 131 Cal Rptr 14, July 1, 1976.

U.S. Protection of Human Subjects Regulation, 45 *CFR* §46, Revised June 18, 1991.

U.S. Rehabilitation Act, Pub. Law 93-112.29, 74 USC, 1973.

In re Yetter, Ct. Com. Pleas, Northampton Co., PA, Ct. Div. (Orphans), 62 Pa. D. & C., 2nd 619, 1973.

11

Health-Care Delivery and Resource Allocation

ALLEN BUCHANAN

SUMMARY

Increasingly, medical ethics involves decisions concerning the allocation of health-care resources and the institutional arrangements for making those decisions. The key concepts of health-care resource allocation and cost need to be defined because they shape the moral and policy discussion. This chapter considers different criteria for evaluating allocation of health-care resources. Two types of models of allocation are examined—efficiency models and ethical models.

In efficiency models of allocation, utility maximization, cost-benefit analysis, and cost effectiveness are the standards for judgment. Efficiency criteria are not by themselves sufficient for evaluating allocations; ethical criteria are also necessary. Two case studies, which present issues involved in rationing chemotherapy and the allocation of human heart for transplantation, illustrate the differences in the two approaches.

Broader issues relating to the ethics of resource allocation also are presented. Among these are the problem of access to health care and controversies over rival specifications of the right to health care, including utilitarian, egalitarian, equality of opportunity, and "decent minimum" views. In addition, it is argued that a comprehensive conception of just health care must address the question of how the cost of providing access for all to an adequate level of care is to be distributed fairly.

Recently, attention has shifted to include beneficence as well as justice. Issues central to approaches that emphasize beneficence include the nature of societal obligation, the freerider problem, the assurance problem, and the enforcement of obligations. Although many strategies have been offered for making ethical evaluations of health-care resource allocation, none, so far, is fully adequate or uniquely attractive.

Virtually every significant problem in medical ethics includes ethical issues concerning the allocation of scarce resources or is shaped by allocation decisions that are subject to ethical evaluation. For example, in deciding whether to prolong the life of a severely disabled newborn, when doing so will involve great financial burdens (for her parents, the hospital, and the public coffers), the decision maker—whether it be a parent, a court-appointed legal guardian, the physician, or a hospital administrator—is in effect choosing to allocate scarce resources to this particular baby rather than to someone else or something else. Unless previous allocation decisions had been made to channel resources into neonatal research and into the construction of the neonatal intensive care units in which the results of research were applied, then the need for the allocation decision that will determine this particular baby's fate would never have arisen.

This chapter is a critical survey of several major views on the ethical evaluation of decisions concerning the allocation of health-care resources, and the institutional arrangements established for making those decisions.

PRELIMINARY ANALYSIS OF KEY CONCEPTS

Health-Care Resources

In the most inclusive sense, health-care resources are any goods or services that can reasonably be expected to have a positive effect on health. Thus, health-care resources include, but are not restricted to, medical resources. Furthermore, health-care goods and services are not limited to those that are produced by persons ordinarily recognized as health-care professionals, such as physicians and nurses. Health-care resources are not just medical drugs, procedures, and treatments; they are also the many resources used for pollution control, shelter, and food required for normal growth and functioning.

Allocation

To *allocate* is to distribute resources among alternative uses. Allocation in this broad sense does not presuppose an allocator (an individual or a group) who deliberately distributes the available resources. Thus, a competitive market allocates social resources through the interactions of individual exchangers, each of whom makes allocation decisions concerning only his or her own resources in the pursuit of his or her own particular ends. Allowing a market for the buying and selling of organs, for example, is just as much an allocation decision as the adoption of an explicit rationing policy that allocates organs according to a criterion of social contribution or personal desert.

Even when an allocation of resources results directly from a social (rather than an individual) decision, the allocation is often a by-product of the pursuit of other goals (rather than an intended result). For example, a law stating that nurse–midwives must be supervised by physicians if their services are to be reimbursed by third-party payers has an allocational effect. It transfers income from nurse–midwives to physicians because the physicians charge nurse–midwives for the service of supervision, and it restricts the available number of practicing nurse–midwives to those who are able to secure such supervision. Similarly, a decision to pump millions of dollars of public funds into cancer centers affects the allocation of physicians among specialty training programs. If more money is available for residencies in oncology than for primary-care residencies, more medical students may become oncologists and fewer may become primary-care specialists. In neither of these examples is it necessary that any decision be aimed at the allocational effect in question. Allocations are subject to ethical assessment, however, regardless of whether they are the objects of explicit allocation decisions.

Cost

In the sense most pertinent to reasoning about allocation, the cost of something may be defined as the value of the most preferred alternative. Suppose that one has to decide how to spend one's weekly entertainment budget. In the order one prefers them, alternatives are (1) seeing the ballet; (2) attending a football game; and (3) going out to dinner. Because one's budget is limited, if the ballet is chosen, one loses the opportunity to attend the game and dine out. Since the game is the next most preferred alternative, its value is the cost of one's decision to see the ballet. In this sense, all costs are "opportunity costs." Given that resources—including time—are limited, deciding to use a resource for one purpose forecloses opportunities for alternative uses.

TYPES OF ALLOCATIONS

Discussions of allocation often utilize a distinction between macro- and microallocation. This distinction is, however, of limited use, and can be misleading unless its relative nature is clearly recognized. A decision by the U.S. Congress to allocate N billion dollars for Medicare and $N + m$ billion for national defense is perhaps the paradigm of a macroallocation decision. A microallocation decision would be, for example, a decision made by a particular physician when she decides to use the one available bed in her burn unit for Mr. Jones rather than for Ms. Smith. There are, of course, many types of allocation decisions that are smaller-scale than the former but larger-scale than the latter.

In response to this complexity, it is tempting to say that whether an allocation is "micro" or "macro" is determined by the *level* of decision-making authority or the level of available resources to be distributed. Talk of levels, however, is misleading to the extent that it encourages the fiction that there is an overall system, of a hierarchical character, within which decisions are interconnected in some principle way. Whether any existing society is this highly structured in its mechanism for allocation may be a matter of controversy, but it is fair to say that the United States, perhaps more so than many industrialized countries, currently lacks anything that could realistically be called an allocation system with regard to health-care resources.

It is perhaps more useful to begin with a classification of fundamental types of allocation problems that leaves open the question of what sort of allocational system, hierarchical or otherwise, will be needed to solve them. James F. Childress offers the following list:

1. What resources (time, energy, money, etc.) should be put into health care and into other social goods such as education, defense, eliminating poverty, and improving the environment?
2. Within the area of health (once we have determined its budget), how much time, energy, money, etc., should we allocate for prevention and how much for rescue and crisis medicine?
3. Within either preventive care or rescue medicine, who [if anyone] should receive resources such as vaccines or artificial hearts when we cannot meet everyone's needs? (Childress 1982)

CRITERIA FOR EVALUATING ALLOCATIONS

Existing, predicted, or proposed allocations may be evaluated on grounds of efficiency, ethics, or both. It is unfortunate that discussions of the ethics of health-care resource allocation typically ignore the efficiency evaluations that dominate the work of real-world policy makers and policy analysts, who in turn often convey the impression that by exclusively employing efficiency criteria they are approaching allocation issues in a nonethical or value-neutral way. Both approaches are mistaken.

Allocation decision processes may also be evaluated ethically and for efficiency. A decision process may be inefficient due to excessive expenditures of material resources (e.g., equipment for information gathering and processing), time, or human resources, or because the cost of the social conflict the process engenders is excessive. Even if an allocation decision is itself ethically unassailable, the process by which it is reached may be challenged from an ethical standpoint for procedural unfairness or on grounds that the decision maker lacked appropriate authority. For example, an adequate ethical evaluation of an allocation decision may require an assessment of the procedural fairness of the decision-making process (from which that allocation issued) because there is no consensus among reasonable persons as to whether the allocation, considered by itself, is ethically acceptable.

Efficiency Criteria

The dominant conception of efficiency among economists is that of *pareto optimality*. A state of a system is pareto optimal if there is no feasible alternative state in which at least one person would be better off and no one would be worse off (Buchanan 1985, 4–13). A move from a state that is not pareto optimal to one that is pareto optimal is a pareto improvement, and the latter state is pareto superior to the former.

Many economists and policy analysts find the paretian conception of efficiency attractive. One important reason for its appeal is that it avoids what many consider insurmountable obstacles to making the interpersonal utility comparisons that would be required if the principle of utility, a criterion of utility maximization, were employed instead. According to the *principle of utility*, allocational states are to be ranked according to how much net, over-all utility they produce. The net, overall utility of a particular allocation is calculated by summing up the net utility for each individual affected. The net utility for each individual is the sum of the benefits that allocation produces for him or her, minus the costs ("disbenefits") to him or her. An allocation maximizes utility if the net, overall utility it produces is at least as great as, if not greater than, the net, overall utility produced by each of the feasible alternative allocations.

To determine whether an allocation maximizes utility, it is necessary to sum up utilities and disutilities (or costs and benefits) for different individuals, and the interpersonal utility comparisons require that we be able to locate every person's state of well-being along a single numerical scale. The obstacle to achieving this is that there does not appear to be a nonarbitrary method for selecting a common zero point or baseline from which different individuals' utilities could be measured, nor a way to determine a common unit of measurement. Even if a utility scale could be constructed for each individual by recording the choices he or she makes among various options, this seems to provide no basis for relating the respective utility scales to one another in a way that allows the needed aggregation (Brock 1973, 245–49; Sartorius 1975).

To ascertain whether an allocation is pareto optimal (or to determine whether a change from one allocation to another would be a pareto improvement), however, it is not necessary to make interpersonal utility comparisons. All that is required is that each person's well-being under a particular allocation be comparable to his or her own well-being under alternative feasible allocations.

Although an allocation may be pareto optimal and still not maximize utility, a move from one allocation to another that constitutes a pareto improvement at least entails an increase in utility because at least one person's utility increases and no one's decreases. Consequently, use of the paretian concept of efficiency can be seen as a kind of second-best alternative to the utility-maximization criterion.

If the paretian conception of efficiency is seen in this way, relying on it as the exclusive or primary standard for evaluating allocations is no more plausible than a similar reliance on utility maximization would be, if the problem of interpersonal utility comparisons were solved. But there are strong objections to the principle of utility, quite apart from the difficulty of interpersonal comparisons.

First of all, it would be a mistake to view the principle of utility simply as a principle of collective rationality that is an uncontroversial extension of the principle of individual rationality prevalent in economic theory. The latter simply defines efficiency as taking the least costly, most effective means to one's end, that is, as individual utility maximization. Some who assume that utility maximization would be the appropriate criterion for evaluating allocation (were it not for the problem of interpersonal comparisons) and who view pareto optimality as a second-best approximation, may be under the impression that the principle of utility is an uncontroversial extension of the principle of individual utility maximization. This, however, is an error. First, if it is assumed that what is rational for an individual is to maximize his or her own utility, whether it is rational for anyone to seek the maximization of overall utility depends on whether, as a matter of contingent fact, the decision is the best way for him or her to maximize his or her own utility. Clearly there are many instances in the real world in which maximizing one's own utility and maximizing overall utility diverge. Whenever they diverge, the economic definition of rationality as individual utility maximization undermines, rather than supports, the claim that overall utility maximization is the rational standard for evaluating allocations.

Second, the principle of utility fares no better if it is understood not as the principle of individual rationality extended to society, but as an ethical principle. To assume that the principle of utility is the appropriate standard for evaluating allocations is to make the ethically controversial assumption that society is to be viewed as an apparatus for maximizing overall utility. Such a view of society may be incompatible with according proper respect to individual persons, who ought not to be regarded merely as contributors to ends that are not their own (Buchanan 1985). A particular allocation, or a complete social system, might maximize overall utility and yet be grossly unfair or unjust, which would violate the most fundamental rights of some individuals. Rawls and others have observed that a system in which some persons were slaves would in fact maximize overall utility, as long as the gains to the masters exceeded the losses to the slaves (Rawls 1971). That the criterion of utility maximization would not only allow but indeed require such a system, if it did in fact produce the most utility, is taken by many to be a telling objection to utilitarianism.

This extreme example illustrates the more general objection that opponents of utilitarianism often raise—that evaluating social arrangements, including allocations, simply according to their tendency to maximize overall utility neglects fairness as a fundamental ethical value. Similarly, utilitarianism has frequently been criticized for ignoring another key ethical value: personal desert. That one individual deserves some good, but another does not, is never itself a reason for the utilitarian to allocate the good to the former person; all that matters is how much utility can be gained.

Ethical objections also apply to attempts to evaluate allocations using the paretian criteria for efficiency. An allocation may be pareto optimal, yet grossly unjust or unfair (for example, it may be impossible to improve the condition of some of the slaves without worsening the condition of some of the slave holders). Similarly, the pursuit of pareto improvements recognizes no role for personal desert as such—all that matters is whether a change can be made that improves the condition of some without worsening the condition of any, regardless of who deserves the benefits conferred.

It follows that policy analysts who evaluate allocations solely by the standard economic (i.e., paretian) criterion of efficiency are either mistakenly assuming that they have avoided controversial ethical issues or are offering a fundamentally incomplete evaluation that must be supplemented by ethical criteria. If the paretian standard of efficiency is employed as the sole criterion for evaluating allocations, what is required is nothing short of a full-scale defense of utilitarianism, which, as we have just seen, is a very controversial ethical theory.

If, on the other hand, the paretian standard is offered not as the sole criterion for evaluation, but as one standard among others, including those that embody ethical values such as justice, fairness, and personal desert, what is needed is a theory, a systematic account, of how much weight should be given to efficiency relative to the other standards of assessment.

Cost-Benefit and Cost-Effectiveness Analyses

In part because the direct and unrestricted use of the utility-maximization criterion requires staggering amounts of information about the consequences of all feasible alternatives, and in part because in the more vexing policy decisions none of the feasible alternatives is likely to be pareto optimal (typically there will be losers as well as winners, no matter what is done), policy analysts have developed other efficiency criteria. The most widely discussed of these are cost-benefit analysis (CBA) and cost-effectiveness analysis (CEA), which M. C. Weinstein and W. B. Stason concisely define and contrast as follows.

> The key distinction is that a benefit-cost [or cost-benefit] analysis must value all outcomes in economic (e.g., dollar) terms, including lives or years of life and morbidity, whereas a cost-effectiveness analysis serves to place priorities on alternative expenditures without requiring that the dollar value of life and health be assessed (Weinstein and Stason 1977).

The preceding definition restricts CBA to a comparison of the health benefits of a particular allocational decision with the costs of implementing that decision. If this restriction were lifted, so that all costs and benefits of a particular decision were compared with all costs and benefits of each feasible alternative, CBA would be identical with the use of the utility-maximization criterion. Although CBA in the sense defined by Weinstein and Stason is narrower than utility-maximization because it only compares health benefits with costs, it nonetheless, in principle, allows quite diverse programs to be ranked. For example, CBA purports to tell whether a program to educate teenage females about prenatal care would produce a greater ratio of health benefits (for pregnant teenagers and the children they bear) to financial costs of the program than the ratio of health benefits (for persons with hypertension) to the costs of a hypertension screening program. According to CBA, resources are to be allocated to those uses that have the highest health benefit-cost ratios.

As should be apparent, the chief objections to utility-maximization apply with equal force to CBA. Even in the narrow sense, CBA requires interpersonal utility comparisons because the cost-benefit ratio for a given allocation is determined by subtracting the total financial cost from the sum of all the health benefits to all persons affected. Similarly, the most obvious ethical objections to utility-maximization apply to CBA, even when restricted to health benefits—neither criterion for allocation takes into account fairness or personal desert.

There are, in addition, special difficulties with the methods that cost-benefit analysts have proposed for assigning a dollar value to lives saved or to life-years gained as a result of the alternative allocations whose cost-benefit ratios are to be compared. The two most common methods are (1) future earnings (or human capital) and (2) willingness to pay.

According to the former, the monetary value of each individual's life, for purposes of calculating a cost-benefit ratio, is his or her total expected lifetime income. Critics of the future-earnings approach point out that it places a higher value (on average) on the lives of men than on the lives of women. The difficulty is not simply that women who work in the home typically receive no reported wages for their labor—this could be remedied by calculating the market value of their domestic services and counting it as income. The real problem is that even when women receive income for their services, they often receive lower pay than men do for performing comparable work. Hence, to value women's lives for purposes of determining allocations of health-care resources according to their expected future earnings simply compounds the unfairness of an already unfair social system.

As we have already seen, to allocate resources strictly according to which allocation has the highest overall benefit-cost ratio is to assume that utilitarianism is the correct ethical theory. Even if this controversial assumption is left unchallenged, however, future earnings are an inadequate measure of the value of human life for purposes of calculating overall utility because the effect an individual's life (or the loss of it) has on overall utility is not equivalent to his or her future earnings. For one thing, an individual's earnings represent (at best) the utility his or her services produce for those who pay for them, not the total utility—or disutility—produced by his or her rendering of those services. In other words, the future-earnings approach does not take into account the effects of "externalities," whether positive or negative, on overall costs or overall benefits. An *externality* is a spillover, or neighborhood effect, or third-party effect of an exchange. For example, air pollution from a chemical plant is an externality (a negative one in that it results in harm to people, wildlife, and plants), a cost that is not reflected in the exchange between the chemical plant and its customers. Even if an individual's future earnings were an adequate approximation of his or her contribution to social utility, it can still be objected that it is unethical to view society as a kind of grand machine for producing ever more utility and human beings as cogs in the machine ("factors of production" in a productive enterprise).

Quite apart from its ethical defects, the future-earnings approach is flawed as an account of how people actually value not only their own lives but the lives of others as well. The value a parent places on her child—and the loss she feels at the child's death—typically has little to do with what the child's lifetime income would have been had he or she survived. Similarly, the value an individual places on his own life typically reflects the value he places on the future experiences and activities he will be deprived of, not the loss of future earnings (Brock 1986). The future-earnings approach, then, is not only ethically deficient, but descriptively inaccurate.

The second method assigns value to a life or to prolongation of a life according to the amount of money the person whose life it is would pay to avoid the loss of his life (or to reduce the risk of losing it) or to prolong it for some specified period. The chief attraction of the willingness-to-pay approach is that it is subject-centered—the value assigned to a life is determined by the preferences of the individual him- or herself, not by others. Unfortunately, however, willingness to pay does not avoid the ethical objection raised earlier against future earnings. It, too, systematically reproduces whatever injustices in the distribution of wealth already exist, because how much a person is willing to pay to avoid death or reduce the risk of death depends on how great his or her resources are. If the current distribution of wealth is unjust or unfair, relying on the willingness-to-pay approach to make allocation decisions is unfair and unjust.

Although the forgoing problems are extremely serious, it would be a mistake to conclude that CBA has nothing of value to bring to decision-making concerning the allocation of health-care resources. Understood in the most general way, CBA is an indispensable procedure for overall practical reasoning, not just for matters of resource allocation. In its broadest outlines, it is simply the attempt to make the gains and losses of alternative courses of action explicit and, to the extent that this is possible, to make them sufficiently commensurate with one another so that at least an approximation of a maximizing strategy can be formulated. Any theory of practical reasoning that recognizes that there is a plurality of goods, that at least some gains are not costless, and that values are at least sometimes roughly commensurate, utilizes CBA in this generic sense, and this includes non-utilitarian ethical theories.

In the latter, moral values that represent constraints on overall utility-maximization can be reflected in the weights that are assigned to different gains and losses. For example, an ethical theory that rejects utilitarianism and takes certain individual rights as fundamental, but that recognizes that rights may conflict, might nevertheless find it illuminating to use a cost-benefit procedure, in the broadest sense, to arrive at reasonable trade-offs between basic rights when they conflict.

The preceding objections to CBA are not to be understood, then, as a rejection of all practical reasoning that attempts to weigh losses against gains and in some sense maximize gains. Instead, they are criticisms of attempts to use specific maximizing techniques that either ignore or beg important ethical questions about the proper scope of maximizing reasoning and the appropriate weight that different values (for instance, fairness versus efficiency) ought to be given when a maximizing procedure is appropriate.

There are two quite different ways to construe the ethical objections to both the future-earnings and the willingness-to-pay approaches. One is to argue that even if one or both adequately captures the economic value of life, attending only to the economic value of life is an insufficient basis for calculating overall benefit, even if we accept the principle that we are to maximize overall benefit in making allocation decisions. In this first view, future earnings and willingness to pay are incomplete measures of the value of lives, where value is objective and commensurate in the way required for a maximizing calculation. On the second reading, a critic of these two approaches can admit that one or both of them adequately captures the economic value of lives and that the only objective and commensurate sense of value is economic, yet also maintain that there are ethical considerations (for example, of fairness) that place limits on the extent to which the value of a person's life (in this objective and commensurate sense) ought to determine his or her share of resources. For the first view, the charge is that willingness to pay and future earnings are inadequate measures of the value of lives; for the second, it is that maximizing value is not the sole consideration in allocating resources.

Unlike CBA, CEA does not require that health benefits, including lives saved or prolonged, be measured by the same units (dollars) as the costs of the allocation of resources that provides those benefits. All that is necessary is that all the health benefits expected from a particular allocation be measured by a common unit, usually "quality-adjusted life-years," and that all costs be measured by a common unit (dollars). CEA allows a ranking of alternative programs for producing a given level of health benefits according to the dollar costs of each for producing the desired effect.

There are three major limitations on the usefulness of CEA. The first, needless to say, is the difficulty of formulating a reasonable, objective concept of quality of life for determining the unit of benefit measurement, the quality-adjusted life-year. Perhaps the chief issue is the extent to which the quality of an individual's life (or of a life-year) is to be understood in a subjective fashion, that is, according to his or her own estimate, or objectively.

The second is simply a variant of the major ethical objection to CBA and to utilitarian approaches more generally—CEA itself recognizes no ethical concerns about how benefits are distributed, except so far as the distribution affects the total benefit produced. In other words, to determine allocations exclusively according to CEA is to beg fundamental allocation questions. CEA might indicate, for example, that a program that establishes mobile coronary care units produces more health benefits for the money than does a liver transplant program, but it cannot indicate what proportion of total social resources should be allocated to health care and what proportion to education or defense. This is a serious limitation because, at the present time, there are many who believe that the health-care sector has been draining a disproportionate share of social resources away from other areas.

ETHICAL CRITERIA

The Need for Ethical Criteria

We have seen that efficiency criteria are not by themselves sufficient for evaluating allocations; ethical criteria are also necessary. Often, allocation decisions, especially those toward the "micro" end of the continuum, are made in a much less systematic way than advocates of CBA or CEA would prefer. But here, too, the need for ethical and efficiency criteria is apparent. Two examples are discussed briefly below: the allocation of human hearts for transplantation and the selective use of cancer chemotherapy. For the former, the ethically controversial nature of the process is apparent—there are not enough transplantable human hearts for everyone who needs one, problematic choices are being made, and the effects of these decisions, if not the decision-making processes themselves, are often exposed to public scrutiny by the harsh glare of the media. For the latter, the usual situation is *not* one in which a limited quantity of a cancer drug is available to a physician and he or she must decide which patients will get it. Nevertheless, ethically controversial decisions are made daily as to which patients will receive certain cancer drugs and in some cases it is clear that the high cost of these drugs plays a role in decision making (though often in indirect and complex ways). Rationing occurs with both human hearts and cancer drugs.

Rationing Chemotherapy

In their controversial book *The Painful Prescription* (subtitled *Rationing Hospital Care*), Aaron and Schwarz contrast the use of cancer drugs for various classes of cancer patients in the United States and England. They note that England spends about 70 percent less per capita on cancer-fighting drugs than the United States does (Aaron and Schwarz 1984, 47), and that the most dramatic difference lies in the tendency of American physicians to treat, and British physicians *not* to treat, patients who have metastatic solid tumors and who have few symptoms that might be relieved by chemotherapy and for whom chemotherapy rarely produces an extension of life and even less frequently a cure. Aaron and Schwarz report that the rate at which American physicians treat such patients is five to six times greater than that for British physicians (Aaron and Schwarz 1984, 48).

British physicians interviewed in the study justified their practice on the grounds that, for this group of patients, the disability and discomfort that are often side effects of chemotherapy are not worth the small chance or benefit. American physicians, in contrast, seemed more frequently to be committed to treating such cancer aggressively, even though they admitted that the prospects for success were very small.

The responses of some British physicians support the hypothesis that financial considerations are playing a role in this pronounced difference in patterns of practice (Aaron and Schwarz 1984, 50). British physicians know that they are custodians of a scarce public resource—that the British National Health Service must operate within a limited budget. American physicians operate under no such overall budget constraint and, as Aaron and Schwarz point out, American cancer specialists under the third-party, fee-for-service system have a strong financial incentive to treat patients aggressively.

However, Aaron and Schwarz neglect to mention that American physicians in some cases are already beginning to find themselves subject to budget constraints that give them incentives to take a harder look at *how much* benefit can reasonably be expected from chemotherapy. The director of an oncology department at a hospital owned by a large Health Maintenance Organization (HMO) in the United States reported that he only ordered extremely expensive new cancer drugs if their expected benefit exceeded a certain threshold—say, a 0.2 probability of "significant" improvement in terms of life extension with "reasonable" quality of life.[1] Unless some such rationing device were employed, he stated, his oncology unit, by using every new cancer drug that promised some net benefit, would bankrupt the entire HMO in a month's time. Although this case comes from an HMO, it could have occurred in any hospital in which close attention is paid to how resources are allocated among different services.

The differences in prescribing patterns for chemotherapy illustrate two important points. First, the question of what level of expected benefits to the patient is high enough in relation to costs to the patient (in terms of side effects) to justify the treatment is *not* a medical question. For persons who

---

[1] This was reported to the author in a personal communication with the director of the oncology unit.

value the extension of their life very highly, gaining a rather small chance of longer survival may be worth considerable disability and discomfort; others may have a more demanding standard for what counts as an acceptable quality of life. Even when all the medical facts are in, a decision about whether, strictly from the patient's standpoint, chemotherapy is appropriate, depends on personal values. Second, the greater the extent to which physicians come to regard themselves as operating under budget constraints—imposed by society or by their own hospital administration, the more likely it is that the cost-benefit threshold they use to determine whether to prescribe expensive drugs will be influenced by broader cost considerations, not by what is best for this particular patient.

As cost-containment pressures mount, one of the most vexing questions concerning the allocation of health-care resources is: How can the physician play an effective role in efforts to ration scarce resources responsibly without undermining his or her traditional and valued role as advocate for the individual patient? Once the fact that rationing decisions are not only morally permissible but morally required for the fair and efficient use of scarce social resources, it will become harder to sustain the illusion that different practices concerning the use of cancer drugs or other expensive therapies simply reflect differences in medical judgment.

Allocating Hearts

The system—or rather the inconsistent patchwork of processes—by which human hearts for transplantation are allocated in the United States is neither efficient nor fair according to any reasonable standard (Mathieu 1988). There are several sources of inefficiency. A study by the national Task Force on Organ Transplantation (a committee appointed by the U.S. Department of Health and Human Services) found that regionalization of heart transplant centers, rather than the current proliferation of centers as individual physicians and medical centers compete for dollars and prestige, would save resources and increase the quality of care (Department of Health, Education, and Welfare 1986). Perhaps just as important, a coordinated, regionalized system of transplant centers would provide better prospects for developing and monitoring more ethical and more efficient procedures for allocating hearts. At present, hearts are sometimes allocated to patients who will almost certainly die even though they receive a heart, despite the fact that there are other potential recipients who have a much better chance of living if they were to receive the heart.

This inefficient—and morally irresponsible—use of the public resources used in the development and deployment of transplant technology can occur because of the defective way in which the human heart allocation "hotline" works. A registered transplant surgeon who wants a heart for his patient may call the hotline and request a heart. The most abusable feature of this system is that the physician who makes the request unilaterally classifies his patient according to a priority classification. In one recent case, a transplant surgeon designated his patient a "priority 1" on the grounds that the patient would die almost immediately if he did not receive a heart. Although this was true, it was in fact not a sufficient reason for bestowing the heart on this patient instead of another. The patient's condition had already so deteriorated that competent medical opinion agreed it was virtually certain that he would die even if he received the heart (Mathieu 1988). An allocation system that allows "urgency"—without consideration of relative expected benefit—to determine priority and that relies on interested parties to make priority classifications can only be expected to waste precious social resources.

Quite aside from the problems of inefficiency, the current processes by which human hearts are allocated also can be criticized as unfair. The chief criticism is that morally arbitrary factors often play a decisive role in determining who lives and who dies. The most obvious of these is ability to pay: most transplant centers require as much as $60,000 "cash up front." Further, some centers give first priority to in-state residents; thus, where one happens to live may mean that one will not get a heart, even if the medical need and potential benefit are greater than that of a person fortunate enough to be living in the right state. Geographical discrimination is especially suspect because millions of federal tax dollars (not state funds) were spent to develop the technology. Some transplant centers are, in effect, selling hearts to the highest bidders—in many cases foreign nationals (chiefly Saudis and Greeks, according to one study) (Mathieu 1988).

Ethicists who recognize the need for a more satisfactory method of dealing with the problem of allocating scarce organs for transplantation have recognized two polar approaches (Rescher 1974). On the one hand, an exclusive concern with efficiency or with producing the most benefit possible requires that allocations be made according to what would maximize quality-adjusted life-years. Such an approach simply assumes the correctness of utilitarianism as a moral theory and is subject to the charge that it disregards all issues of fairness. Perhaps most important, it can be argued that a strictly utilitarian system for allocating scarce organs fails to show proper regard for the equal worth of persons, a worth that cannot be equated with contribution to social utility.

Some who reject utilitarian allocation systems on the latter ground suggest that the only way to show proper regard for equal moral status or worth of persons is to give them equal chances to receive the scarce good, either by using a fair lottery method in which each has an equal probability of winning, or by using a first-come, first-serve system to approximate the randomness of a lottery. The latter proposal is clearly flawed: The poor would be disadvantaged by a first-come, first-serve system not only because they tend to be less educated and informed about medical matters but also because they are less likely to see a physician and be advised of the need to get in line for a transplant.

The lottery method (assuming the lottery is fair) would avoid this problem and could be seen as showing equal respect for persons, but it goes too far in eschewing entirely all considerations of how much benefit an allocation will produce. Unless some initial threshold of expected benefit to the patient is used as an eligibility requirement for participation in the lottery, use of a randomizing method will mean that lives of extremely poor quality will be prolonged, perhaps only briefly, at the expense of much longer lives of higher quality.

One ethicist has suggested that a three-tiered system for allocating hearts would better express the conviction that both efficiency (or maximizing benefit) and equal respect for persons are important values (Mathieu 1988). First, potential recipients would be selected according to a standard of *medical suitability* (that is, the minimal expected benefit threshold). Only if their expected benefit (in terms of quality-adjusted life-years) exceeded a specified threshold would they be placed on the list of potential recipients. Second, those among the first group whose need was most urgent—those who would die soon unless they receive a heart—would be given top priority. Third, if the number of available hearts were greater than the number of people in the top priority group, the remainder of those who passed the medical suitability test would receive hearts on a first-come, first-serve basis.

This sketch of a system is not intended to solve all the problems of allocation for hearts—it does not address the issue of whether a person whose immune system rejects a first heart should receive another, for example, nor does it address the objection that a first-come, first-serve method may discriminate against the poor. But it does illustrate how one system might incorporate both efficiency and fairness (or equity) considerations in a coherent way.

An alternative would be to rate each potential recipient according to expected benefit (number of quality-adjusted life-years), but allow expected benefit to be decisive only if there is a difference in expected benefit that exceeds some rather high threshold. In effect, such a system would show strong—not unlimited—regard for the equal worth of persons by allocating hearts randomly unless some nonrandom allocation would produce a very marked increase in benefit (Brock 1988). Although both the allocation models would be an improvement over the current arrangements inasmuch as each recognizes that both efficiency and fairness are relevant values, neither by itself avoids the perplexing issue of exactly what the trade-off should be when the two values are in conflict.

The Ubiquity and Inescapability of Rationing

Although politicians sensitive to public opinion and hospital administrators vulnerable to lawsuits are loathe to admit it, rationing of health-care resources is not limited to exotic therapies like transplants. *Rationing*—which means the withholding of care expected to be of net benefit—occurs throughout every health-care system and is unavoidable. Rationing is a necessity because resources are finite and because there are other goods worth pursuing besides health care. To use the language of economics, the opportunity costs of attempting to provide everyone with all the health care that is expected to be of any net benefit are unacceptable.

It is important to understand that rationing is not confined to government health-care systems. In a purely private insurance system, health care is rationed according to ability to pay, with the result that those who are at greatest risk for illness may not be able to afford any health care. Regardless of the type of system, rationing takes a number of forms, some overt and dramatic, as in the allocation of scarce organs for transplantation, others subtle and even hidden. For example, an HMO administrator, recognizing that the elderly use more care on average and are less able to travel considerable distances to receive care, may decide to build a new clinic in an area with fewer elderly people. Thus, the choice of location has the effect of rationing care by limiting utilization. Or, a managed care organization may require patients to clear a number of hurdles (e.g., seeing a nurse practitioner first, then a primary care physician, before gaining access to a specialist) and work their way through a waiting list as a way of limiting utilization.

One of the most perplexing and urgent issues we now face in health care is the question of *who* should make rationing decisions. Different forms of delivery assign responsibility for rationing to different agents at different locations within the institutional structure. In the British National Health Service, a consensus on rationing policies develops among medical specialty groups through interaction with regional health authorities, but the public appears to have little opportunity for input and may not even know that rationing is occurring. In sharp contrast, Oregon recently instituted an explicit rationing program for Medicaid services, utilizing rationing criteria that were developed through a political process with a rather high degree of public participation. At this point, it is not clear whether the trend will be toward broader democratic participation in rationing decisions or toward a complex array of highly localized, largely hidden, and for the most part unaccountable rationing processes. The question of whether, or to what extent, rationing policies should be developed through democratic processes, whether directly participatory or representative, raises profound issues of political ethics.

There are two general ethical issues concerning rationing in health-care delivery systems. The first is the fairness of the system of rationing as it affects patients. A system that arbitrarily concentrates the burdens of rationing on certain classes of individuals (for example, the elderly, as in the example above) or the poor (as some critics of the Oregon Medicaid rationing plan have complained) is ethically defective.

The second issue is the fairness of the rationing system toward the providers of care who must comply with the system. Increasingly, physicians in the United States complain that the rationing policies they are required to implement create unacceptable conflicts of interest and compromise their role as patient advocates.

Depending on who the agents of rationing are and the location of rationing decisions within the system, different health-care delivery systems will exacerbate or ameliorate the problem of conflict of interest for providers. For example, in a highly competitive health-care environment, administrators, through the use of various penalties and rewards, will exert pressure on physicians to limit utilization of care. Thus, a physician who orders more tests than the average physician of the same specialty working in the organization may be told that his or her contract will not be renewed, but one who is especially successful in limiting utilization may receive a year-end bonus. Obviously, in such a situation conflicts can occur between the physician's interest in remuneration, professional advancement, and job security, on the one hand, and the commitment to providing the best care available to each patient, on the other. A system that minimizes the strains of commitment on physicians and reduces the incentives for behavior that puts patients at risk is ethically preferable.

The "Access Problem" and the Ethical Evaluation of Large-Scale Allocation Patterns

Ethical theorizing about large-scale allocation patterns has arisen in part from the recognition that "macro" decisions shape "micro" problems and that piecemeal approaches (such as those sketched in the discussion of the preceding two examples) are inadequate. In addition, two powerful social factors motivate the search for coherent ethical criteria for evaluating large-scale allocation patterns. First, there is the growing perception that the rapid rise in health-care expenditures constitutes a "crisis"—and that serious cost containment measures are a necessity. Second, there is the sobering recognition that from 30 to 37 million Americans lack any health-care coverage, either through private insurance or public programs such as Medicare and Medicaid, and that as many as 22 million more have coverage that is inadequate by virtually any reasonable standard (President's Commission 1983). Systematic theorizing is needed (1) to determine when differences in access to health care for various individuals or groups constitute ethically objectionable inequalities, and (2) to determine which cost containment measures are ethically acceptable.

RIGHTS TO HEALTH CARE

Until very recently, the prevailing view has been that to resolve the important large-scale allocation issues in health care, it is necessary to determine whether there is a moral right to health care, and if so, what its content is. However, this assumption is now being challenged by persons who maintain that it is unduly restrictive to limit the discussion to matters of justice and, more specifically, of individual rights. Their point is that allocations may be criticized for being uncharitable or ungenerous even if they are not unjust and violate no one's right. Just as respecting others' rights is not the whole of moral virtue for an individual, so justice, even if it is the first virtue of social institutions, is not the sole virtue.

Positions on the right to health care range from the denial that there is a moral right to health care to the claim that there is a strong egalitarian right, a right of each to an equal share of health resources. Another view holds that the right to health care is derivative and is based exclusively on considerations of utility-maximization. The opposing thesis is that the right to health care is independent of and overrides all appeals to utility-maximization. To appreciate these disagreements over the existence or scope of a right to health care it is first necessary to clarify the general import of the assertion that a person has a right to something. The distinctive features of such "right" are typically said to be as follows (Buchanan 1984b, 63; Feinberg 1979, 87):

1. If Jones has a right to X, he has a valid claim or entitlement to it. This is not captured by saying that Jones would benefit from X or that Jones's having it is desirable (to him or others). Because to have a right is to have a basis for making a claim to the thing in question, the appropriate posture for the right-holder is not that of the supplicant pleading for a favor, but rather that of someone demanding what is due to him or her.
2. Consequently, if Jones' right is violated, it is not merely that an unfortunate or less than morally optimal situation has occurred; in addition, Jones has been wronged by those who failed to fulfill their obligations and is therefore the appropriate recipient of compensation or restitution.
3. If Jones has a right to X, someone or some collectivity (society, the government as the agent of society) has an obligation to make X available to Jones.
4. The existence of Jones's right provides a strong prima facie justification for enforcing these obligations if necessary.

Many discussions of rights assume a fifth feature:

5. A valid right-claim overrides appeals to utility maximization; in other words, the mere fact that failing to respect the right would maximize utility is not itself a sufficient reason for doing so (Dworkin 1977, 184–205).

Writers who focus on the fifth feature sometimes fail to point out that it is quite compatible with viewing rights as being derivative from and ultimately justified by appeals to utility maximization.

A Utilitarian (Derivative) Right to Health Care

Utilitarianism purports to be a comprehensive moral theory, of which a utilitarian theory of justice, including an account of justice in health care, would be only one part (Buchanan 1981, 4–5). There are two main types of comprehensive utilitarian theory: act and rule utilitarianism. Act utilitarianism defines rightness with respect to particular acts—an act is right if and only if it maximizes net utility. Rule utilitarianism defines rightness with respect to rules of action and makes the rightness of particular acts depend on the rules under which those acts fall. A rule is right if general compliance with that rule (or with a set of rules of which it is an element) maximizes net utility, and a particular action is right if it falls under such a rule.

The most prevalent form of the theory, sometimes called *classic utilitarianism*, (Buchanan 1981)[2] defines the rightness of acts or rules as maximization of aggregate utility. The aggregate utility produced by an act or by general compliance with a rule is the sum of the utility produced for each individual affected. *Utility* is defined as pleasure, satisfaction, happiness, or as the realization of preferences, as the latter are revealed through individuals' choices.

The distinction between act and rule utilitarianism is important for a utilitarian theory of justice because rule utilitarianism must include an account of when institutions are just. Thus, institutional rules may maximize utility even though the rules do not direct individuals as individuals or as occupants of institutional positions to maximize utility in a case-by-case fashion. For example, it may be that a judicial system that maximizes utility will do so by including rules that prohibit judges from deciding a case according to their estimates of what would maximize utility in that particular case. Thus the utilitarian justification of a particular action or decision may not be that it maximizes utility, but rather that it falls under some rule of an institution or set of institutions that maximizes utility.

Some utilitarians hold that principles of justice are the most basic moral principles because the utility of adherence to them is especially great. According to this view, utilitarian principles of justice are those utilitarian moral principles that are of such importance that they may be enforced, if necessary. Some utilitarians also hold that among the utilitarian principles of justice are principles specifying individual rights, in which the latter are thought of as enforceable claims that take precedence over appeals to what would maximize utility in the particular case.

---

[2]The discussion of utilitarianism, and some material on libertarianism and on Rawls's theory, is drawn from Buchanan's essay "Justice: A Philosophical Review" with permission from D. Reidel Publishing Co.

A utilitarian moral theory, then, can include principles of rights that themselves prohibit or trump appeals to utility maximization, as long as the justification of the principles is that they are part of an institutional system that maximizes utility. In cases in which two or more rights principles conflict, considerations of utility may be invoked to determine which rights principles are to be given priority. Utilitarianism is incompatible with rights only if rights exclude appeals to utility maximization at all levels of justification, including the most basic institutional level. Rights founded ultimately on considerations of utility are called *derivative* rights, to distinguish them from rights in the strict, fundamental sense.

Whether an overarching total institutional system that maximizes net utility will include a right to health care will depend on a wealth of empirical facts not deducible from the principle of utility itself. A utilitarian system of derivative rights will designate certain goods as being the goods that make an especially large contribution to the maximization of net utility. It is reasonable to assume, on the basis of scientific empirical data as well as commonsense experience, that health care, or at least certain forms of health care, would be among them. Consider, for example, perinatal care, broadly conceived as including genetic screening and counseling (at least for special risk groups), prenatal nutritional care and medical examinations for expectant mothers, medical care during delivery, and basic pediatric services in the crucial months after birth. If empirical research indicates (1) that a system of institutional arrangements that maximizes net utility would include such services and (2) that such services can best be ensured if they are accorded the status of a right, with all that this implies, including the use of coercive sanctions where necessary, according to utilitarianism, there is such a derivative right. The strength and content of this right relative to other derivative rights is determined by the utility of various forms of health care relative to one another as compared with other kinds of goods.

It has been argued that utilitarianism is not capable of providing a secure foundation for a universal right to health care—a right to at least some minimal core of health-care services for everyone (Buchanan 1984a, 60). Certain classes of individuals might be excluded from virtually all health-care services. The class of newborns with Down syndrome (formerly called Mongolism), for example, might well be excluded from the "decent minimum" of health care (and other goods and services), which others should receive as a matter of derivative right on utilitarian grounds. These retarded individuals, who often also suffer from serious physical disabilities, tend to require a rather large outlay of social resources over the course of their lives. Relative to the costs of caring for them, the contribution these individuals make to social utility may not be large, at least so far as we are limited to a concept of contribution that permits quantification. If this is the case, utilitarianism will permit—indeed will require—that these individuals be excluded from the right to health care.

To understand why this is taken to be a serious criticism of utilitarianism, two points require emphasis. The first is that these infants are generally capable of enjoyment, purposeful activity, and meaningful interpersonal relationships, and can often attain something approximating a normal life span. In these respects, they are unlike more severely disabled individuals, such as those who become permanently comatose due to disease or trauma, anencephalics (babies born with no brain above the brain stem or with no cerebral cortex), or even profoundly demented patients with Alzheimer's disease. If utilitarianism only rendered problematic the claim that the latter sorts of individuals have a right to health care, it would be significantly less ethically problematic because the moral status of such individuals, our obligations to them, and even their capacity to benefit from our aid are more dubious.

Second, utilitarian calculations may require that the Down syndrome babies (or other groups of moderately disabled people) be excluded, not just from extremely expensive, exotic medical technology, but also from the most basic care. In sum, utilitarianism may mandate that even for basic and relatively inexpensive goods and services, what is guaranteed for most should not be provided for some, even though their needs are as great and they would benefit very much.

Criticism of the utilitarian account of the right to health care is simply an application of the more general objection that utilitarianism fails to provide a secure foundation for any of the most important moral rights as rights of all, not just some, persons. Rawls has argued that the case for equal, basic, civil and political rights for all should not depend, as it does according to utilitarianism, on contingent assumptions about what will in fact maximize overall utility. He also contends that this deficiency, as well as utilitarianism's inability to accord proper recognition to the values of fairness and desert, stems, ultimately, from its failure to take seriously the "separateness of persons" (Rawls 1971). According to utilitarianism, the ultimate objects of moral concern in the universe are desires or preferences, not the persons (or even sentient organisms) whose desires or preferences they are. For the utilitarian, persons are mere receptacles or loci for utility.

The fundamental ethical objections to utilitarianism as a general theory count heavily not only against the attempt to base a right to health care on strictly utilitarian grounds, but also against exclusive reliance on the principle of utility as a guide to more limited allocation decisions both within and outside health care. None of this, however, supports the more extreme conclusion that utilitarian considerations should have no weight whatsoever in allocating health-care resources. In virtually every ethical theory other than libertarianism (in its more extreme forms), and in commonsense moral thinking, maximizing overall utility is often a weighty consideration, even when it is not the sole or even the preponderant factor. This is hardly surprising, assuming that ethics is concerned in some fundamental way with human welfare.

Libertarianism: The Challenge to All Welfare Rights, Including the Right to Health Care

There are a number of different types of theories that are sometimes called libertarian, but Robert Nozick's is often taken to be paradigmatic.[3] Nozick begins by assuming, not arguing for, a very strong right to private property, a right to exclusive control over whatever one can attain through voluntary exchanges in the market (assuming that both parties in fact own what they exchange), through gifts voluntarily bestowed by others, and by appropriating previously unowned things by "mixing one's labor" with them, so long as (1) one's appropriation does not worsen the condition of others by creating a situation in which they are "no longer . . . able to use freely [without exclusively appropriating] what [they] . . . previously could" or (2) one properly compensates those whose condition is worsened in the way specified in (1) (Nozick 1974).

Apart from the special case of rectifying past injustices, Nozick's view strictly prohibits any coercive efforts to redistribute wealth, even for the purpose of providing the most minimal welfare rights, including all forms of a right to health care. The legitimate role of the state, according to this view, is restricted to the protection of so-called negative rights. The state may wield its coercive power only to protect citizens from assault, theft, and fraud, and for national defense.

According to Nozick, the competitive market with private property is the only social structure compatible with respect for these individual rights. Consequently, for Nozick, there is no need for a theory of the just allocation of resources in general, including health-care resources. Resources will be allocated by market processes; insofar as people exchange or give what they have rightfully acquired, whatever allocation of resources that results is just.

Nozick's libertarianism has been effectively criticized on a number of grounds, but two major objections are especially potent. First, it has been noted that Nozick fails in his attempt to show that every principle of justice that requires redistribution either (1) is either intuitively unjust or (2) would require unacceptable disruptions of people's expectations by frequently appropriating their holdings for the sake of preserving the overarching pattern of distribution specified by the principle.

To support the first prong of his attack on redistributive principles of justice Nozick tries to persuade us that it is counterintuitive to think that injustice could arise merely from voluntary exchanges among people, each of whom owns what he exchanges, and that, consequently, any principle of

---

[3]This statement may be misleading because Nozick's view is more extreme than that of some who are frequently labeled libertarians, such as F. A. Hayek, who admit that enforced contributions to provide a minimal welfare safety net are sometimes justifiable.

justice that requires allocations arising from such exchanges to be overturned must be unjust.

As several critics have pointed out, however, Nozick's intuitions will not be shared by anyone who takes seriously the problem of cumulative harms. Once the cumulative negative effects on both welfare and liberty are appreciated, the need to avoid or minimize the negative externalities can provide strong ethical grounds for limiting the individual's right to acquire and exchange goods—and thus for challenging the virtually unlimited private property right Nozick merely assumes without argument. For example, strictly voluntary exchanges of property may lead to such extreme concentrations of wealth that the rich are able, even through largely legal means, to undermine the civil and political liberties of the poor (Cohen 1978).

The second prong of Nozick's attack is weak as well. It is true that a very demanding principle of justice that required, for example, strict equality in resources, might necessitate frequent redistributions that would be intolerably coercive and disruptive. It is much less plausible to argue, however, that *all* redistributive principles suffer from this defect. Implementing a principle requiring only that everyone is to have a decent minimum of certain basic goods, including food, shelter, and a core set of important health-care services, need not result in frequent or severe disruptions. Long-standing, publicized laws specifying predictable tax obligations can be and are used to fund such a core of welfare goods.

Another major objection to Nozick's libertarianism turns against him his own provocative suggestion that the ultimate foundation for his strong right to private property (and hence for the denial of welfare rights it entails) is an appreciation of the central role of autonomy in the leading of a meaningful life. This vague suggestion seems to backfire on Nozick. An autonomous person who wishes to lead a meaningful life—which for most of us would not be a life in which poverty limits our aspirations to securing the next meal, finding shelter for the night, and coping with suffering and disability due to health problems that could have been avoided—will require at least a modicum of material resources, including access to health care. An autonomous person values opportunity, and our opportunities can be limited not only by deliberate interferences by others but also by lack of resources, by illness, and by disability.

Libertarians such as Nozick have a reply to the charge that justice as they see it shows too little concern with the human welfare and with the material resources for meaningful, autonomous living. They emphasize that justice is not the whole of morality and that the harsh effects of the libertarian ban on enforced redistribution can be moderated by voluntary adherence to principles of beneficence. However, an examination of approaches to health-care allocation that rely chiefly on principles of beneficence (or "humanity," or "charity"), rather than on principles of justice, shows serious obstacles exist to efficient, coordinated voluntary redistribution, which libertarians tend to overlook.

Rawls's Theory and the Right to Health Care

In his widely acclaimed book, *A Theory of Justice,* John Rawls offers a new and highly sophisticated version of the traditional theory of the social contract, as developed by Hobbes, Locke, Rousseau, and Kant. Although Rawls supplies several distinct lines of justification for the principles of justice he advances, the hypothetical contract argument is the most distinctive:

> The principles of justice for the basic structure of society are the principles that free and rational persons concerned to further their own interests would accept in an initial position of equality as defining the fundamental terms of their association. These principles are to regulate all further agreements; they specify the kinds of social cooperation that can be entered into and the forms of government that can be established. This way of regarding the principles of justice I shall call justice as fairness (Rawls 1971, 11).

One of the chief functions of this hypothetical choice situation, which Rawls calls the *original position,* is to capture a particular conception of impartiality or fairness. Thus, the parties in the original position must choose principles of justice from behind a "veil of ignorance" that deprives them of information about their own socioeconomic class, race, or gender—facts that might bias their choice by enabling them to tailor the principles to their own particular advantage. The basic idea is that fair principles of social cooperation are those that would emerge from a choice situation that is fair to all individuals as autonomous persons who have a highest-order interest in being free to choose and revise their ends and to pursue them effectively.

Rawls produces a number of arguments to show that the parties would agree on the following principles of justice:

First Principle:
Each person is to have an equal right to the most extensive total system of equal basic liberties compatible with a similar system of liberty for all.

Second Principle:
Social and economic inequalities are to be arranged so that they are both:
   a. to the greatest benefit of the least advantaged, and
   b. attached to offices and positions open to all under conditions of fair equality of opportunity.

Rawls calls the first principle *The Principle of Greatest Equal Liberty.* The second principle includes two parts. Part *a* is the *difference principle,* which states that social and economic inequalities are to be arranged so that they are to the greatest benefit of those who are least advantaged. Part *b* is the *principle of fair equality of opportunity*, which states that social and economic inequalities are to be attached to offices and positions that are open to all under conditions of fair equality of opportunity.

A vast literature on Rawls's theory and a number of serious criticisms of his view have emerged. It has often been noted, for example, that the difference principle would be chosen in the original position only if, as Rawls assumes, the choosers have such an extreme aversion to risk that all they care about is avoiding a situation in which, should they turn out to be among the worst-off, they have a lesser share of primary goods than they would have if they were the worst-off in some other arrangement. In other words, they care only about minimizing losses should they turn out to be among the worst-off; they do not care about reaping the higher gains they might make if they were among the better-off under a less egalitarian principle. Once this implausibly strong assumption about the attitude toward risk is dropped, it can be argued that a principle requiring only that everyone be guaranteed a "safety net" or decent minimum of welfare goods, rather than the difference principle, would be chosen.

Even if this and other major objections to Rawls's general theory can be met, however, it is far from clear that Rawls's theory as he himself presents it, contains the conceptual resources for justifying a right to health care that is specific enough to provide a useful goal for policy. To understand the limitation on Rawls's theory, let us suppose that health care is either itself a primary good covered by the difference principle or that health care may be purchased with income or some other form of wealth that is included under the difference principle. In the former case, depending on various empirical conditions, the best way to satisfy the difference principle might be to establish a state-enforced right to health care. But whether maximizing the prospects of the worst-off will require such a right and what the content of the right would be depends on what weight is assigned to health care relative to other primary goods included under the difference principle. Similarly, a weighting must also be assigned if we are to determine whether the share of wealth one receives under the difference principle would be sufficient for both health-care needs and for other ends. Until we have some solution to the weighting problem, Rawls's theory can shed only limited light on the question of priority relations between health care and other goods and among various forms of health care.

It is important to see that the informational constraints imposed by Rawls's veil of ignorance preclude a solution to the problem of weighting health care against other primary goods because the solution depends on facts about the particular conditions of the society in which the notions in question would be applied. At best, Rawls's hypothetical contractors would choose a kind of "placeholder" for a principle establishing a right to health care, on the assumption that the content of the right can only be filled out at later stages of agreement in the light of specific information about their particular society.

However, nothing in Rawls's concept of rational decision suggests that once relevant, concrete information is available, rational persons will agree on a single assignment of weights to the primary goods. It follows that Rawls's theory does not itself supply any content for the notion of a right to health care. Instead, at best, it lays down a very abstract structure within which the content would be worked out through the democratic political processes specified by the list of equal basic liberties. Given this, Rawls's theory advances us very little beyond the idea that there is a universal right to health care (Buchanan 1984a, 61–62).

Equality of Opportunity as the Basis for a Right to Health Care: Norman Daniels's Rawlsian Theory

In his book *Just Health Care*, Norman Daniels develops a substantive account of the right to health care by relying on Rawls's principle of fair equality of opportunity. Although Daniels offers no justification for that principle, he indicates that he believes that Rawls's contractarian derivation of it is plausible and also contends that there is a considerable consensus, at least within liberal democratic political philosophy, that equality of opportunity is a central element of justice (Daniels 1985).

According to Daniels, the right to health care is derived from the following principle of fair equality of opportunity:

> Basic institutions that affect the allocation of health care resources
> are to be arranged so that, as far as is possible, each person is to enjoy
> his or her fair share of the normal opportunity range for individuals
> in his or her society.

The normal opportunity range for a society is the full set of individual life plans that it would be reasonable for individuals in that society to pursue, assuming that they enjoy "normal species functioning." Although Daniels makes it clear that normal species functioning as he understands it is a strictly objective, biological, nonnormative concept, he does little to say just what it encompasses. However, he does state that disease and disability are to be understood as departures from normal species functioning (Daniels 1985, 28).

For Daniels, an individual's fair share of the normal opportunity range is that set of life plans that it would be reasonable for that individual to pursue, given his or her particular "talents and skills," were the development of those talents and skills not impeded by departures from normal species functioning; that is, by disease or disability (Daniels 1985, 34), or by features of the social system (such as discriminatory hiring practices and inequalities in the social class into which one is born) that are arbitrary from a moral point of view. The allocation of health-care resources, then, is one important tool for ensuring that everyone has fair equality of opportunity, because health-care resources serve to prevent, minimize, or compensate for departures from normal species functioning and because departures from normal species functioning (i.e., disease and disability) constitute one important barrier to fair equality of opportunity understood as having one's fair share of the normal opportunity range.

Daniels's account is designed to help answer two important questions central to an ethical theory of health care–resource allocations: (1) What makes health care morally special? and (2) How should various kinds of health care be ranked relative to one another in terms of priority? The answer to the first question is that health care affects the attainment of normal species functioning and that lack of the latter is one important barrier to fair equality of opportunity. The answer to the second is that those kinds of health care that have the greatest impact on preventing, minimizing, or compensating for departures from normal species functioning should have the highest priority, at least at the level of designing basic health-care institutions, including mechanisms for allocation.

There are, however, several serious problems with Daniels's approach quite apart from objections to the more general Rawlsian account of justice on which it builds. First, and perhaps most important, Daniels's fair equality of opportunity principle, especially if it is given lexical priority over all principles of distributive justice (other than a principle distributing basic liberties, like Rawls's first principle), seems to place too great a demand on overall social resources in the name of implementing a right to health care. What it requires is that we continue to pump social resources into health care as long as doing so continues to bring individuals closer to the ideal of normal species functioning—which is nothing less than a life free of disease and disability, because the latter are defined as departures from normal species functioning. The only constraint on the imperative to channel all available resources into health care is that doing so must not undermine other efforts needed to achieve fair equality of opportunity by eliminating impediments to one's fair share of the normal opportunity range other than disease and disability (and with satisfying a lexically prior principle of greatest equal liberty).

The objection is that the demand for fair equality of opportunity, understood according to Daniels's principle, makes the health-care sector a kind of "black hole" capable of sucking in almost unlimited quantities of social resources because, especially for persons with grave disabilities and diseases, there is virtually no limit to how much could be done, granted continuing technological advances, to bring such persons closer to the goal of normal species functioning. For example, being born blind, mentally retarded, and deaf is surely one of the most severe impediments to being able to pursue effectively that set of life plans that it would be reasonable for one to pursue in this society, given the talents and skills one would have, were the development of one's talents and skills not impeded by disease or disability. If this is so, efforts to remedy or compensate for these severe departures from normal species functioning should have high priority in overall efforts (inside and outside the health-care sector) to ensure that every individual enjoys equality of opportunity. The commitment to providing such resources might be so demanding that honoring it would amount to a virtually unlimited right to health care.

Second, Daniels's principle not only seems to create an excessive drain on resources, it also does not appear to provide guidance as to how we are to make priority decisions within efforts to achieve fair equality of opportunity through allocation of health-care resources. It is silent on the question of whether we should first try to improve the condition of the worst-off—persons whose disease or disability is so severe that they are the furthest from the ideal of normal species functioning—even if doing this means that the better-off will get access to virtually no health-care resources, or whether everyone is to receive at least some of the basic health-care resources.

It is important to understand that Daniels's view that the normal opportunity range is society-relative does little to blunt the force of the black-holes objection. The normal opportunity range is society-relative, for Daniels, in the sense that whatever life plans are reasonable for various people in a society to pursue will be influenced by the resources, cultural attitudes, and so forth, of the society in question. But in response to a critic who pointed out that the distribution of health-care resources that exists in a particular society will also determine which life plans it is reasonable to pursue (Buchanan 1984a, 64), Daniels explicitly states that the normal opportunity range is that array of life plans it would be reasonable for people to pursue in the society if they enjoyed normal species functioning, that is, if they were free of disease and disability. And normal species functioning, Daniels emphasizes, is not society-relative (Daniels 1985, 28–29). Thus, even if everyone in a particular society suffered from a certain disease, say a kind of anemia, having that disease would still be a departure from normal species functioning and would be an impediment to everyone's attaining his or her fair share of the normal opportunity range because the normal opportunity range is that set of life plans that would be reasonable to pursue in that society in the absence of departures from normal species functioning. As Daniels puts it:

> The anemia in this case is a disease which keeps each individual from adequately carrying out *any* life plan that otherwise would be reasonable in his society. Remember, our reference point is normal species-functioning functional organization, not functioning in a certain society (Daniels 1985, 55).

A third problem with Daniels's fair equality of opportunity principle is that it, like Rawls's narrower principle concerning access to offices and positions, is based on the fundamental belief that opportunity should not be limited by "morally arbitrary" factors. Yet again, like Rawls's principle, it arbitrarily takes an individual's talents and skills as a fixed baseline. In Daniels's case, the baseline is hypothetical—the talents and skills one would have were their development not impeded by disease or disability. The problem is that, as Rawls and Daniels both admit, there are factors other than disease and social position that influence the development of talents and skills, but that are equally arbitrary from a moral point of view. The most obvious of these is one's normal genetic endowment. Neither Rawls nor Daniels gives any reason why efforts to achieve fair equality of opportunity should not deal directly with this important, "morally arbitrary" determinant of opportunity. Moreover, new advances in genetic engineering may soon make such an extension of their notions of fair equality of opportunity technically feasible. Daniels believes it to be an advantage of his theory that it takes skills and talents (as they would be, absent the effects of disease and disability) as the baseline for determining fair share of the normal opportunity range and ". . . does not require us to 'level' all differences among persons" (Daniels 1985, 52). However, the same fundamental concern to eliminate the influences of morally arbitrary factors on opportunity that leads Daniels to require that resources be used to minimize departures from normal species functioning and the effects of socioeconomic class position also seems to require the use of resources for increasing the opportunity of those who are not genetically disabled or diseased but who are, nonetheless, at a genetic disadvantage relative to the more fortunate.

Less Systematic Accounts of the Right to Health Care

Some ethicists have attempted to approach the right to health-care issue in a somewhat less systematic fashion. Instead of undertaking the ambitious task of first developing a comprehensive theory of justice and then drawing its implications for the right to health care, they have operated mainly at the middle level of ethical theorizing and have offered one or more general principles concerning the distribution of health care and provided less formal arguments for them, arguments that do not rely on complex theoretical backdrops.

An Egalitarian Right to Health Care

Writers who advocate an egalitarian right to health care have generally taken the less formal approach (Gutman 1983). They contend that the right to health care is not to be understood simply as a guarantee of a certain safety net, decent minimum, or core set of basic health-care services. Instead, they advance a much stronger claim of rights—everyone having equal need for a health-care service or resource is to have equal access to it. In some cases, this alleged egalitarian right to health care is advanced as a corollary of a more general egalitarian welfare right—all resources are to be distributed so as to approximate, as nearly as possible, a condition in which everyone's net welfare over a lifetime is equal (Menzel 1983, 21; Veatch 1981, 264–268).

Such a view can be criticized in two ways. On the one hand, those who provide a more systematic account of a less egalitarian right to health care can appeal to the strengths of the background theory from which that is derived and point to the lack of a well-articulated supporting theory for the egalitarian right. On the other hand, the egalitarian position on the right to health care can be criticized using two less formal sorts of arguments. The first attacks the more general egalitarian welfare rights principle by noting that it would be irrational for anyone—including the worst-off—to insist on equality if allowing certain inequalities would improve everyone's situation. Suppose, for example, that it is true that a system that gave higher salaries to physicians than to most other workers would stimulate more intelligent and able people to become physicians, with the result that a higher quality of medical care would be available to all. Without a convincing systematic theory to support egalitarianism, it is difficult to see why anyone would find such an arrangement objectionable, as long as the greater income of physicians did not have negative effects that outweighed the gain in quality of care to persons who have lesser salaries.

Of course, the egalitarian might object by saying that there will be a preponderance of negative effects in most real-world cases in which income differentials (or other inequalities) are allowed for the sake of increasing benefits for the worst-off—those with higher incomes will wield undue political influence, the self-esteem of the lower-paid will suffer, and so forth. This defense of the general egalitarian principle is in a sense, however, a retreat from it. What it amounts to is the claim that, even though inequality is acceptable and perhaps even preferable to equality in principle, striving for the goal of equality is a more appropriate practical goal in an imperfect world.

The second objection is directed against those who do not hold that there is an egalitarian right to welfare goods in general but only an egalitarian right to health care. The egalitarian right to health care requires that no one is to have access to any health care that is not also available to everyone else in similar need. The objection takes the form of a dilemma (President's Commission 1983, 18–19). Either the level of health care to which everyone is entitled—and more than which no one is allowed to have—is set as high as is technically possible or it is set lower. If the former, then the commitment to providing everyone with the very best care technically possible for every condition will place an unacceptable strain on overall social resources and the loss of opportunities to secure important non-health-care needs would be too great.

If, on the other hand, the equal level of health care is set sufficiently below the technically possible optimum to avoid irrational allocation of overall resources, so long as there are inequalities in income and differences in preferences for health care, some people will be prohibited from purchasing higher levels of or better quality health care, even though they wish to do so with their own resources. Such a situation would be inefficient because lifting the stricture that levels of health care must be equal would allow a pareto improvement—those who are better-off and have a preference for more or better care would gain by being allowed to satisfy it, and the worse-off would not lose so long as they received an adequate share of the non-health-care benefits that could be reaped by keeping the level of health care guaranteed to all lower than the technically possible optimum. Quite apart from the objection on grounds of inefficiency, an egalitarian right to health care that sets the level lower than the technically possible optimum would require unacceptable interferences with individuals' liberty to use their after-taxes income to purchase the health care they desire, but would permit them to use their money for luxury goods such as fine wines or antique cars, perhaps much more questionable choices.

The Right to a Decent Minimum or Adequate Level of Health Care

The force of the objections to the claim that there is an egalitarian right to health care helps to explain the popularity of the view that, although there is a right to health care, it is a limited right, a right to a decent minimum or adequate level of care. Such a position has several attractions (President's Commission 1983, 20). First, the notion that people have a right to a decent minimum or adequate level, rather than to *all* health care that produces any net benefit, clearly acknowledges that, because not all health care is of equal importance, allocational priorities must be set within health care and that resources must also be allocated to goods other than health care. Second, this position is also consonant with the intuitively plausible conviction that our obligations to the less fortunate, although fundamental enough to be expressed in the language of rights, are nonetheless *not unlimited*. Third, the decent minimum is a floor beneath which no one should be allowed to fall, not a ceiling above which the better-off are prohibited from purchasing services if they wish. Thus, this position avoids the troublesome interferences with individual liberty, which an egalitarian right requires (President's Commission 1983, 20).

The chief objection to this way of understanding the right to health care is that it is virtually devoid of content. The chief import of the claim—that the right to health care is the right to a decent minimum or adequate level of care—is negative. It indicates only that neither a right to all care that is of any net benefit nor to only all technically possible care is appropriate. Beyond this cautionary function, little is conveyed, unless a reasonable way of filling out the content is supplied.

Although it acknowledges the inadequacies of various ad hoc proposals for specifying the adequate level of care, the President's Commission offers little by way of a concrete alternative. At one point, the report offers the apparently plausible suggestion that the fundamental idea behind the notion of an adequate level is the belief that everyone is to have access to

". . . enough care to achieve sufficient welfare, opportunity, information, and evidence of interpersonal concern to facilitate a reasonably full and satisfying life" (President's Commission 1983, 20). Unfortunately, this statement, in effect, takes back much of what was said about the obligation being a limited one because some individuals are so badly off that enormous amounts of resources could be spent in attempting to ensure them of ". . . a reasonably full and satisfying life." Further, there may be considerable disagreement over what counts as a "reasonably full and satisfying life." This is simply the notion of quality of life that crops up elsewhere in medical ethics—a mask for sharply conflicting values.

In an attempt to provide practical content to the notion of a decent minimum of care while avoiding an unlimited obligation that would raise the specter of the black holes problem, Alan Gibbard has proposed a seemingly simple but ingenious hypothetical choice procedure or thought experiment (Gibbard 1983, 153–178). To determine which health-care services should be included in the decent minimum, Gibbard asks us to think of a person as choosing among different lifetime health-care insurance policies, each of which represents a different mix of preventive and curative services, medical and nonmedical services, and so forth. Because different persons would choose different policies tailored to their own particular health-care needs if they could predict them, it is necessary to impose a veil of ignorance— a set of informational constraints—upon the choosers. Gibbard suggests that it would be necessary to think of a person as choosing among policies before his or her own conception because, from conception on, our health-care prospects diverge. Granted this restriction, the rational choice of an insurance policy would be based on general statistical information about overall morbidity and mortality rates for one's society.

Before a determinate choice could be made, however, another parameter of the choice situation must be specified—the chooser must know his or her budget, what his or her total disposable wealth is. The choice of a particular health-care insurance policy will then depend not only on one's estimate of the comparative health-care benefits of the different policies, but also on how much one values the health-care benefits in question relative to benefits that could be obtained by using one's resources on goods and services other than health care.

The fundamental limitation on this strategy for specifying the ethically required decent minimum, of course, is not simply that it yields a determinate outcome if a fixed budget for the individual is assumed, but what that budget should be is itself an ethical question. Gibbard frankly acknowledges this when he describes his thought experiment as a way of giving content to the guaranteed decent minimum of health care once we know what the appropriate guaranteed income share is. In other words, until we know what individuals have a right to, by way of the allocation of income, we cannot determine how health-care resources ought to be allocated. So it seems that we have merely substituted the problem of specifying one kind of decent minimum for another. Further, there is also a problem of circularity—whether something is a fair income share (or an adequate level of income) depends on whether it would be sufficient for providing adequate levels of various important goods, including health care. Both these objections point to the conclusion that the rational health-care insurance chooser approach cannot settle the most fundamental ethical issues concerning the allocation of health-care resources and fails to provide a fully satisfying response to the objection that the notion of a right to a decent minimum or adequate level of care is too vague to be of much practical value (Baily 1986).[4]

Indeed, once the problem of vagueness is appreciated, it may even become difficult to distinguish between the decent minimum view and the egalitarian view that its proponents reject. Those who believe that there is an egalitarian right to health care but who are not committed to across-the-board egalitarianism presumably hold that there is something special about health care that requires it to be distributed equally even if (some) other goods need not be. But if health care means all forms of health care, then this is a most implausible position, because, at best, only some of the most important forms of health care could have this special status. Consequently, the claim that there is an egalitarian right to health care should be understood as meaning that everyone is to have equal access to some especially important subset of health-care services and resources. Until these are specified, and until it is determined whether they exceed those included in a decent minimum, it will not be possible to distinguish between the egalitarian view and the decent minimum view. After all, the right to a decent minimum is an egalitarian right—everyone is to have equal access to whatever it is that constitutes the decent minimum. Without a clearer specification of what the decent minimum includes, it is possible to distinguish between it and the claim that there is an egalitarian right to health care only if the latter is taken in an unrestricted sense, as meaning that everyone is to have equal access to all beneficial forms of health care that anyone else is getting (assuming equal need).

Fair Financing as an Element of Distributive Justice in Health Care

Remarkably enough, theorists of the right to health care have usually proceeded as if distributive justice concerned only the question Who is to get what? and have neglected the question Who is to pay how much, for whom? In other words, discussions have focused on only one aspect of distributive justice, the nature and justification of the right to health care, and

---

[4]It would be a mistake, however, to conclude that the idea of an adequate level has no useful policy implications. See M. A. Baily. "Rationing Health Care: Defining the Adequate Level."

they have neglected the issue of fair financing, the just distribution of the costs of providing that health care to which individuals are supposed to have a right.

Different systems for ensuring a right to health care for all distribute costs differently. For example, a single-payer system, such as the Canadian national health insurance system, finances the right to health care from taxes. If the taxation arrangements are progressive, the financing of the right to health care is just, at least if it is assumed that a just distribution of costs requires those with greater resources to bear a larger portion of the costs. On the other hand, if, as in some health-care reform plans now under consideration in the United States (including President Clinton's plan), everyone is required to pay the same dollar amount in premiums for the standard benefit package to which all are supposed to be entitled, the distribution of costs is regressive. (A janitor making $15,000 a year will pay the same premium as the chief officer of a major corporation, even though the latter earns 20 times as much money). Similarly, a system that has uniform rates for deductibles or co-payments (regardless of ability to pay) will be to that extent regressive in its distribution of costs. A co-payment of $20 will have a much greater impact on a poor person than it will have on a rich person. Clearly, the comprehensive ethical evaluation of a health-care delivery system must consider the distribution of costs as well as the distribution of benefits.

When theorists of the right to health care have mentioned the distribution of costs, they have tended to assume that the question of the content of the right to health care can be answered independently of and before the question of who pays how much for whom. Yet if, for reasons noted above, the right to health care should not be understood as an unlimited right to *all* care that is expected to be of any net benefit, but rather a right to an adequate level or decent minimum of care, the assumption proves false. Part of what should go into determining how generous the adequate level or decent minimum of care should be is how burdensome ensuring the amount of care will be on those who must pay for it. An extremely generous package of benefits to be ensured for all might impose excessive burdens on the better-off, even if the financing arrangements were strictly progressive. Thus, the question of what the right to health care includes cannot be answered without considering how the cost of providing care is to be distributed.

It is worth noting that, even if a systematic discussion of just cost distribution has been lacking in theories about distributive justice in health care, the topic has not been ignored in the area of health-care policy, albeit it has not been dealt with systematically in that area. For example, the primary justification given for instituting the Medicare program (1965) was that, without subsidized insurance, the elderly were forced to bear an excessive cost in securing health care. The argument was not that the elderly absolutely could not afford to obtain care, but that the cost they would have to bear to obtain it was unacceptable. Because it is financed from general tax revenues, the Medicare program represents a political judgment that others should pay a share of the costs of providing health care for the elderly.

BENEFICENCE RATHER THAN JUSTICE: OBLIGATIONS WITHOUT RIGHTS

Partly because of dissatisfaction with the forgoing attempts to settle major allocation questions by an appeal to principles specifying a right to health care, and partly because of a growing perception that justice is not the only ethical value bearing on allocation, some recent works have begun to focus instead on principles of beneficence or charity. The President's Commission argues for a societal obligation to provide an adequate level (or decent minimum) of care for all and that the ultimate responsibility and authority for seeing that this is achieved lies with the federal government (President's Commission 1983, 3–6). The Commission approach, like that advocated in an earlier article by Buchanan, rejects a premise that has guided much of the ethical literature on allocation—the assumption that any policy for allocating health-care resources that involves nonvoluntary transfers of wealth from the better-off to the worse-off is justifiable only if it can be shown to be based on a moral right to health care. Uncritical subscription to this assumption has led, quite naturally, to the belief that very little can be said about the ethical evaluation of the current pattern of health-care resource allocation in the absence of a convincing defense of the claim that there is such a moral right. This in turn would require clear adjudication between rival theories of justice.

There may be an even more fundamental—and even less thoroughly examined—assumption that underlies the exclusively rights-based approach to allocation issues. This is the view that the government is morally justified in using coercion (in this case to enforce transfers of wealth) only for purposes of guaranteeing moral rights. The latter view is a very strong and usually inadequately defended assumption about the sole condition under which the use of state power is morally legitimate.

Implicit in the Commission's approach is the thesis that, even if it is true that the need to guarantee rights is the strongest and most obvious moral justification for enforcing allocation policies, it is not the only justification. The Commission argues that, because of the special moral significance of health care (or, rather, of some forms of it), because health-care needs are often to a significant extent underserved, and because health-care needs are typically so unpredictable, costly, and unevenly distributed among people that it is implausible to expect everyone to be able to meet them using only their own resources, society has a moral obligation to provide an adequate level of care or set of health-care services to those who cannot provide them for themselves. In effect, the Commission contends that this obligation is of such fundamental moral importance that it may be enforced, if necessary, regardless of whether there is a corresponding individual right to an adequate level of care.

The general line of argument can be fleshed out in a more systematic and convincing way (Buchanan 1984a, 1985, 1987).[5] The basic premises employed are the following:

1. The provision of at least some of the more important forms of health care to the needy can be viewed as a collective good, and strictly voluntary schemes for securing them may succumb to familiar obstacles to successful collective action—in particular, the freerider problem and the assurance problem.
2. In some cases, enforcement of obligations to contribute is both necessary and sufficient for the successful provisions of collective goods, including important forms of health care for the needy.
3. The fact that enforcement is necessary and sufficient for achieving such a morally fundamental collective good as the provision of the most important forms of health care to the needy is a strong prima facie justification for enforcement, independently of whether the individuals who will receive the good have an antecedent moral right to it.

Whether this strong prima facie justification is a decisive justification all things considered depends on a number of factors. Is use of enforcement compatible with avoiding unacceptably dangerous concentrations of power in the government? Can a system of enforced contributions be achieved— one that fairly distributes the burden of providing for the needy among the better-off and that avoids unpredictable, arbitrary, and excessively burdensome appropriations of individuals' wealth? Only if these questions can be answered affirmatively can the prima facie justification become a decisive justification.

The attractiveness of this line of argument becomes clearer once premises 1 and 2 are explicated. Without an effective enforcement mechanism, strictly voluntary compliance with duties to aid the needy may founder due to the fact that a system of aid is a collective good. Even if rational individuals agree to a system of duties to contribute to the good, they may find it rational to defect from it, to be freeriders, as long as compliance is voluntary. The situation has an incentive structure similar to that of a many-person prisoners' dilemma. Each individual may reason as follows: Either enough others will contribute to the good in question, regardless of whether I contribute, or they will not. Because my contribution is a cost to me, the rational thing for me to do is not to contribute, so long as I will be able to partake of the good regardless of whether I contributed.

---

[5]The argument is drawn from Buchanan (1987), with permission of the journal *Ethics*.

It might be replied that, in fact, individuals will not behave thusly because their desire to maximize their own utility will be constrained by altruism. The extent to which individuals observe moral constraints on their individual utility-maximizing behavior is an empirical issue. But this much seems clear: Because altruism is generally limited, the scope of duties to aid that we can expect people to fulfill voluntarily is probably considerably narrower than that of duties they would discharge if those duties were enforced.

The freerider problem arises on the assumption that the good at which each individual aims is accurately described as the provision of aid to the needy. If this is the goal, the individual may withhold his contribution if he believes that the needy will be provided for by others or that they will not, regardless of whether he contributes. And there are several different ways in which one may benefit from the attainment of this good without having contributed to it. Some may derive satisfaction or avoid discomfort simply by knowing that the needy are provided for. Others may view the provision of aid to the needy as instrumentally good—it makes for a more stable social structure, in which those who have wealth and power may enjoy them in greater security, and it increases overall productivity by enabling more people to work. Indeed, it is often said that the major social welfare programs initiated in western Europe in the late nineteenth century were motivated chiefly by the latter sorts of considerations rather than by a sense of justice or a direct concern for the well-being of the needy.

On the other hand, the freerider problem will not block successful collective action if a sufficient number of people desire to provide for the needy, rather than simply desiring that the needy be provided for. If I regard the good to be attained as "a system of aid to the needy to which I contribute," then, of course, I cannot partake of that good without contributing to it.

Whether a sufficient number of people will be effectively motivated by the desire to be charitable to achieve a particular goal of collective charity (rather than simply by the desire that charity be done) is an empirical question whose answer will vary from case to case, depending on the psychology of the individual involved. But even if an individual does not himself wish to take a free ride on the contributions of others to a system of aid to the needy, he still may be unwilling to render aid to the needy unless he has assurance that others (with resources as great as or greater than his) will also render aid to those in need. He may be unwilling to contribute without assurance that others will do so for either or both of two distinct reasons: (1) He may conclude that it is better to expend his "beneficence budget" on an act of independent charity toward some particular person in need, rather than risk contributing to a collective charity in which the threshold of contributions needed for success is not reached; (2) his commitment to being charitable may be limited by a requirement of fairness or reciprocity. That persons who are strict individual utility maximizers may fail to achieve systems of aid that are public goods is hardly surprising. What is striking is the more general conclusion that collective action to create and maintain systems of aid may falter even if some individuals are significantly altruistic.

Whether enforcement will be necessary to achieve goals of collective charity does not appear to admit of a general answer. Under certain rather strong conditions, strictly voluntary contributions may suffice. However, in the case of systems of aid that are collective goods, as with collective goods generally, there seem to be no strictly voluntary strategies that will work in all circumstances. If this is so, and if enforcement is justified in any such cases, it is not the case that enforcement of a duty to contribute is justified only where there is an antecedent moral right to a share of the good in question, whether it be national defense or a system of health care for the needy.

The non-rights-based or enforced beneficence approach has four important advantages. First, it represents, in effect, a kind of end run around the conceptual impasse created by the deadlock of rival theories of distributive justice in health care because it provides an ethical basis for evaluating current allocations and for designing new allocation policies without having to adjudicate decisively among such theories. Indeed, the enforced beneficence arguments can be seen as providing moral support for establishing a legal right to health care in the absence of a clear justification for a moral right on which to found the legal right.

Second, obligations of beneficence are traditionally understood to be limited by the proviso that rendering aid to the needy is not to be unduly burdensome to the benefactor. Consequently, the enforced beneficence approach avoids objections to which more demanding egalitarian concepts of the right to health care are vulnerable.

Third, the notion of enforced beneficence gains some plausibility from the widespread acceptance of the legitimacy of arguments for enforcement to secure more familiar collective goods, such as national defense. It is well known that freerider problems, assurance problems, or both can block voluntary contribution to such goods and there is a rather broad agreement that enforced contribution is at least sometimes justifiable.

Fourth, the enforced beneficence approach can be seen as a step toward rectifying two unfortunate biases of much of contemporary ethical thinking, both within and outside medical ethics—a tendency to proceed as if morality were limited to justice and a propensity to concentrate exclusively on matters of individual, rather than collective, responsibility and action, which thereby glosses over problems of social coordination.

On the other side of the ledger, there are two main difficulties with the enforced beneficence view. Perhaps the most important is that the obligation of beneficence in health care may be so vague that it, like the alleged right to a decent minimum, may not provide sufficient guidance for substantive policy decisions. In addition, a systematic, societywide effort to specify and coordinate obligations to contribute may seem to run contrary to what many take to be a distinctive feature of those obligations of beneficence that do not have correlative rights. Such obligations, often called *duties of charity*, are traditionally thought to allow a broad sphere of discretion for the bene-factor, who may choose either the form his aid will take or to whom it will be given, or both. If a coordinated, enforced system of contributions to the needy is to avoid this objection, the system must be designed in such a way as to allow a significant exercise of autonomy for benefactors, either within the system or outside it.

CONCLUSION

The foregoing critical survey has exposed a number of serious difficulties with each of the main strategies for making ethical evaluations of health-care re-source allocation. None of the strategies has emerged as fully adequate or uniquely attractive. Such a result should prompt neither surprise nor pessi-mism. Systemic thinking about these difficult issues has barely begun. Only in the past few years have economists, other policy analysts, and those who actually make policy begun to recognize that ethical issues are unavoidable and that they are not merely matters of taste, but that they can be reasoned about. Similarly, systematic ethical theorizing about matters of distributive justice is also a relatively recent phenomenon, and the hard work of teasing out the concrete implications of such general theories for real-world alloca-tion problems is in its infancy.

DISCUSSION QUESTIONS

1. What resources (time, energy, money, etc.) should be put into health care and into other social goods such as education, defense, eliminating pov-erty and homelessness, and improving the environment? Are health-care professionals appropriate persons for making these allocational decisions?

2. Within the area of health care (once we have determined its bud-get), how much time, energy, money, etc., should we allocate for preven-tion and how much for rescue and crisis medicine? Are health-care profes-sionals appropriate persons for making these decisions?

3. Within either preventive care or rescue medicine, who (if anyone) should receive resources such as vaccines or artificial hearts when we can-not meet everyone's needs?

4. Often, because of their conditions, the sickest and most needy pa-tients are not the ones who would benefit the most from health-care inter-ventions. For example, the worst-off heart patients may not benefit from a heart transplant as much as patients who are in somewhat better physical condition. Under ethical principles of utility and justice, who should receive the scarce resource?

5. If health care is to be allocated at least in part on the basis of need, do people who have great need because of voluntary lifestyle choices have high-priority claims on scarce resources or, because of their lifestyle choices, have they waived their claim on these resources?

REFERENCES

Aaron, H., Schwarz, R. *The Painful Prescription: Rationing Hospital Care.* Washington, DC: The Brookings Institution, 1984.

Baily, M. A. "Rationing Health: Defining the Adequate Level." In George Agich and Charles Begeley, Eds., *What Price Health?* Dordrecht, Holland: D. Reidel, 1986.

Brock, D. W. "Recent Work in Utilitarianism." *Am Philos Q* 10(1973): 8, 15.

———. "Ethical Issues in Recipient Selection for Organ Transplantation." In D. R. Mathieu, Ed., *Organ Substitution Technology: Ethical, Legal, and Public Policy Issues.* Boulder, CO: Westview Press, 1988: 86–99.

Buchanan, A. E. "Justice: A Philosophical Review." In E. E. Shelp, Ed., *Justice and Health Care.* Dordrecht, Holland: D. Reidel, 1981: 3–21.

———. "The Right to a 'Decent Minimum' of Health Care." *Philos Pub Aff* 13 (1984a): 55–78.

———. "What's So Special About Rights?" *Soc Philos Policy* 2 (1984b): 63.

———. *Ethics, Efficiency, and the Market.* Totowa, NJ: Rowman & Allanheld, 1985.

———. "Justice and Charity." *Ethics* 97 (1987): 558–575.

Childress, J. F. "Priorities in the Allocation of Health Care Resources." In T. L. Beauchamp and L. Walter, Eds., *Contemporary Issues in Bioethics,* 2nd ed. Belmont, CA: Wadsworth, 1982: 417–423.

Cohen, G. A. "Robert Nozick and Wilt Chamberlain: How Patterns Preserve Liberty." In J. Arthur and W. H. Shaw, Eds., *Justice and Economic Distribution.* Englewood Cliffs, NJ: Prentice Hall, 1978: 246–262.

Daniels, N. *Just Health Care.* Cambridge: Cambridge University Press, 1985.

Department of Health, Education and Welfare. *Report of the Task Force on Organ Transplantation.* Washington, DC: U.S. Department of Health and Human Services, 1986.

Dworkin, R. *Taking Rights Seriously.* Cambridge: Harvard University Press, 1977.

Feinberg, J. "The Nature and Value of Rights." In D. Lyons, Ed., *Rights.* Belmont, CA: Wadsworth, 1979: 143–158.

———. "The Nature and Value of Rights." In *Rights, Justice, and the Bounds of Liberty.* Princeton, NJ: Princeton University Press, 1980: 143–158.

Gibbard, A. "The Prospective Pareto Principle and Equity of Access to Health Care." President's Commission, *Securing Access to Health Care, Vol. 2: Appendices: Sociocultural and Philosophical Studies.* Washington, DC: U.S. Government Printing Office, 1983: 153–178.

Gutman, A. "A Principle of Equal Access." President's Commission, *Securing Access to Health Care, Vol. 2: Appendices: Sociocultural and Philosophical Studies.* Washington, DC: U.S. Government Printing Office, 1983: 51–66.

Mathieu, D. R., Ed. *Organ Substitution Technology: Ethical, Legal, and Public Policy Issues.* Boulder, CO: Westview Press, 1988.

Menzel, P. T. *Medical Costs, Moral Choices.* New Haven: Yale University Press, 1983.

Nozick, R. *Anarchy, State, and Utopia.* New York: Basic Books, 1974.

President's Commission. *Securing Access to Health Care, Vol. 2: Appendices: Sociocultural and Philosophical Studies.* Washington, DC: U.S. Government Printing Office, 1983.

President's Commission for the Study of Ethical Problems in Medicine and Biomedical and Behavioral Research. *Securing Access to Health Care, Vol. 1: Report,* 1983.

Rawls, J. A. *Theory of Justice.* Cambridge: Harvard University Press, 1971.

Rescher, N. "The Allocation of Scarce Exotic Livesaving Therapy." In S. Gorovitz et al., Eds., *Moral Problems in Medicine.* Englewood Cliffs, NJ: Prentice Hall, 1976: 522–535.

Sartorius, R. E. *Individual Conduct and Social Norms.* Belmont, CA: Dickenson, 1975.

Veatch, R. M. *A Theory of Medical Ethics.* New York: Basic Books, 1981.

Weinstein, M., Stason, W. "Foundations of Cost-Effectiveness Analysis for Health and Medical Practices." *N Engl J Med* 296 (1977): 716–721.

12

Death and Dying

DAN W. BROCK

SUMMARY

Some of the most controversial moral issues and arguments in current medical ethics involve decisions about terminally ill patients and about what it means to be dead. The traditional criterion for determining death, that is, the permanent cessation of heart and lung functions, has been supplemented by the contemporary criterion of cessation of brain function. Now some are maintaining that only the higher brain must be destroyed for a person to be dead. The medical as well as judicial and conceptual changes that have occurred must be understood before we can know what it means for a person to be dead.

For those persons who are still alive we need an ethical framework for life-support decisions. The authoritarian (paternalistic) model of the physician–patient relationship is contrasted in this chapter with the more patient-centered model aimed at promoting patients' well-being while respecting their self-determination. The role that quality-of-life considerations should play in life-sustaining treatment decisions is explored. Decision-making procedures for the incompetent patient are developed together with the moral principles that should guide these decisions so as to respect patients' wishes, or if they are not known, serve their best interests. Advance directives that can be used to state one's wishes about treatment and select a surrogate decision maker are explained.

The ethical framework presented for life-support decisions allows patients or their surrogates to weigh the benefits and burdens of treatment from the patient's perspective and to refuse any treatment. However, just because life itself is at stake some employ additional distinctions for these decisions. The chapter explores in some detail differences between withholding and withdrawing life support; killing and allowing to die; ordinary versus extraordinary treatment; whether forgoing life support constitutes suicide, physician-assisted suicide and voluntary active euthanasia, and pain relief that hastens death.

Finally, three issues are discussed that raise special policy concerns—decisions about critically ill newborns, forgoing life-sustaining nutrition and hydration, and limits on physicians' responsibilities to provide futile treatment.

In recent decades medicine has gained dramatic new abilities to prolong life. Patients with kidney failure can be placed on renal dialysis; patients who have suffered cardiac arrest can sometimes be revived with advanced life-support measures including drugs, electric shock, airway intubation, and closed or open heart massage; patients with pulmonary disease can be assisted by mechanical ventilation on respirators; patients unable to eat or drink can receive nourishment and fluids intravenously or with tube feedings; and patients with failure of a vital organ can obtain an organ transplant. These are only some of the most dramatic and well-known additions to medicine's armamentarium for staving off death in the gravely ill. Although these and other life-sustaining treatments often provide very great benefits to individual patients by restoring or prolonging functioning lives, they also have the capacity to prolong patients' lives beyond the point at which they desire continued life-support or are reasonably thought to be benefited by it. Thus, where once nature took its course and pneumonia was the "old man's friend," now increasingly someone must decide how long and by what means a life will be prolonged, and when death will come. This chapter addresses some of the principal moral issues and arguments in current debates about life support. Below, we address very briefly a related issue: the definition of death.

THE DEFINITION OF DEATH

The traditional criterion for determining death until recent years was the permanent ceasing to function of the heart and lungs. When a person stopped breathing and his or her heart stopped beating for more than a few minutes the loss of function was irreversible and the patient was declared dead. The loss of oxygen to the brain would quickly produce irreversible brain damage and loss of all cognitive function. However, the advent in recent years of new medical technology and, most important, of respirators, has enabled modern medicine to continue artificially patients' heart and lung function when they would no longer function unassisted. As already noted, this can often save lives that previously would have been lost and sometimes permit the patient to recover a normal level of functioning. In a few other cases, however, heart and lung function can be restored or continued by these artificial means after brain function has been partially or completely destroyed, for example, from prolonged loss of oxygen or severe trauma to the brain. Such cases have forced a rethinking of the criteria for the determination of death (President's Commission 1981).

The other factor that has led to a rethinking of the definition of death is the need to secure organs for transplantation. Unless an individual can survive the loss of an organ taken for transplantation, the so-called dead donor rule has precluded taking a donor's organ before the donor has died. But if the determination of death must await the ceasing of heart and lung function, the donor's organs will typically be so damaged that they are not usable for transplantation. Thus, the brain-death criterion for death is needed so that the removal of organs of an individual who has died is possible while the person's heart and lung function are maintained.

This rethinking has led to a widely acknowledged additional criterion for death, the complete and irreversible loss of all brain function, or so-called brain death. This criterion allows a patient who has suffered complete and irreversible loss of brain function to be declared dead even if the patient's respiration and circulation are being continued by artificial means. A single unitary concept of death is retained, for example, "permanent cessation of the integrated functioning of the organism as a whole," or "irreversible loss of personhood" (Capron and Kass 1972, 102–104). What has been introduced is an additional criterion, namely, the complete and irreversible loss of all brain function, for use when this concept of death applies to a particular individual. Of course, once this additional criterion has been accepted, the practical question then is precisely which medical tests and procedures establish the loss of brain function. The answer is a matter for medical determination given a particular level of medical knowledge and technology, and it will change over time (President's Commission 1981). This chapter considers the principal area of philosophical controversy between so-called whole-brain and higher-brain formulations in the new criteria for the determination of death.

The new definitions adopted by state courts and legislatures, as well as by various official bodies that have studied the matter (such as the President's Commission), have adopted the whole-brain formulation. In this formulation it is loss of functioning of the whole brain, either as the integrating mechanism of the body's major organ systems or as the hallmark of life itself of the human organism, that is required for death. To quote from the President's Commission:

> When all brain processes cease, the patient loses two important sets of functions. One set encompasses the integrating and coordinating functions, carried out principally but not exclusively by the cerebellum and brainstem. The other set includes the psychological functions which make consciousness, thought, and feeling possible. These latter functions are located primarily but not exclusively in the cerebrum, especially the neocortex (President's Commission 1981, 38).

Thus, the whole-brain formulation includes both the loss of integrating functions that make natural respiration and circulation possible as well as the functions that make consciousness, thought, and feeling possible. The higher-brain formulations focus exclusively on the latter functions. In this view, it is consciousness, thought, and feeling that is necessary to personhood, and when they have been irreversibly lost the *person* has died or permanently ceased to exist (Green and Wikler 1980; Veatch 1975). Anyone dead by the whole-brain formulation is obviously dead by the higher-brain formulation, but not vice versa. In particular, brain injury that can result from stroke or trauma may permanently destroy all capacity for consciousness, thought, and feeling, but may allow respiration and circulation to continue, either assisted or unassisted. This is essentially the condition of patients in so-called persistent vegetative states such as Karen Quinlan and Nancy Cruzan, who were able to breathe on their own for a number of years before they died.

There is not space here to explore the deep philosophical questions about the nature of personhood and personal identity that divide whole- and higher-brain formulations. Some version of the higher-brain formulation is supported by most accounts of personhood, but also at issue is whether the appropriate criterion is the death of a person, which would seem to be the issue of moral concern, or the death of a human being or organism. Because the determination of death is principally a legal determination, practical considerations of social and legal policy are also relevant. Use of the higher-brain conception requires being willing to declare as dead individuals whose body's circulatory and respiratory functions remain intact; that is, those whose bodies are still breathing on their own. It would also require practical methods of discrimination of brain function that permit determinations of the permanent loss of higher-brain function while some lower-brain or brain-stem function persists, and to do so with the very high degree of certainty reasonably required for any declaration of death.

Because public and legal policy has, for the present, mainly settled on the whole-brain concept, we shall assume that concept in the discussion that follows. It is emphasized that, according to this concept, patients such as Karen Quinlan or Nancy Cruzan who suffered a permanent loss of consciousness and of all capacity for thought and feeling have *not* died. Such patients may, however, constitute a unique class of patients for decisions about forgoing life support because the permanent loss of all consciousness may imply the lack of any possible interest in continued life.

AN ETHICAL FRAMEWORK FOR LIFE-SUPPORT DECISIONS

Any account of morally appropriate procedures and content for life-support decisions presupposes a broader account of medical treatment decision making generally and of the physician–patient relationship. These broader issues are addressed more fully in Chapter 7. Here, we set out only briefly the issues in a general account of treatment decision making and of the physician–patient relationship that could guide life-support decisions. It is too easy to exaggerate the shift in actual practice regarding medical treatment decision making that has taken place in recent decades and to reduce discussions of models of physician–patient relations to caricatures. However, it is widely agreed that it was common historically to view the physician–patient relationship as one in which the physician directed care and made decisions about treatment and the patient's role was to comply with the

"Doctor's orders." Patients were told only as much about their condition and treatment as was necessary to comply effectively with treatment.

This is sometimes called the authoritarian or paternalist model of the physician–patient relationship. It reflects the medical training, knowledge, and experience possessed by the physician but not by the average patient, as well as the anxiety, fear, dependency, and regression experienced by some critically ill or dying patients. Moreover, if the end of medicine is seen as the preservation of the patient's health and life by the treatment of disease, it is not surprising that physicians are viewed as possessing the necessary expertise to determine which treatment best does this. With the dramatic increases in recent decades in medical knowledge and expertise, as well as the many new modes of treatment now possible from advances in medical technology, the case for the physician as primary treatment decision maker now seems stronger. Yet the weight of argument and opinion has shifted substantially toward securing an enlarged, indeed principal, role in treatment decision making for the patient (President's Commission 1982). Why has this happened? One reason is a new concept of the ends of medicine and of the proper form of the physician–patient relationship (Katz 1984; President's Commission 1982; Siegler 1981).

There are many ways of more precisely formulating the new concept. One prominent version sees the goals of health-care decision making as the promotion of patients' well-being while respecting their self-determination (President's Commission 1982). How is this different from promoting and preserving patients' health and life? What best promotes health and life is naturally thought to be an objective factual matter, an empirical question, one not dependent on a particular patient's preferences and values. So understood, what best promotes patients' health and preserves their lives is a factual matter about which the physician, not the patient, possesses expertise. Why then is a central role necessary for the patient in deciding on treatment?

To view the end point of the health-care process as the patient's well-being, instead of as health and life in general, is not to deny that physicians seek to beneficially affect patients' health and life. Rather, it is to stress that health and life extension are ultimately of value in the service of the broader, overall well-being of the patient. They are of value insofar as they facilitate the patient's pursuit of his or her overall plan of life—the aims, goals, and values important to the particular patient. In many instances the decision of which alternative treatment best promotes a patient's well-being, including the alternative of no treatment, cannot be objectively determined independent of the patient's own preferences and values.

In the case of life-support decisions, when the forgoing of life support is under serious consideration, it is usually because (1) the patient is critically or terminally ill and likely to die soon no matter what is done, and (2) because the quality of the patient's life is seriously limited by the effects of disease, disability, and sometimes the treatment itself. Whether treatment and continued life under such severely constrained conditions are better than no more life must depend in significant part on how the particular patient views his or her life under those conditions. The physician is in the best position to predict the specific outcomes of different treatment alternatives and their effects on the patient, but the patient is in the best position to evaluate what importance should be given to any particular effect, such as the discomfort and restrictions on communication caused by intubation, or the restrictions on activities caused by dialysis. It is well established that different persons evaluate the importance of such burdens significantly differently—some tolerate intubation or dialysis relatively well if it allows their lives to be prolonged; others find that the limitations make life no longer worth living.

There is no single right answer to how such conditions should be valued; there are only the actual answers that real persons give for themselves. This is why many have urged that health-care decision making should be a process of shared decision making between physician and patient (Katz 1984; President's Commission 1982; Siegler 1981). Each brings something to the decision-making process that the other lacks, and the communication is necessary to decisions that best serve the patient's well-being: The physician brings knowledge about the likely outcomes of alternative treatments; the patient brings knowledge of the personal aims, ends, and values by which to evaluate those outcomes. Thus, even if treatment decision making aims only to serve the patient's well-being, shared decision making (a process of conversation between the physician and patient) is necessary to identify the best alternative.

In this more recent view of health-care decision making, the other value that should guide the process is the patient's self-determination or autonomy. Self-determination can be understood as the interest each person has in making important decisions that shape and affect one's life for oneself and according to one's own aims and values (Dworkin 1988). Respecting people's self-determination helps give them control and responsibility for the lives they lead and the kind of persons they become. In health care, involving patients in important treatment decisions and leaving them free to refuse any proffered treatment respects their self-determination. If people's interest in self-determination is important in ordinary medical care, surely it is more important in decisions about life support that determine when and under what conditions their lives will end. Valuing self-determination requires respecting both patients' own concept of their well-being (the subjective aspect of well-being noted above) and patients' interest in participating in the decision-making process about their care.

Both values of patient well-being and self-determination support a process of shared decision making between physician and patient in which the patient retains the right to refuse any offered treatment. Shared decision making does not preclude, but instead can foster, the important trust traditionally and commonly bestowed by patients on their physicians; nor is it incompatible with patients asking their physicians to make some decisions for them. There is a crucial moral difference, however, between patients transferring their right to decide to a trusted physician or family member and patients deferring to physicians because decision making is considered physicians', not patients', business. The ultimate right to select among available treatments, and to refuse any treatment, rests with the patient because it is the patient's body, and in turn the patient's life, that bears the principal effects of any treatment instituted.

This increased role for the patient in a process of shared decision making has not, of course, gone unchallenged and unprotested (Kass 1985; Sider and Clements 1985). Some commentators have insisted that the proper goal of medicine is objective (as opposed to subjective) promotion of health; for example, health defined in terms of species function. They argue that physicians are in the best position to determine what will best serve this goal and physicians should not be guided solely by the patient's preferences. Many physicians no doubt also share this resistance to any incursion on their traditionally dominant decision-making role. Nevertheless, the debates generally have not made clear to what extent, if any, these commentators would limit a competent patient's right to refuse any life-sustaining treatment. Disagreement probably more often concerns whether a physician must accede to a request, either from a competent patient or more likely from an incompetent patient's family, for life-sustaining treatment that the physician believes is inappropriate. All generally agree that no physician should be required or forced to provide treatment that he or she believes is not within the bounds of acceptable medical practice, but a substantive difference may remain about how these boundaries should in a particular case be defined and how responsive they should be to patient or family preferences. (We pursue this issue further in the section below on futility.)

The account of decision making about life-sustaining treatment based on the values of patient self-determination and well-being empowers the competent patient, or the incompetent patient's surrogate, to weigh the benefits and burdens of alternative treatments, including the alternative of no treatment, according to the patient's perspective (President's Commission 1983a; Hastings Center 1988). If the competent patient, or the incompetent patient's surrogate, judges that the overall benefits and burdens of employing life support are worse for the patient than the alternative of forgoing treatment with its expectation of death, that choice is to be respected. It essentially involves a judgment by the patient or surrogate that the expected duration and quality of the continued life possible for the patient are so bad that on balance they are worse than no further life at all.

It should be noted that, in this view, carefully limited quality of life considerations *do* quite properly and inevitably play a role in the assessment of alternatives and of their overall benefits and burdens. For most persons, whether the continued life made possible by a particular life-sustaining treatment is, on balance, wanted and a benefit will depend at least in part on the quality of that life. What is important is that the assessment should be of the quality of life *to the patient*. This view does not sanction giving weight to how the patient's continued life may affect the quality of other's lives, for example by making the patient a burden to others. Nor does it sanction any judgments that some people's lives are not socially or economically worth sustaining because they are of low quality. The proper question is whether the patient's present and anticipated quality of life is sufficiently bad to make it, according to him or her, worse than no more life at all. This is a very narrowly constrained role for quality-of-life considerations that is fully compatible with respecting patients' self-determination and their own view of their well-being.

THE INCOMPETENT PATIENT

Our account of life-support decision making thus far largely assumes that the patient is competent to make such decisions. Of course, this is often or even usually not the case when forgoing life-sustaining treatment is seriously at issue. The effects of illness and disease, as well as of treatments themselves, commonly compromise or eliminate patients' abilities to participate in decision making. Someone else then has to decide for them. This portion of the chapter is concerned with ethical issues concerning life support and discusses the moral principles that can guide decision making for incompetent patients (Buchanan and Brock 1989).

The most direct way for incompetent patients to participate in decisions about their care in a manner serving their well-being and self-determination is through use of advance directives. There are two principal forms of advance directives: instructional directives, which state the patient's wishes about treatment; and proxy directives, which name a surrogate to decide for the patient. Living wills are the best known form of instructional directive. Durable Powers of Attorney for Health Care combine the functions of designating a surrogate and giving instructions to the surrogate about the patient's wishes concerning treatment. Nearly all states in the United States now give legal force to advance directives, and the federal Patient Self-Determination Act requires all health-care institutions to inform patients about their rights to have them. Nevertheless, advance directives are at best only a partial solution to the problem of decision making for incompetent patients for several reasons. First, and probably most important, only a small proportion of incompetent patients for whom such decisions must be made now have advance directives, and even with increased efforts to publicize advance directives and their value, most patients will probably not have them in the foreseeable future.

Second, to ensure the patient's competence when they are made, advance directives are usually made well in advance of the circumstances in which they are to be applied. Thus, they are inevitably framed in somewhat vague and general terms, and commonly make use of phrases like "if I am terminally ill and death is imminent, no further artificial or extraordinary means to prolong my life shall be employed," and so forth. Although such instructions can provide others with general guidance as to the patient's wishes regarding life support, they inevitably leave much discretion to those who must interpret them in the patient's specific circumstances. At what point is death imminent? Are antibiotics extraordinary means? Even when patients have advance directives, others must unavoidably play the important role of interpreting them. This has led many persons to conclude that Durable Powers of Attorney for Health Care are more helpful than Living Wills.

A third difficulty is that, as a way to guard against possible well-intentioned misuse or ill-intentioned abuse by others of advance directives, the conditions bringing the directives into legal effect are sometimes narrowly limited. For example, the condition that death be imminent on many natural interpretations restricts the directive so that it does not apply in many of the circumstances in which decisions about life support must be made. But this legal limitation need not restrict their use because it is rarely the case that such directives are taken to court to enforce action in accordance with them. Instead, their function has been to serve in a more informal way as evidence of what the patient would have wanted in the circumstances.

In the absence of any advance directive, others must decide for the incompetent patient. The principle guiding such decisions most in accord with promoting the patient's well-being, as he or she views it, while also respecting his or her self-determination, is the principle of substituted judgment (Buchanan and Brock 1989). This principle directs the surrogate decision maker to attempt to decide as the patient would have decided in the circumstances that now obtain if he or she were competent. This essentially directs the surrogate to use his or her knowledge of the patient's preferences and values relevant to this decision, even if these preferences and values are different from most people's or the surrogate's, in determining what the patient would have wanted.

In the absence of any information about what the particular patient would have wanted, for example, because there are no available family or friends of the patient, it is generally accepted that the principle guiding decisions should be the best interests principle. This principle directs the surrogate to decide about life support in a manner that best serves the patient's interests. Lacking any knowledge of this particular patient's wishes, such decisions inevitably involve asking what most reasonable persons would want for themselves in the circumstances.

It is widely agreed that the surrogate decision maker who is to apply these principles should usually be the patient's closest family member. The presumption for the family member as surrogate is usually based on at least three reasons. First, in most instances the family member is the person whom the patient would have wanted to make necessary decisions. Second, in most cases the family member both knows the patient best and cares most about the patient and, thus, is usually the person best able to secure what the patient would have wanted. Finally, the family in our society is commonly accorded a significant degree of authority to care for its dependent members.

It should be emphasized that these considerations only establish a presumption for the family member as surrogate. They do not imply that the family member is always the appropriate decision maker, but only that in most cases a family member is a better surrogate than anyone else who might generally be consulted. When the reasons supporting the family member as surrogate do not hold in a particular case, for example, because there is evidence the patient would have wanted a different surrogate, because there is a serious conflict of interest between the patient and the family member, or because the patient and family member have been estranged for many years, someone else should serve as surrogate. The physician may then have a positive obligation to ensure that the family member is removed as surrogate, through appeal to the courts if necessary.

There are a number of points of controversy concerning surrogate decision making that we shall merely note here. One concerns the proper procedures and standards for determining whether the patient is incompetent to decide for himself or herself. In cases of questionable competence, this is a complicated matter (see Chapter 7). Very roughly, what is needed by a patient is adequate capacity to understand relevant information about alternatives and their consequences, together with the ability to apply one's own values to those alternatives and to select one as best (Buchanan and Brock 1989). A second point of controversy is when and to what extent the interests of others such as family members or broader societal interests should be given weight in decision making for an incompetent patient. Third, in what cases and to what extent is it desirable or should it be required to involve others in the surrogate decision-making process? For example, when and how might institutional ethics committees within hospitals and other health-care delivery institutions become involved (Fost and Cranford 1985; Rosner 1985), and when is court review of decisions desirable? Despite these and other areas of controversy about surrogate decision making for incompetent patients, however, the fundamental ethical framework discussed above for the competent patient that appeals to the values of patient well-being and self-determination can also be extended to the incompetent patient.

SOME ADDITIONAL CONTROVERSIAL MORAL CONSTRAINTS ON FORGOING LIFE SUPPORT

Many of the principal moral disputes about life-sustaining treatment do not focus on the broad issues discussed above of the proper role of patients or surrogates in health-care decision making and of the proper form of the physician–patient relationship. Instead, the disputes are more specific to life-sustaining treatment and reflect the important fact that death is typically the direct and expected result of forgoing such treatment. The disputes have taken several forms. First, are there special constraints on what is morally permissible regarding life support because life and death are directly in the balance? For example, although it may be morally permissible not to start a particular life-sustaining treatment, is it also equally permissible to stop the treatment once it has begun? Would doing so be to kill the patient, not merely to allow him to die, and if so, would it therefore be wrong? If life-sustaining treatment can be withdrawn with the expectation that death will result, is physician-assisted suicide or euthanasia also permissible, for example, by giving a lethal injection to a terminally ill and suffering patient who voluntarily requests it?

These are only some of the special issues and distinctions that we shall consider below and that are important in the debates about moral limits on acceptable action concerning life-sustaining treatment because life and death are in question. Since the prohibition of the intentional killing of an innocent human being is one of our society's strongest moral and legal norms, it is hardly surprising that these issues should be difficult and controversial.

A second area of substantial recent concern is whether there are morally important differences between different kinds of treatment that would make forgoing some treatments impermissible in circumstances in which forgoing others would be permissible. For example, some persons believe food and water should never be withheld though treatments like mechanical ventilation and dialysis may be. Third, many persons find morally important differences between different kinds of patients, justifying either greater restrictions on withholding life support, or greater latitude in doing so. Examples of each sort include critically ill newborns and patients in a persistent vegetative state. Finally, we shall address the debate about whether physicians must provide futile care when patients or families demand it. In the remainder of this chapter we shall work somewhat systematically through these moral issues in the care of the dying.

One issue not addressed is the economic costs of care of the dying (Emanuel and Emanuel 1993). Whether costs are excessive (Bayer et al. 1983) and whether substantial cost savings are possible are controversial. The precise nature, basis, and scope of a general social obligation to ensure access for all to an adequate level of health care, including life-sustaining care, is also controversial and complex (President's Commission 1983b). These issues are addressed in detail in Chapter 11. However, although 40 million in the United States remain without health insurance, we assume here that ability to pay should not be a general moral criterion limiting access to life-sustaining care.

Withholding and Withdrawing Life Support

Some people believe that although patients or their surrogates may refuse to start any life-sustaining treatment they judge to be excessively burdensome or without benefit, it is not morally permissible to stop life support once it has begun. Alternatively, even if such treatments can sometimes be stopped once begun, it is often held that it is a graver matter requiring weightier reasons to stop; stopping is at least sometimes not permissible in circumstances in which it would be permissible not to start. This accurately reflects some medical practice in which, for example, physicians who are prepared to honor patients' or their families' requests for Do Not Resuscitate or Do Not Intubate orders nevertheless, in similar circumstances, are reluctant to stop respirators on which patients are dependent for life. Physicians commonly feel more responsible for a patient's death that results from stopping the patient's respirator than from not starting it. But is there good reason to treat withdrawal of life-sustaining treatment as morally different and more serious than withholding such treatment? Consider Case 12.1.

CASE 12.1

A very gravely ill patient is brought into a hospital emergency room from a nursing home and sent to the intensive care unit (ICU). The patient begins to develop respiratory failure that is likely to require intubation very soon. At that point, the patient's family members and longstanding attending physician arrive at the ICU and inform the ICU staff that there had been extensive discussion about future care with the patient when he was unquestionably competent. Given his grave and terminal illness, as well as his state of debilitation, the patient had firmly rejected being placed on a respirator under any circumstances, and the family and physician produce the patient's advance directive to show this.

Most would hold that this patient should not be intubated and placed on a respirator against his will, and most ICUs would probably not do so. Suppose now that the situation is exactly the same except that the attending physician and family are slightly delayed in traffic and arrive 15 minutes after the patient has been intubated and placed on the respirator. Can this difference be of any moral importance? Could it possibly justify ethically a refusal by the staff to remove the patient from the respirator? Do not the very same circumstances that justified not placing the patient on the respirator now justify taking him off it? Do not factors like the patient's condition, prognosis, and firmly expressed competent wishes morally determine what should be done, not whether we do not start, or fifteen minutes later stop, the respirator? Why should the stop/not start difference matter morally at all?

Cases such as this have led many to conclude that the difference between not starting and stopping, or withholding and withdrawing, life-sustaining treatment is not in itself of any moral importance (President's Commission 1983a; Rachels 1975; Steinbock 1980). Put differently, any set of circumstances that would morally justify not starting life-sustaining treatment would justify stopping it as well. If this is correct, the fact noted above, that persons feel more responsible for the patient's death when they stop life support and are as a result more reluctant to stop than not to start, suggests that many people's natural reactions lead them to act in ways that they themselves believe are not morally defensible and that conflict with their own considered moral judgments. Consequently, this may be a situation in which physicians and others should be especially reflective about their behavior because their unreflective natural reactions may lead them morally astray. In practice, one often gains a reason that one did not have earlier to stop a treatment once it has been tried. Very often there is considerable uncertainty about how well a patient will do or what progress he or she will make with a particular form of life support such as mechanical respiration. The treatment is usually worth trying to see whether it has the hoped-for positive effect. When it does not have the hoped-for positive effects, and so no longer holds out the reasonable but uncertain prospect of benefits to the patient, there is then a reason to stop the treatment, a reason that did not exist earlier not to start the treatment.

Does it matter that some physicians and families are unwilling to stop treatments such as respirator support in circumstances in which they would be willing not to initiate it, even if there is no significant moral difference between the cases? For patients, there are at least two serious bad effects of reluctance to stop life support. The first and most obvious is patient overtreatment. Life-sustaining treatment will be continued beyond the point at which it is reasonable to believe that the patient either is benefited by or still wants or would want the treatment. This is wasteful of what is commonly very costly care but, more important, it fails to respect the patient's self-determination while often inflicting unnecessary emotional distress on patients, families, and others.

The less obvious effect is at least as serious. A common fear of patients, families, and physicians is that the patient will be "stuck on machines." To avoid this outcome, parties involved in decision making may be reluctant to try life-sustaining treatment when its benefits are highly uncertain. This has the effect of denying life-sustaining treatment to some patients for whom it would have proved to be of genuine and substantial benefit, and is indeed a serious harmful consequence of the reluctance to stop life support once it is in place. Time-limited trials of therapies, such as ventilator support, should be more commonly employed. In trials it is clearly understood that the trial, if unsuccessful, can be terminated so as to allay this otherwise reasonable fear of patients and families of losing control of treatment and being stuck on machines.

If the difference between stopping and not starting a life-sustaining treatment is thought to be of moral significance, it is then important how some common cases are to be classified. For example, with any therapy that involves multiple courses of treatment over time, such as dialysis or many medications, a decision to forgo further treatment plausibly might be construed either as stopping the overall course of treatment or as not starting the next course of dialysis or dose of medication. That such cases might be plausibly interpreted either as stopping or not starting should give further pause about resting much moral importance on which is done.

Killing and Allowing to Die

The distinction between stopping and not starting a life-sustaining treatment corresponds in general to the distinction between acts and omissions leading to death. Ambiguities also abound about whether decisions to forgo a life-sustaining treatment should be classified as an act or an omission. Does the positive decision to forgo treatment make doing so an action, or does the content of the decision not to start a treatment make it an omission? However these distinctions are more precisely drawn, if there is no moral importance to whether a life-sustaining treatment is stopped or not started, it would seem to follow that it is not morally significant according to this view whether it is an act or omission of the physician that leads to death. This implication is increasingly widely accepted (*Barber and Nedjl* 1983; *Conroy* 1985; Wanzer et al. 1985; Hastings Center 1988). Yet the distinction between acts and omissions leading to death is also commonly understood to be the basis for the distinction between killing and allowing to die. Some commentators have gone on to accept, or to explicitly argue, that killing is in itself no different morally than allowing to die, although, of course, that position remains controversial (Glover 1977; Steinbock 1980; Kamm 1993). The "no difference" position is compatible with many or most actual acts of killing being morally worse, all things considered, than most cases of allowing to die.

Although this view has been accepted by many philosophers and bioethicists, many health-care personnel, patients, and their families strongly resist it. For many, the view that killing is both wrong and also worse than allowing to die is a deeply and powerfully held view. But the positive decision actively to turn off a life-sustaining treatment such as a respirator seems to be an action, not an omission, which leads to death, and so, in this view, it is considered a killing, not a case of allowing to die. This line of reasoning uncovers a more general concern about whether all stopping of life support might be killing and therefore morally wrong. In assessing this question, it is important to be clear, first, about the meaning of the claim that killing is *in itself* no different morally than allowing to die. The claim is that the mere fact that one case is an instance of killing, another of allowing to die, does not make one any worse morally than the other, or make one justified or permissible but the other not. This is not to say that any particular instance of killing may not be morally worse than some instance of allowing to die. It *is* to say that if the killing is worse, it is because of its other properties such as the motives of the killer, whether the victim consented, and so forth, that differentiate it morally from the particular instance of allowing to die.

Second, it is important to distinguish whether common instances of stopping life support should be understood as killing or as allowing to die from whether, if they are killings, they are for that reason morally wrong. Most commentators who have argued that stopping life-sustaining treatment is killing have insisted as well that it is not therefore wrong; some killing, including stopping life support, is morally permissible and justified.

Are standard cases of stopping life-sustaining treatment killing or allowing to die (Brock 1993; Rachels 1975)? A physician who stops a respirator at the voluntary request of a clearly competent patient who is terminally ill and undergoing unrelievable suffering would commonly be understood by all involved as allowing the patient to die, with the patient's underlying disease the cause of death. If done with the consent of the patient, and with the intent of respecting his self-determination while promoting his well-being as he views it, it would be held by many to be morally justified. Let us agree that it can be morally justified, but is it allowing to die? Suppose the patient has a greedy nephew who stands to inherit his money and who has become impatient for the old man to die so that he will get the money. Thinking that his uncle is prepared to continue on the respirator indefinitely, that his physicians would not be willing to stop it in any case, and that his inheritance will be exhausted by a lengthy and expensive hospitalization, he slips into the room, turns off the respirator, and his uncle dies. The nephew is found out, confronted, and replies, "I didn't kill him, I merely allowed him to die; his underlying disease caused his death." Surely this would be dismissed as specious nonsense. The nephew deliberately killed his uncle. However, it does seem that he did exactly what the physician did in the other case. Both acted in a manner that caused the patient's death, expected it to do so, and might have performed the very same bodily movements in doing so.

If the nephew killed his uncle, doesn't the physician kill his patient as well? Of course, the physician acts with a different and proper motive, with the patient's consent, and in a professional role in which he is authorized to carry out the patient's wishes concerning treatment. The differences in motive, consent, and social role make what he does, but not what the nephew does, morally justified. That is not to say, however, that what he does, and whether he kills or allows to die, is any different from the nephew—only that his killing was justified, but the nephew's was not. One can kill or allow to die with or without consent, with a good or bad motive, and in or not in a social or legal role that authorizes doing so. This general line of reasoning, then, accepts that standard cases of stopping life-sustaining treatment are sometimes correctly understood as killing, but rejects any inference that they therefore must be wrong.

One explanation of why this account is resisted is that many physicians and others use the concept of killing as a normative concept to refer to unjustified actions causing death. In this view, killing may occur in medicine accidentally or negligently, but physicians do not knowingly and deliberately

kill their patients; put flippantly, physicians do not understand killing patients to be part of their job description. Yet, of course, physicians do stop
life support in cases like the above and believe, quite rightly, that they can
be justified in doing so. Thus, there is a powerful motive to understand what
is done as allowing to die, not as killing. Common though this way of thinking may be, it is mistaken. It is a mistake to suppose that all killing must be
unjustified, either morally or in the law. Killing in self-defense is an example
of justified killing outside of medicine, and stopping life support appears to
be one within medicine.

There is another explanation of why standard cases of stopping life support are thought to be allowing to die and not killing. In the case of a terminally ill patient, a lethal disease process is already present. A life-sustaining
treatment such as use of a respirator may then be thought of as holding back
or blocking the normal progress of the patient's disease. Removing the artificial intervention is then viewed as standing aside and allowing the patient
to die by letting the disease process proceed unimpeded. This may be a plausible explanation of why stopping life-support is commonly understood to
be allowing to die, but if it is to be any more than a metaphorical account, it
must at the least explain why the nephew does not also allow to die. It is not
clear how this is to be done consistent with the way killing and allowing to
die are distinguished over a broad range of cases. Even if stopping life support is understood as allowing to die along these lines, killing may still not
be, in itself, morally different from allowing to die.

Is Forgoing Life Support Suicide?

Parallel to the concern that stopping life-support systems is killing and therefore wrong is the concern that any forgoing of life support is suicide or assisted suicide and therefore wrong. Courts in particular try to distinguish
forgoing life support from suicide, probably to insulate physicians, families
and other health care personnel from possible liability under laws prohibiting assisting in a suicide. The 1985 New Jersey Supreme Court decision in
Conroy summarizes well the reasoning of many courts and others:

> . . . declining life-sustaining medical treatment may not properly be
> viewed as an attempt to commit suicide. Refusing medical inter-
> vention merely allows the disease to take its natural course; if death
> were eventually to occur, it would be the result, primarily, of the
> underlying disease, and not the result of a self-inflicted injury. In
> addition, people who refuse life-sustaining medical treatment may
> not harbor a specific intent to die, rather, they may fervently wish
> to live, but to do so free of unwanted medical technology, surgery,
> or drugs, and without protracted suffering. . . . Recognizing the right
> of a terminally ill person to reject medical treatment respects that
> person's intent, not to die, but to suspend medical intervention at
> a point consonant with the "individual's view respecting a personally

preferred manner of concluding life." The difference is between self-infliction or self-destruction and self-determination (*Conroy* 1985).

Although this way of distinguishing forgoing life support from suicide may seem plausible, it is at least problematic in some cases. The judgment of a person who competently decides to commit suicide is essentially that "my expected future life, under the best conditions possible for me, is so bad that I judge it to be worse than no further continued life at all." This seems to be in essence exactly the same judgment that some persons who decide to forgo life-sustaining treatment make. The refusal of life-sustaining treatment is their means of ending their life; their intent is to end their life because of its unacceptable prospects. Their death now when they otherwise would not have died *is* self-inflicted, whether they take a lethal poison or disconnect a respirator. There need be, of course, no underlying lethal disease process present when a person commits suicide, whereas there must be when life-sustaining treatment is refused, but that need only mean that the person with a lethal disease thereby has an additional means of ending his or her life; there is no reason to think that a person subject to a lethal disease process therefore could not commit suicide.

The court's reasoning, at the most, distinguishes some but not all cases of forgoing life-sustaining treatment from suicide, although it should be adequate to protect all instances from falling under legal statutes concerning assisting in suicide. Even if at least some instances of forgoing life-sustaining treatment are suicide, it does not follow that they are morally wrong. The very same reasoning offered earlier in support of a competent patient's moral right to refuse any life-sustaining medical treatment applies in any cases in which doing so may be suicide. The patient's self-determination and well-being support the moral permissibility of his or her declining *any* life-sustaining treatment, including any instance that might reasonably be construed as suicide. Cases of competent decisions to decline life-sustaining treatment that constitute suicide are commonly instances of rational and morally permissible suicide. Moreover, in virtually all states, committing or attempting suicide is not legally prohibited.

Ordinary and Extraordinary Treatment

A different way of distinguishing some forgoing of life support as impermissible is with the distinction between ordinary and extraordinary treatment. This distinction has had special importance in cases of incompetent patients who are unable to decide about life support for themselves and so must have others decide for them. It is often held that the surrogate decision maker can decide to forgo only extraordinary treatment for the patient. Many court decisions have also made reference to extraordinary treatment in endorsing the legal permissibility of forgoing life support, though often in passing and without any analysis of how ordinary and extraordinary treatment are to be distinguished.

There are two important questions regarding this distinction. First, what is the difference between treatments that the distinction is thought to mark? Second, is that difference of sufficient moral importance to mark a difference between the morally permissible and impermissible? With regard to the first question, it is clear that many different meanings have been intended. Among the differences that the distinction is thought to mark are: treatment that is usual, for example for a given condition, as opposed to unusual; treatment that employs high technology, artificial means as opposed to relatively simple means; treatment that is highly invasive as opposed to relatively non-invasive; treatment that is very costly as opposed to relatively inexpensive; treatment that is heroic in the sense of a "long shot, last ditch" attempt to keep the patient alive when other more ordinary means have failed.

Because there are so many interpretations of this distinction, confusion about what a particular user intends by it is inevitable unless its meaning is made explicit, as it usually is not. However, for any possible interpretation like those just mentioned, it is important to ask our second question. Why does this difference, for example whether treatment employs high technology as opposed to relatively simple means, determine whether forgoing it is morally permissible or impermissible? High-technology respirators or dialysis treatments promise to some patients benefits that clearly outweigh their burdens; a competent patient would choose them. For other patients, the life they continue may be of such limited duration and poor quality that the patients would competently choose to forgo them. Why should it be morally important to whether the choice is justified that a treatment is common or unusual, employs high technology or is simple, is invasive or noninvasive, and so forth?

Instead, what is relevant is the overall balance of benefits and burdens of the treatment to a particular patient, according to that patient's own values. Interpretations of the difference between ordinary and extraordinary treatments such as those noted above seem to appeal to differences that are not in themselves morally important, but instead are important only insofar as they affect the benefits and burdens of treatment to the patient.

All these common and commonsense interpretations of the ordinary–extraordinary difference may misunderstand it. The distinction probably originated within Roman Catholic moral theology in which extraordinary treatment was understood, roughly, as treatment that was excessively burdensome for the patient (McCormick 1974). When treatment was judged by the patient (or by others acting as surrogates for an incompetent patient) to be excessively burdensome, it was held that neither patient nor surrogate were obliged to begin or continue it. But to determine whether a treatment is *excessively* burdensome, it is necessary to weigh its burdens against whatever benefits it promises.

This interpretation of the ordinary–extraordinary difference simply appeals to the patient's assessment of the benefits and burdens of treatment and endorses the patient's right to refuse treatment he or she judges to be excessively burdensome. It thus can constitute no further moral constraint on a patient's right to refuse such treatment that it must be extraordinary and not ordinary. *Extraordinary treatment* is here only the label placed on treatment that has already and independently been determined to be excessively burdensome. The assessment of benefits and burdens, not any independent ordinary–extraordinary difference, is the criterion of whether any treatment is justified. "Ordinary" and "extraordinary" merely label the conclusions of that determination; they play no substantive role in making it. Thus, it is misleading to suppose that a list of all treatments, some ordinary, others extraordinary, could be compiled that could help determine which should be employed with any particular patient. A treatment that is ordinary for one patient in particular circumstances can be extraordinary for another or for the same patient in different circumstances. Any kind of treatment could be beneficial to some patients but not to others. Although the ordinary–extraordinary distinction in this interpretation plays no positive or substantive role in an assessment whether to employ or to forgo a treatment, its use does have one serious bad effect. The many possible and natural understandings of the ordinary-extraordinary distinction mean its use in decision making about life support almost inevitably leads to confusion as different parties understand different things by it. Reasons of this sort have led many recent commentators to conclude that, except within particular religious traditions where its meaning is clear, the distinction is unhelpful and best avoided in decision making about life support (*Conroy* 1985; President's Commission 1983a).

Physician-Assisted Suicide and Voluntary Active Euthanasia

If competent patients are morally entitled to refuse any life-sustaining treatment, should they also be permitted in similar circumstances to have others, such as their physicians or family members, directly end their lives, or assist them in directly ending their lives, by a lethal injection or medication? We have deliberately avoided using until now the term *euthanasia* because of its strong emotionally laden connotations, but it is this sort of direct and active killing that is commonly understood as euthanasia. The very same values of patient well-being and self-determination that support a patient's right to refuse any life-sustaining treatment appear also to support physician-assisted suicide or voluntary euthanasia in some circumstances. Does this show that if one accepts that forgoing life support is morally permissible, one must accept physician-assisted suicide and voluntary euthanasia as well?

In the increasingly intense public and professional debates on the issue, many have endorsed physician-assisted suicide but not euthanasia. Are the two importantly different morally? The only difference between them need be who performs the final physical act of administering the lethal dose—the physician or the patient. In both, the choice should rest fully with the patient, who can change his or her mind until the time the process is irreversible. This small difference in the parts played by the physician and the patient seems not to support a substantial moral difference between them. At most, physician-assisted suicide might provide in some cases slightly stronger evidence of the patient's resolve. Of course, some believe there is an obvious and important moral difference—in assisted suicide, the patient kills himself or herself, whereas, in euthanasia, the physician kills the patient. But this is misleading at best. In physician-assisted suicide, the patient and physician collaborate in a joint effort to kill the patient for which both are responsible. Physician-assisted suicide and voluntary euthanasia are not substantially different morally—the arguments for and against them generally apply equally to both.

It is important to distinguish two levels at which the morality of assisted suicide and euthanasia can arise. The first is whether any specific instances of euthanasia are morally permissible. The second is whether public and legal policy should permit euthanasia. Many opponents of a public policy making euthanasia legally permissible nevertheless grant that there are particular cases in which it is morally permissible. For example, consider the case of a terminally ill and imminently dying patient with a form of cancer that causes him very great and unrelievable suffering. With his competence not in question, the patient implores his physician to end his suffering by giving him a lethal injection. It seems cruelly perverse to hold that if a life-sustaining treatment were in place we should honor the patient's request to remove it and let him die, but that otherwise we cannot intervene and must leave him to suffer in pain until nature takes its course. How could assisted suicide or voluntary euthanasia be morally wrong in a case such as this?

Some would respond that deliberate or intentional killing of innocent persons is always wrong, even if done for an otherwise good end, such as relieving suffering. If our argument above was correct, that some cases of stopping life support are both intentional killing and morally justified, then we have already established that some killing of persons is not morally wrong. But even if all forgoing of life support is allowing to die, but all euthanasia is deliberate killing, it does not follow that euthanasia must be wrong. To see this, we need to ask why killing is morally wrong in cases that are uncontroversially wrong. A plausible answer is that it deprives the victim of a very great and desired good—future life, and all that the person killed would have been able to do in that future life. But in cases of assisted suicide or voluntary euthanasia, the patient wants death, not future life, and judges the best future life possible for him or her to be a burden, not a good. The values of patient self-determination and well-being do not oppose, but support, assisted suicide and euthanasia. Thus, the reasons that make paradigm cases of wrongful killing wrongful do not apply to assisted suicide and euthanasia. Nevertheless, even if assisted suicide and euthanasia are morally justified in some cases, it could be bad public policy to permit them.

There is space here to give only examples of some of the more important good and bad consequences likely from making assisted suicide and voluntary euthanasia legally permissible. What are the more important good consequences? One has already been cited, the relief of dying patients' suffering when only death will provide that relief; James Rachels called this the argument from mercy (Rachels 1975). But there are not great numbers of patients undergoing severe suffering that can only be relieved by directly killing them. Modern methods of pain management make it possible to control the pain of nearly all such patients without the use of lethal means, though sometimes at the cost of so sedating the patient that interaction and communication with others is limited or no longer possible. Most cases in which such suffering is not in fact relieved are due to wrongful failure to employ effective methods of available pain management, not to a prohibition of assisted suicide or euthanasia. But even with adequate pain relief, some dying patients would prefer active steps to end their lives to "letting nature take its course." Moreover, public opinion polls consistently show that a majority believes assisted suicide and euthanasia should be available to patients who want it. Although few people would ever exercise the choice to use assisted suicide or euthanasia, many more would get the important reassurance that, should they want them, they would be available. Finally, some patients would have a more peaceful, humane, and dignified death. Denying this alternative to patients who want it has a cost that should not be borne lightly in a society that values self-determination highly in its moral, political, and legal traditions.

Opponents of permitting assisted suicide or euthanasia cite a number of potential bad consequences. For example, they argue that assisted suicide and euthanasia are incompatible with the fundamental moral and professional commitments of physicians as healers to care for patients and protect life (Gaylin et al. 1988). Public trust in the profession's commitment to fight with the patient against disease and death might be undermined if physicians also became "the angels of death." Physicians themselves might also find the role of administrator of euthanasia in uneasy conflict with their role as medical caregivers to the sick and dying, and their capacity to care effectively for the dying might be undermined. Moreover, opponents fear that permitting assisted suicide and euthanasia would weaken society's commitment to provide optimal care for dying patients, especially frail and vulnerable elderly patients, in an era of cost containment in health care. But perhaps the most common and influential worry of opponents is expressed in the so-called slippery slope argument (Kamisar 1958). Even if we begin by permitting assisted suicide and euthanasia in the few cases in which such direct killing might be justified, we would inevitably end up permitting it in a great many other cases in which it would be wrong. It is the first step on the path to the Nazi policy of killing the old and the weak and the socially disfavored and must be firmly resisted. Since this path is slippery and steep, we must stay off it altogether.

What is to be made of this argument? If the factual claim is true that any relaxation of the prohibition of assisted suicide or euthanasia must inevitably lead to the Nazis' final solution, then all will agree that the prohibition must be firmly maintained. What is controversial, however, is how serious and likely is the risk of abuse. There are few data regarding such risks and what data there are are controversial. For example, both proponents and opponents of assisted suicide and euthanasia cite the example of the Netherlands, the only country in which the practices are legally permitted, in support of claims that the practices can or cannot be adequately limited and controlled (Van der Maas 1991). It is uncontroversial, however, that the likelihood of abuse depends on the procedures and safeguards that are built into any policy proposal and practice. More extreme versions of the slippery slope, those that see the practice as leading to the Nazi euthanasia program, lack credibility; we can and do make very clear and firm distinctions, for example, between voluntary and involuntary euthanasia, and the values supporting the former in no way support the latter. More likely is that over time the practice might be extended from competent patients to surrogates choosing for incompetent patients, just as has happened with forgoing life support. But even if this occurred, it would not be all bad, just as extending authority to surrogates to forgo life support for incompetent patients has not been entirely, or even overall, for the worse.

Reasonable people disagree both about the likelihood of these and other good and bad effects occurring from an authorization of assisted suicide or voluntary active euthanasia, as well as about the relative moral importance of them. I believe that these and other considerations, on balance, do support a carefully controlled practice permitting physician-assisted suicide and voluntary euthanasia. Different persons, however, can reasonably reach different conclusions about whether this trade-off, on balance, argues in favor of or against permitting assisted suicide and euthanasia, but it is on the basis of such considerations that the policy question ought to be decided.

Intended versus Merely Foreseen Consequences

Some have seen a different issue at stake in assisted suicide and euthanasia. They argue that the intentional killing of innocent human beings is morally wrong, but actions from which a person's death is foreseen, though not intended, may sometimes be morally permissible (Fried 1978). This is the distinction embodied in the Roman Catholic Doctrine of Double Effect, sometimes also characterized as the difference between direct and indirect intention (Frey 1975). It is important not merely in its potential implications for active euthanasia but also for the issue of providing adequate relief of suffering to the dying. The following cases illustrate both implications. It sometimes happens that, in the final stages of some terminal cancers, levels of medication (usually morphine) necessary to control pain reach levels that seriously risk depressing the patient's respiration and hastening his or her death. In such cases physicians often administer morphine at the patient's request with the intention or goal of relieving the patient's suffering, but foresee, though not intend, the patient's likely earlier death from respiratory depression. Most physicians, on the other hand, would not give a lethal injection of potassium chloride (which causes cardiac arrest and death) at the patient's request to end the patient's suffering if morphine were unavailable or unavailing. Apart from what is legally permitted, is there an important moral difference between the two cases?

Many think that the important difference lies in the physician's intentions. No fully adequate analysis exists of the concept of intention. Nevertheless, it does seem that the patient's earlier death is intended only in the morphine, not in the potassium chloride, case. In each case, however, the physician's aim is to respond to the patient's request to end his suffering. The difference appears to be that in the potassium chloride case the means used to do so is to kill the patient; only through his death is the suffering ended. In the morphine case the administration of morphine is the means to the end of relieving the suffering and earlier death is merely a foreseen side effect. The end sought is the same in each case, and the difference is that the death is the means to the end in one case and the foreseen consequence of achieving the end in the other.

Can this difference be of sufficient moral importance to make the one morally permissible and the other prohibited? Many have argued that it cannot (Bennett 1981). In each case, the physician's end or motive of relieving suffering at the request of the patient is the same. In each case, it is causally impossible to end the patient's suffering without acting in a way that will cause his death. In each case, both the patient and physician are prepared to end the suffering even at the cost of the patient's earlier death. The relief of suffering is judged to be of sufficient importance to justify acting in a way that leads to death. These seem to be the essential value judgments involved and they do not differ in the two cases. The difference in intention seems to be one of causal and temporal structure—in one, the death precedes and brings about the end and relief of suffering; in the other, it temporally follows and is a causal consequence of achieving the end. It is hard to see why this difference in causal and temporal structure should have much, or any, moral importance. It is tempting to reply that in the morphine case one would have given the morphine even if respiratory depression and death would not have followed, but that the point of the potassium chloride was to cause death. However, if somehow potassium chloride would have relieved the suffering without causing death, one would have given it as well. In each case, in the circumstances that existed, it was necessary to act in a way that the physician knew would lead to the patient's death as a way to relieve his suffering.

There is a difference in the two cases in the certainty with which the earlier death will occur. It may never be completely certain that the dosage level of morphine is sufficient to cause death, and none would deny that this is a morally significant difference in the two cases. However, in some instances this difference in probability may be extremely small and so not support a

great moral difference between the two cases. In any event, this is a difference in the risk of a bad outcome and not of intentions. Critics of the
foreseen/intended distinction have argued that physicians are reasonably held
equally morally responsible for all the foreseen consequences of their actions,
regardless of whether intended, because all such consequences are under
their control. In this perspective, in both cases it is a matter of weighing the
relative benefits and burdens to the patient of relieving his suffering and shortening his life. If the patient judges that relief of suffering is paramount, the
physician would be morally justified in acting in either the morphine or
potassium chloride case. For the reasons of public policy discussed above it
may be wise, nevertheless, not legally to authorize the performance of direct voluntary euthanasia as in the potassium chloride case. It is important
to emphasize that this would not be because the two cases are in themselves
significantly different morally, but because of public policy concerns about
the one and not the other. It is important to emphasize also that the general
right of the patient to decide about treatment includes the right to have adequate pain medication, even if that may shorten his life. The relief of suffering is a longstanding, central, and fully legitimate aim of medicine.

SOME CASES OF SPECIAL POLICY CONCERN

Many of the issues addressed in this chapter are of very great public and
policy concern. We have sought to cover the principal questions involved
in the development of an overall ethical framework for decisions about life
support. Of course, no such framework can be applied in any mechanical
fashion to yield conclusions in particular cases. A framework is only that,
and it must be applied and interpreted with sensitivity and understanding
to the unique features and details of any actual case. Nevertheless, the ethical
framework should be applicable across the broad class of life-support cases.
There are, however, three issues of special current concern that raise some
questions not yet addressed: seriously ill newborns, life-sustaining nutrition and hydration, and futility.

Seriously Ill Newborns

Several cases of forgoing life support for seriously ill newborns have been
front-page news during the past decade. Public and government attention
was focused in this area a number of years ago in the so-called Baby Doe
case in Bloomington, Indiana, when an infant who suffered from Down syndrome was allowed to die after its parents refused to permit surgery to repair its esophagus so that it could take nourishment. The federal government
promulgated the Baby Doe Rules, which went through extended negotia-
tions and court challenges. These rules essentially require that all medically
indicated treatment be provided to an infant unless the infant is irreversibly

comatose; the treatment would merely prolong the dying of the infant and would be futile in terms of its survival; or the administration of the treatment would itself be virtually futile and inhumane. However these regulations are in fact interpreted by individual physicians and families, it is clear that their intent, both symbolic and for practice, was to exclude the use of considerations about an infant's expected quality of life from decisions about its treatment and to limit severely parents' and physicians' discretion in decisions to forgo life support for such infants.

Although the fundamental ethical framework developed above for life-support decisions generally applies to newborns, there are a few issues that are especially prominent with newborns (Singer and Kuhse 1986; Weir 1984). One is already implicitly noted in the Baby Doe regulations. What role, if any, should the infant's expected quality of life play in decisions about treatment? As discussed earlier, a narrowly constrained role for quality-of-life considerations is inevitable if competent patients, or incompetent patients' surrogates, are to be free to decide whether a life-sustaining treatment and the life that it makes possible are, on balance, a benefit or excessively burdensome for the patient. Using this standard, few infants will have prognoses so poor that continued life is reasonably deemed not in their interests. The clearest cases are probably when the infant's life will be short and filled with substantial and unrelievable suffering and when the infant has suffered such severe brain damage as to preclude any significant social or environmental interaction. Other cases of very severe disabilities are more controversial and problematic, in part because of the wide variation in the weight adult patients give to such considerations and the fact that infants do not yet have preferences or values of their own.

A second issue is the relevance, if any, of the effects on others, such as the parents, of continued life support for the newborn. As a general matter, our society rejects the involuntary sacrifice of one person's well-being or life for the benefit of others. The very high value we give to the protection of human life suggests that life-sustaining treatment for a seriously ill newborn should rarely if ever be forgone because of the burdens its continuing existence would place on others. Moral rights not to be killed are commonly understood to protect an individual from being killed, whatever the effects on others of the individual continuing to live. Nevertheless, it would be callously insensitive to deny the often overwhelming long-term burdens placed on the parents of severely impaired newborns, particularly in light of the often inadequate social and medical support services available to them. This issue reflects a fundamental difference between utilitarian moral principles, which weigh all the effects of a decision about treatment, including the effects on others besides the patient, and moral rights, which exclude, or at least largely exclude, effects on others from consideration when a person's right to life is in question. As a practical matter, in most cases in which the parents judge the infant to be an excessive burden on them, they have the alternative of giving up the child for adoption or placing it under the care of the state.

A third issue concerns the moral status of infants. Should they have the very same moral (and legal) protections as adults, particularly in light of common views on the moral permissibility of aborting fetuses? Birth seems an arbitrary point at which to draw a great difference in the moral permissibility of killing. Some commentators consider newborns closer morally to unborn fetuses than adults, or as somewhere between the two (Tooley 1983). Unborn fetuses, however, in this view are often considered replaceable and permissibly killed—for example, when found by amniocentesis to have serious disabilities or conditions—as a way to try again for a normal pregnancy. This general issue concerns whether infanticide might be morally permissible in at least some circumstances in which killing an adult person would not be.

Finally, there is the policy issue of what review mechanisms, if any, are needed for parents' and physicians' decisions to forgo a life-sustaining treatment for a newborn. There are at least two important reasons to believe that conflicts of interest between seriously ill newborns and their parents may be more common than in most other cases of surrogate decision making for incompetent patients. First, the strong bonding that exists between parent and older child or between family members has not yet occurred with newborns, which can result in a weaker commitment of the parent to the infant's well-being. Second, the often enormous burdens of caring for the infant if life-sustaining treatment is continued will fall largely on the parents. Thus, serious conflicts of interest may be sufficiently likely in decisions to forgo life-sustaining treatment of newborns to warrant some form of regular review, for example, by hospital ethics committees, so-called infant care review committees, or even the courts.

These are some of the issues of special importance in life-support decisions for newborns, but it bears emphasis that the fundamental ethical issues are not different from those with adults.

Life-Sustaining Nutrition and Hydration

The moral permissibility of a competent patient, or an incompetent patient's surrogate, deciding to forgo treatments such as respirator support or kidney dialysis has become fairly widely accepted by the public and health care professionals, as well as in recent court decisions. More recently, concern has focused on the provision of artificial nutrition and hydration through the use of nasogastric tubes, intravenous lines, surgically inserted tubes, and so forth. Must nutrition and hydration, or food and water, always be continued, or may it too permissibly be forgone (Lynn 1986)?

If nutrition and hydration are considered part of treatment, the same ethical framework discussed above for other kinds of life support can be applied. That framework calls for an assessment of the benefits and burdens to the patient of continuing nutrition and hydration as opposed to discontinuing it. For nearly all patients, that assessment will favor continuing them, but in a few cases it does not do so (Lynn and Childress 1983). The process of providing nutrition and hydration can itself involve substantial unavoidable burdens for some patients—for example, when patients' disease states make taking in nutrition the cause of significant discomfort or when patients' dementia and resultant confusion requires physically restraining them to prevent their removing feeding tubes. In a very few other cases the quality of the life continued by nutrition and hydration may be substantially and unalterably burdensome or without benefit to patients. Against possible burdens of continuing nutrition and hydration must be weighed the benefits and burdens of discontinuing it. For most patients, discontinuing nutrition and hydration would result in substantial subjective distress and is not likely to be in their interests even if death might otherwise be welcome to them. Once again, however, for a few patients in the final stages of certain terminal diseases or in a persistent vegetative state in which all conscious experience is irretrievably lost, withholding nutrition and hydration and the patient's subsequent death hastened by a weakened physical state or by dehydration does not result in additional suffering. The assessment of the benefits and burdens to a particular patient of continuing life-sustaining nutrition and hydration will, in most cases, favor doing so, but there can be no assurance that this must always be so.

This conclusion has been challenged on several grounds; for example: (1) human life is of infinite value and so deliberately shortening it can never be a benefit to the victim; (2) a patient's choice to forgo food and water is suicide, and therefore wrong; (3) life is a gift of God that we are not at liberty to destroy. The first two objections are really general challenges to forgoing any life support, not nutrition and hydration in particular. The third appeals to religious views, which could quite properly guide the choices of those individuals who share the particular religious faith, but should not form the basis for public policy in a pluralistic society.

A further concern about permitting the forgoing of nutrition and hydration centers on its symbolic meaning together with worries about abuse (Siegler and Weisbard 1985). The provision of food and water is one of the very first acts of concern, caring, and support that each person receives as he or she enters the world. Throughout life, feeding the hungry is properly invested with great moral importance and starvation is associated with suffering and strong moral repugnance. This deep concern with not permitting suffering or death from starvation in general serves us well, and, in this view, we should be extremely reluctant to do anything that might weaken it. This is especially so because many patients who might be endangered by any weakening of the requirement to provide food and water are debilitated and vulnerable, unable to protect themselves and to assert their own interests. Permitting the withholding of food and water risks the deliberate killing of the vulnerable and burdensome on morally unacceptable grounds such as the economic costs of sustaining their lives. Moreover, many see any withholding of food and water as only a very small step from active voluntary, or

even involuntary, euthanasia and oppose the former for fear that it will inevitably lead to the latter.

Like all slippery slope arguments based on a worry about potential abuse
of a specific authorization, reasonable persons may disagree on several counts.
Is it possible to discriminate clearly between cases in which withholding food
and water is morally justified from those in which it is not? Can we develop
procedures for making such decisions that would provide adequate safeguards
against abuse? Given such procedures, how likely are abuses and are they
sufficiently serious to outweigh the benefits of withholding food and water
that is excessively burdensome or without benefit to the patient? Courts
that have addressed the issue of withholding nutrition and hydration have
been sensitive to the need for procedures with strong safeguards against
abuse, but have nonetheless generally held that artificial measures for provision of nutrition and hydration are not in principle different than other
treatments, such as use of respirators that artificially provide oxygen to the
patient (*Conroy* 1985; *Cruzan* 1990; *Barber and Nedjl* 1983). All fall under a
patient's general moral and legal right to decide about and to refuse any
medical treatment.

Futility

In recent years, conflicts between physicians and patients or their families
about life support have increasingly shifted from physicians who are unwilling to accept patients' or families' decisions to forgo treatment, to patients
or families demanding treatment that physicians consider futile (Tomlinson
and Brody 1990; Troug et al. 1992). The debate about futility began over
cardiopulmonary resuscitation (CPR) and whether it must be offered and
made available to all patients who want it, even if their physicians deem it
futile (the debate has spread from CPR to other life-sustaining treatments).
The debate has touched broader questions as well, such as the nature of the
physician–patient relationship and the appropriate decision-making authority of patients and families. Although it is now generally accepted that patients or their families can refuse any treatment, their choice of treatments
is typically thought to be from among medically accepted or indicated alternatives. When physicians are not asked to stand back and withhold or withdraw treatment by the patient or family, but instead are asked to join with
the patient in a collaborative effort to provide treatment, it seems reasonable that what is done should be acceptable to both patient and physician.

It has seemed to many only common sense that treatment that is truly
futile need not be offered or provided. Much of the debate has centered
on how futility should be defined. Some have sought to specify a narrow
physiological notion of futility—treatment is futile when it is known with
high medical certainty that it cannot produce the physiological effect that
is being sought. The judgment about futility in this narrow sense seems to
be an empirical or factual matter about which physicians should be expert,

and so which might plausibly be left to their judgment and decision. Others have pointed out that it is difficult to exclude all value questions from even this narrow notion of futility—how certain is certain enough, and what are the legitimate aims for which a treatment can be used? Some proponents of establishing futility as a basis for refusing patients' or families' demands for treatment have defended a broader, evaluative understanding of futility. For example, some have argued that treatment is futile if it will only preserve unconscious life or if it will not end dependence on intensive care, or if it will not prevent imminent death or only delay it a very short time. Here, the treatment does have a physiological effect, but the effect is judged not, or too slight, a benefit to the patient. A different sense of evaluative futility is when there is a possible benefit, which need not be slight, but the probability of achieving it, while not zero, is considered too unlikely to warrant using the treatment. Finally, some have mixed economic considerations into futility, holding that treatment is futile if its benefits do not justify its costs.

The more the understanding of futility is expanded to include evaluative judgments, such as whether the hoped for effect is likely enough, or is a significant enough benefit, the more morally problematic it becomes for the physician's values to be substituted for the patient's. One central issue in the futility debate has been whether it can be defined narrowly enough not to result in physicians reclaiming unwarranted treatment decision-making authority that is appropriately left with patients or their surrogates. It is also not just a matter of how the term is defined but of developing an institutional practice with sufficient protections against physicians using the appeal to futility to deny patients treatment that should be available to them. Some have argued that this task is sufficiently difficult that physicians should instead focus their efforts on full and frank discussions with patients, families, or both, of the burdens and risks to the patient of procedures such as CPR, together with the lack of expected benefit when that is the case. Further discussion and communication, not taking decision-making authority from patients or their surrogates and reserving it to physicians, may be the best approach to the unrealistic expectations of patients or families and their demands for futile treatment.

CONCLUSION

We have sought in this chapter to address many of the most difficult and troubling ethical issues arising in decisions about life-sustaining treatment. Many of those issues are complex and no widespread agreement yet exists on them. There is, however, a central core of widespread agreement that is worth repeating and underlining. A competent patient, or an incompetent patient's surrogate, is ethically entitled to assess the benefits and burdens of any proffered treatment according to the patient's own aims and values and to accept or reject the treatment. The quite broad agreement on this seemingly simple principle should in no way be taken to imply, however, that the decisions themselves in concrete cases are simple or uncontroversial for those involved in them. There is much truth in the view that the particular circumstances and details of each case make it unique. No simple principles can be mechanically applied in a way that makes for easy choices. Decisions about life and death are inevitably and quite properly difficult and troubling and require sensitive, thoughtful, and wise judgment from all involved.

DISCUSSION QUESTIONS

1. What criteria for death should be used for anencephalics or patients in a persistent vegetative state? Are these patients dead, based on whole-brain concepts of death? On higher-brain concepts of death?

2. When, if ever, should life be prolonged for competent patients against their wishes? Why?

3. Is there any morally significant difference between starting a treatment such as a ventilator and stopping once it has been started? Should physicians have an obligation to withdraw treatment when patients or surrogates withdraw their consent to it? Should physicians have to pull the plug?

4. In what cases and to what extent should it be required to involve others (i.e., institutional review boards, ethics committees, the courts) in the surrogate decision-making process?

5. What are the medical and moral differences, if any, between killing and allowing to die, withholding and withdrawing treatment, euthanasia and suicide?

REFERENCES

Books and Articles

Bayer, R., et al. "The Care of the Terminally Ill: Morality and Economics." *N Engl J Med* 309 (1983): 1490–1494.

Bennett, J. "Morality and Consequences." In S. M. McMurrin, Ed., *The Tanner Lectures in Human Value II*. Salt Lake City: University of Utah Press, 1981.

Brock, D. W. *Life and Death: Philosophical Essays in Biomedical Ethics*. New York: Cambridge University Press, 1993.

Buchanan, A. E., Brock, D. W. *Deciding for Others: The Ethics of Surrogate Decision-Making*. New York: Cambridge University Press, 1989.

Capron, A. M. "The Authority of Others to Decide About Biomedical Interventions with Incompetents." In W. Gaylin and R. Macklin. *Who Speaks for the Child?* New York: Plenum Press, 1982.

Capron, A. M., Kass, L. "A Statutory Definition of the Standards for Determining Human Death: An Appraisal and a Proposal." *U Penn L Rev* 87 (1972): 102–104.

Dworkin, G. *The Theory and Practice of Autonomy.* Cambridge, MA: Cambridge University Press, 1988.

Emanuel, L. L., Emanuel, E. J. "Decisions at the End of Life: Guided by Communities of Patients." *Hastings Cent Rep* 23, no. 5 (1993): 6–14.

Fost, N., Cranford, R. "Hospital Ethics Committees: Administrative Aspects." *JAMA* 253 (1985): 2687–2692.

Frey, R. "Some Aspects to the Doctrine of Double Effect." *Can J Philos* 5 (1975): 259–283.

Fried, C. *Right and Wrong.* Cambridge: Harvard University Press, 1978.

Gaylin, W., Kass, L., Pellegrino, E., Siegler, M. "Doctors Must Not Kill." *JAMA* 259 (1988): 2139–2140.

Glover, J. *Causing Death and Saving Lives.* New York: Penguin Books, 1977.

Green, M., Wikler, D. "Brain Death and Personal Identity." *Philos Public Affairs* 9 (1980): 105–133.

Hastings Center. *Guidelines for the Termination of Treatment and Care of the Dying.* Briarcliff Manor, NY: The Hastings Center, 1988.

Kamisar, Y. "Some Non-Religious Views Against Proposed Mercy Killing Legislation." *Minn L Rev* 42 (1958): 969–1042.

Kamm, F. *Morality/Mortality.* Oxford: Oxford University Press, 1993.

Kass, L. *Toward A More Natural Science: Biology and Human Affairs.* New York: Free Press, 1985.

Katz, J. *The Silent World of Doctor and Patient.* New York: Free Press, 1984.

Lynn, J., Ed. *Forgoing Life-Sustaining Food and Water.* Bloomington: University of Indiana Press, 1986.

Lynn, J., Childress, J. "Must Patients Always Be Given Food and Water?" *Hastings Center Rep* 13 (1983): 17–21.

McCormick, R. "To Save or Let Die: The Dilemma of Modern Medicine." *JAMA* 229 (1974): 172–176.

President's Commission for Ethical Problems in Medicine. *Defining Death.* Washington, DC: U.S. Government Printing Office, 1981.

———. *Making Health-Care Decisions.* Washington, DC: U.S. Government Printing Office, 1982.

———. *Deciding to Forgo Life-Sustaining Treatment.* Washington, DC: U.S. Government Printing Office, 1983a.

———. *Securing Access to Health Care.* Washington, DC: U.S. Government Printing Office, 1983b.

Rachels, J. "Active and Passive Euthanasia." *N Engl J Med* 292 (1975): 78–80.

Rosner, F. "Hospital Medical Ethics Committees: A Review of Their Development." *JAMA* 253 (1985): 2693–2697.

Sider, R., Clements, C. "The New Medical Ethics: A Second Opinion." *Arch Intern Med* 145 (1985): 2169–2171.

Siegler, M. "Searching for Moral Certainty in Medicine: A Proposal for a New Model of the Doctor-Patient Encounter." *Bull NY Acad Med* 57 (1981): 56–69.

Siegler, M., Weisbard, A. "Against the Emerging Stream." *Arch Intern Med* 145 (1985): 129–131.

Singer, P., Kuhse, H. *Should This Baby Live?* New York: Oxford University Press, 1986.

Steinbock, B., Ed. *Killing and Letting Die.* Englewood Cliffs, NJ: Prentice Hall, 1980.

Tomlinson, T., Brody, H. "Futility and the Ethics of Resuscitation." *JAMA* 264 (1990): 1276–1280.

Tooley, M. *Abortion and Infanticide.* Oxford: Oxford University Press, 1983.

Troug, R., Brett, A., Frader, J. "The Trouble with Futility." *N Engl J Med* 326 (1992): 1560–1564.

Van der Maas, P., et al. "Euthanasia and Other Medical Decisions Concerning the End of Life." *Lancet* 338 (1991): 669–674.

Veatch, R. M. "The Whole-Brain Oriented Concept of Death: An Outmoded Philosophical Formulation." *J Thanatol* 13 (1975): 13–30.

Wanzer, S., et al. "The Physicians' Responsibility Toward Hopelessly Ill Patients." *N Engl J Med* 310 (1984): 955–959.

Weir, R. *Selective Non-Treatment of Handicapped Newborns.* New York: Oxford University Press, 1984.

Cases

Barber and Nedjl v. Superior Court, 195 Cal. Rptr. 484 (Cal. App. 2 Dist. 1983).

In re Conroy, 486 A.2d 1209 (N.J. 1985).

Cruzan v. Director Missouri Dept. of Health, 110 S.Ct. 2841 (1990).

In re Quinlan, 70 N.J. 10, 355 A. 2d 647 (1976).

13

AIDS and Ethics

RONALD BAYER

SUMMARY

The acquired immunodeficiency syndrome (AIDS) is the first serious epidemic disease to strike industrial nations in more than a generation. It poses such a wide range of ethical issues that it comprises a summary of the controversies in biomedical ethics. These issues fall into three major groups.

First, AIDS raises the ethics of prevention and protection. A consensus supporting voluntary testing and screening has gradually emerged. Efforts to isolate persons with human immunodeficiency virus (HIV) infection and limit contacts between those infected and others—both lay and professional—have been challenged as unnecessary constraints on human freedom. Confidentiality in reporting of diagnoses has been defended, but recently has also been challenged, especially by those concerned about infected persons who appear to be willfully engaging in behavior that exposes others to significant risk. Coercive controls such as quarantine and statutes criminalizing behaviors linked to the spread of AIDS have been adopted in some jurisdictions, but enforcement has been very limited.

Second, AIDS raises questions of the ethics of research. The emergence of active, organized groups of patients has changed the dynamic of the research enterprise. Persons with HIV infection have provided leadership in reconceptualizing research from a risk from which one should be protected to a potential opportunity to gain access to possible benefits of experimental agents.

Finally, AIDS raises questions about the care of persons with HIV infection. Health-care workers, for the first time in recent history, have had to confront questions about the danger of their occupations. Gradually, a duty of the health-care professional to provide care has been established. At the same time, controversy continues about the duty of the infected health-care worker to warn patients and take precautions to limit patients' exposure. In addition to the problems of right of access that surround the specific infection, AIDS presents serious problems for those excluded from adequate health-care insurance.

AIDS links advanced technological societies with the poorest nations of the world in a common struggle that is likely to present serious problems at the international level of right of access to a future vaccine or therapy. AIDS compels us to recognize that health and disease are always shaped by cultural and political forces as well as by the state of scientific knowledge.

As the first serious epidemic disease to strike advanced industrial nations in more than a generation, acquired immunodeficiency syndrome (AIDS) has posed an extraordinary array of ethical challenges. Among the issues that have drawn attention are the duty of physicians to care for those who are in need, the limits and significance of medical confidentiality, the obligation to seek informed consent before testing and commencing treatment, the functions of counseling infected individuals about their duties to partners, assisting women who are infected as they are compelled to make reproductive decisions, the clash between the canons of research and the canons of care, the limits of acceptable underwriting by insurance companies, and, finally, the rights of individuals with costly medical conditions to leave their countries of residence.

Despite the extraordinary context of the epidemic during the past decade, what is striking about the issues that have been pressed to the fore is that they are not new. What *is* new is the intensity of the discussion, the broad participatory nature of the debate, the political forces called into play, the demands they have made, and the solutions they have sought to fashion.

As a lethal illness, spread in the context of the most intimate relationships, and as a public health threat, AIDS has forced us to confront questions regarding the appropriate role of the state in limiting morbidity and mortality. As a disease of the socially vulnerable, human immunodeficiency virus (HIV) infection and AIDS have compelled people to face issues involving the role of the state in protecting the weak at moments of social stress. As a disease that has affected large numbers of poor individuals without adequate health insurance, AIDS has required us once again to consider what justice demands in terms of the protection of all against the costs associated with illness. Thus, the roles of government in advancing the public health, defending the weak, and ensuring access to health care have all been called upon by the AIDS epidemic.

In this chapter, three broad topics are considered: the ethics of prevention and protection, the ethics of research, and the ethics of care.

THE ETHICS OF PREVENTION AND PROTECTION

AIDS is a blood-borne, sexually transmitted disease. As such, it is transmitted by infected persons to those who are uninfected during homosexual or heterosexual sexual intercourse, through needle sharing by drug users, and by pregnant women to their fetuses. Early in the epidemic, infection was also transmitted through blood transfusions and to those dependent on the clotting factor for hemophilia. In short, the spread of AIDS began as a behaviorally transmitted disease. In the absence of a vaccine, transmission of HIV infection can only be interrupted through modifications in behavior. Those who are infected must wear condoms during sexual intercourse; intravenous drug users must not share needles. The risk of pediatric AIDS can be eliminated completely only if infected women do not bear children.

It is these biological facts that provide the foundations for public health strategies designed to prevent AIDS. It is these facts that raise profound questions about the moral responsibilities of persons with HIV infection to behave in ways that limit the prospect for spreading a lethal disease and of the state to shape policies that facilitate radical modification of sexual and drug-using behavior.

Among the bitterly fought issues raised in this context has been the question of whether AIDS education should stress the moral responsibilities of those who are infected or the importance of self-protection for the uninfected. Of even greater moment has been the political controversy provoked by the centrality of educating gay men and illegal drug users about how they should modify their behaviors to protect themselves and others. Social conservatives opposed to homosexuality and all extramarital sex have objected to the "legitimization" in the name of public health of what they believe is immoral behavior. Indeed, during the Reagan and Bush administrations, they were successful in imposing restrictions on the language and content of messages designed to inform and shape AIDS-related behaviors. Similarly, those who viewed illegal drug use as morally reprehensible opposed educational efforts designed to instruct intravenous drug users about how they might continue to use drugs without placing themselves at risk for a lethal infection.

It was against such resistance that the U.S. Surgeon General, gay rights leaders, political liberals, and most public health officials had to struggle in the formative period of the AIDS epidemic. For them, the conservative resistance represented a profoundly mistaken strategy, one in which the language of morality had been mobilized to defend policies that would lead to enormous suffering.

In the end, the political limits imposed on AIDS prevention efforts were limits on the state's first responsibility to protect the vulnerable. It is no accident that those who bore the burden of that failure were gay men, drug users, African Americans, and Latinos. This, then, was the context within which public health efforts took shape in ways that were quite remarkable.

In the United States as well as in other nations bounded by the liberal tradition, both ethical considerations and pragmatic concerns have contributed to the adoption of public health strategies to control the spread of HIV infection that may be broadly defined as voluntaristic—stressing mass education, counseling, and respect for privacy (Bayer 1991a). This approach stood in stark contrast to the public health response to other infectious and sexually transmitted diseases. Indeed, both in the United States and elsewhere what might be termed "HIV exceptionalism" has dominated public health policy (Bayer 1991b). This general consensus has affected policies on testing for HIV infection, the protection of confidentiality, and the use of the coercive powers of the state to restrict persons whose behaviors are thought to pose a risk of HIV transmission.

Testing and Voluntarism

From the outset, the test developed to detect an antibody to the AIDS virus—first used on a broad scale to screen blood donations—was mired in controversy. Uncertainty about the significance of the test's findings and about the quality and accuracy provided the technical substrate of disputes that inevitably took on a political and ethical character because issues of privacy, communal health, social and economic discrimination, coercion, and liberty were always involved. Public health officials saw in the test a valuable tool for fostering behavioral change. Others, primarily gay rights leaders, saw it as a great threat.

Out of the controversies that whirled about the antibody test, there emerged a broad consensus in the mid-1980s. Except for clearly circumscribed circumstances, testing was to be done under conditions of voluntary, informed consent only after counseling that outlined both the benefits and risks of testing, and the results were to be protected by stringent confidentiality safeguards. In the United States, to underscore the importance of protecting the privacy of tested individuals, the option of anonymous testing was made broadly available. Only voluntary testing, it was believed, could contribute to the overarching goal of behavioral change. The voluntarist consensus was supported by gay rights leaders (American Association of Physicians for Human Rights unpublished report 1985), civil libertarians (North California Branch, ACLU 1986), bioethicists (Bayer, Levine, and Wolfe 1986), public health officials (Association of State and Territorial Health Officials 1985), and by professional organizations representing clinicians (American Medical Association 1987). But as broad as the consensus was, it was also fragile, because it was based on differing interests and commitments. It was a consensus shaped by the relative impotence of medicine in the epidemic's first years.

Advances in therapeutics and a wide range of clinical trials for which the infected were eligible changed the outlook for patients with HIV infection. Those who formerly urged those at risk for infection to exercise great caution before seeking to know their antibody status began to encourage voluntary confidential or anonymous testing. A growing number of clinicians sought to loosen the requirements for specific informed consent before HIV-antibody testing occurred, to "return AIDS to the medical mainstream."

Given the traditions of medicine, such impatience was not surprising. But ethicists have continued to argue for the centrality of consent (Levine and Bayer 1989). A number of arguments have been put forward in this regard. First, as much as the clinical picture has begun to change, there is no definitive therapeutic course for HIV-infected, but otherwise asymptomatic, individuals. At the same time, the prospect of stigma and discrimination have remained a threat to the social well-being of HIV-infected persons. Under these conditions, the arguments for specific informed consent have been considered as important as ever. But ethicists have gone further, arguing that even if the clinical picture improved dramatically, the moral basis for insisting on informed consent before HIV testing would not change. Their conclusions are derived from the well-established principle that competent adults have the right to determine whether to undergo treatment or to terminate treatments already begun. The principle that limits the paternalistic authority of the physician to order therapies in the interest of the patient, it has been argued, extends to the authority to order tests that would serve as the basis for commencing treatment.

But if those concerned with respect for the autonomy of the patient have continued to assert that physicians should exercise restraint, they have also begun to claim that the physician's ethical responsibility to provide appropriate care also requires physicians to routinely offer HIV-antibody testing to those patients whose social histories suggest some increased possibility of infection. In some contexts, it has been suggested that the HIV test be offered to all patients. Only by being offered such tests can patients have the opportunity to learn whether they are infected and exercise their right to choose whether to begin therapy or enter available clinical trials.

More complex is the question of whether the current situation justifies the routine or mandatory screening of infants born to mothers at risk for HIV infection (Faden, Geller, and Powers 1991). Many pediatricians have asserted that the early identification of infected newborns provides an opportunity to initiate aggressive intervention, including the prophylactic administration of zidovudine (AZT), or the early commencement of prophylaxis for *Pneumocystis carinii* pneumonia. Others have been more skeptical of what can be done for asymptomatic infants. Because antibody testing identifies the existence of an infected mother, the mandatory testing of newborns is, in fact, the mandatory testing of women who have given birth. Indeed, until recently it was not possible to distinguish between truly infected babies and those that merely carried maternal antibody. Only when the child was 18 months of age was it possible to clarify the child's true status. More recently, it has become possible to identify infection in newborns much earlier. From an ethical perspective, before such identification can be permitted without consent, it is necessary to demonstrate more than a hypothetical benefit to the infant.

The debate over newborn testing takes place against a background of widely accepted mandatory or routine testing of newborns for other diseases to permit the identification of those in need of special treatment (Faden, Holtzman, and Chwalow 1982). Screening in these instances is held to represent a legitimate exercise of the state's power to protect the vulnerable. Screening for phenylketonuria (PKU) is a good example of such testing. For PKU a definitive diagnostic test, a definitive therapeutic intervention, and an imperative to act quickly are the conditions that provide the empirical and moral grounds for the routine screening of newborns without first seeking parental consent.

None of these conditions now prevails in the case of HIV. Therefore, there is, from an ethical perspective, no basis for mandatory newborn screening. Were a therapy for such infants available, the clinical and ethical bases for making a claim on behalf of the vulnerable child would exist. Such developments might well be sufficient to establish the grounds for testing without previous parental consent.

Despite the enormous attention devoted to the question of newborn testing in the late 1980s and early 1990s, that issue will, in all likelihood, be superseded by pressure to identify HIV-infected pregnant women. The pressure will stem from a remarkable research finding in early 1994 that showed a radical reduction in HIV transmission from infected pregnant women to their fetuses when AZT was administered during pregnancy and delivery and to the newborn for 6 weeks after birth. In the wake of this finding, obstetricians and pediatricians began to assert that the regime surrounding testing should be liberalized so that all infected women could be identified and offered treatment. Almost no one called for mandatory testing during pregnancy (although such testing for syphilis already occurs) because it was recognized that even if unwilling pregnant women with HIV were identified, it would be ethically, legally, and pragmatically impossible to impose therapy on them. Instead, many physicians asserted that the stringent requirements of informed consent, with pretest counseling, be replaced with a strong recommendation to undergo testing with an informed right of refusal. How much would remain of the informed portion of such a right of refusal can only be imagined.

Screening for Safety

Because AIDS represented the first major infectious threat with which advanced industrial societies had to contend in almost a generation, and because the causative agent was not identified until 3 years after the first case reports, it is not surprising that it provoked considerable social anxiety. How was it spread? Who posed a risk? Who was endangered? That AIDS was a disease of socially marginal, and not infrequently despised, individuals only intensified the urge toward discrimination. Employers, landlords, school personnel, and even the staff of some health-care institutions evidenced a willingness to exclude those with the disease. With the discovery of HIV, and the development of a test that could detect antibody to the virus, the potential scope for discriminatory activity increased, despite the epidemiological evidence about how infection was spread.

In the United States, the Centers for Disease Control and Prevention (CDC) moved swiftly to contain the irrational impulse toward exclusion. At the end of 1985, guidelines to prevent the spread of HIV infection in schools

(CDC 1985) and the workplace (CDC 1985) were issued. Early in 1986, detailed guidelines for health-care workers on preventing the spread of infection while engaged in invasive procedures were published (CDC 1986). In each instance, the goal was to convey information, provide protection, and prevent panic. The message was clear: HIV could not be casually transmitted, and so there were no public health grounds for exclusion of infected individuals who otherwise were capable of performing their expected functions. There were, thus, no grounds for mandatory testing for HIV. In the context of the health-care setting, universal blood and body fluid precautions would protect workers not only from HIV but from the far more infectious hepatitis B. Screening could only provide illusory protections.

Although there are still shameful occurrences of efforts to exclude or isolate school children with AIDS or HIV infection, and although cases of discrimination by employers continue to occur, they are almost universally deplored as irrational, unscientific, and ethically retrograde.

The situation in health care has not been so clear cut. The relatively few cases of transmission that have occurred as a result of needle sticks, and the even smaller number of transmissions linked to blood splashes (CDC 1988), have provoked distress among health-care workers, especially among surgeons, obstetricians, nurses, and emergency room personnel. Persons whose work regularly brings them into contact with their patients' blood have felt vulnerable. On rare occasions they have asserted the right to refuse to care for the infected (Abel 1987). Far more frequently, such clinicians have publicly challenged the adequacy of the recommendations for universal blood and body fluid precautions. Instead, they have demanded the right to know whether their patients are infected, and the right to screen on a routine or mandatory basis for HIV infection. The level of vigilance demanded by the threat of a lethal infection could not, they have argued, be maintained at all times. The conflict between public health officials who have declared that universal precautions are sufficient and clinicians who have asserted that they are not has not abated; indeed, it has intensified. A deep fissure has thus emerged, which has ruptured the broad alliance that had existed within the medical profession.

Paralleling this debate has been the unresolved question of the appropriate measures to protect patients from HIV-infected clinicians. Debate on this matter has been driven by the single, still unexplained case of a Florida dentist to whom the only cases of HIV infection in patients linked to a clinician have been traced. Some have argued that although professionals have a moral duty to assume some risks—especially risks that are quite small—in caring for their patients, patients do not have an equivalent duty to expose themselves to even small risks when being cared for (Gostin 1989). Dismissing as irrational those who would deny all infected health-care workers, whatever their functions, the right to engage in clinical work, many have asserted that physicians whose invasive work can place their patients at some risk ought not to engage in those procedures. But if those who know themselves to be infected with HIV have such professional duties, are there correlative institutional obligations to identify the infected, to exclude them from certain functions? Are they obligated to screen health-care workers, and if so, at what frequency? Might concern about protecting patients provide the basis for mandatory screening and surveillance after so much effort to forestall such programs? And if screening and surveillance were to be adopted, what would be the impact on an anxious social climate?

In thinking about these issues it would be useful to underscore the apparent tension between the ethics of informed consent and the ethics of protecting the vulnerable from discrimination. The ethics of informed consent has increasingly been shaped by a commitment to the view that patients should be able to determine, for themselves, the level of risk that is acceptable in the context of medical practice. Such a view rejects the standard of the reasonable person or the physician in determining which risks should be revealed to a patient for his or her consideration. In short, the standard is subjective. The ethics of antidiscrimination practice and policy is profoundly different. It rejects subjectivity; it views subjectivity as the fount of irrationality. From that perspective, personal views about risk cannot override the rights of those with particular disabilities to work. A refusal, for example, to hire a person with limited hearing loss because of a belief that such an individual would represent some remote theoretical risk would never be countenanced under the American with Disabilities Act and the ethical norms that inform the Act. Thus, the understanding of the problem posed by the HIV-infected surgeon or dentist will very much depend on whether it is defined essentially as one that implicates the ethics of informed consent or the ethics of disability rights.

In years to come, new controversies over screening will surely arise. In each of these conflicts, those who confront each other will predictably seek to appropriate the mantle of value-free decision making and will charge that those with whom they disagree have deserted the standards of science. On some occasions, the risk posed by the infected will be understood to be so small and the implications of screening and exclusion so burdensome that even the most cautious will find it hard to justify compulsory testing and the imposition of restrictions; on other occasions, the choices will not be clear cut. But in each case, more than "science" will be involved. Decisions about screening policy will reflect the balance of moral commitments to privacy, reason, and communal well-being.

Confidentiality and Its Limits

There is perhaps no ethical issue involving AIDS that has received more attention than that of confidentiality. That gay men and those who have spoken on their behalf have placed such great stress on confidentiality should come as no surprise. A history of oppression and the existence of antisodomy laws have made the protection of privacy a critical feature of the struggle for social survival. But the call for the protection of confidentiality has come as well from the U.S. Surgeon General (1986), the Centers for Disease Control and Prevention (1985), the Institute of Medicine and the National Academy of Sciences (1986), the Presidential Commission on the HIV Epidemic (1986), and public health officials across the nation (Association of State and Territorial Health Officials 1985). For them, the protection of confidentiality is critical to the strategy to encourage mass behavioral change and to the goal of encouraging people to come forward for testing and counseling.

In states that were profoundly affected by AIDS, public health officials pressed for the enactment of especially stringent legislative and administrative safeguards. The centrality of confidentiality to the pursuit of public health objectives provided an explanation for the unique decision in states with relatively high AIDS case counts not to require reporting of the names of individuals with HIV infection to public health registries, despite the fact that AIDS itself has been a reportable condition in all states since 1983. Although the late 1980s and early 1990s witnessed a gradual shift on this policy matter, concern for the privacy of those who are infected with HIV has continued to influence policy makers in many states.

But what of the role of confidentiality in the clinical setting? What are the moral responsibilities of a physician when an HIV-infected patient refuses to inform identifiable, unsuspecting past or current partners about the dangers of infection (Dickens 1988)? The relevance of the legal and ethical controversies surrounding the Tarasoff decision, in which the California Supreme Court ruled that "the protective privilege ends where the public peril begins," are quite obvious (*Tarasoff* 1976). In the case of past partners, concern has centered on the possibility that an unknowingly infected individual might act as unwitting agent of transmission to yet others or might lose the opportunity to commence early therapeutic intervention. In the case of current partners, the focus has been on the possibility of preventing the transmission of HIV to an as yet uninfected individual. As these issues were considered, it became clear that the process of warning past sexual partners did not require the identification of the source of potential infection. No public health goal would be served by breaching the cloak of anonymity of the index case. When an infected individual refused to warn a current partner, the situation posed graver difficulties. Without revealing the source of potential infection, it was possible that no effective protective warning could be made.

Informing the dispute about how it might be best to proceed has been a deep concern about the consequences that could well follow were it to be widely believed that physicians would routinely breach confidentiality when presented with a patient who refused to warn past or current partners about the risk of HIV infection. Would the consequence be a reduction in clinical candor? Would patients be discouraged from seeking to know their HIV status? Would they be less accessible to the efforts of clinicians to convince them of the importance of warning those who might be at risk? In sum, would breaching confidentiality to warn unsuspecting individuals result in a net loss from the perspective of public health?

Beginning in the latter part of 1987, a number of efforts were made in the United States to resolve the issues associated with the warning of unsuspecting third parties. At the end of 1987, the American Medical Association (AMA) issued a broad set of statements on the ethical issues posed by the AIDS epidemic (1987). In that document the AMA addressed the issue of warning in a forthright manner. Physicians were to try to convince patients of their obligation to warn the unsuspecting. If they failed in that task, they were to seek the intervention of public health officials. Only if public health officials refused or were unwilling to take on the responsibility of warning would it be the obligation of the physician to act directly.

When the Presidential Commission on the HIV Epidemic addressed this issue in mid-1988, it too endorsed the notion that physicians should have the right to breach confidentiality in order to warn the unsuspecting, despite the centrality of confidentiality to its overall strategy (Presidential Commission on the Human Immunodeficiency Virus Epidemic 1988). Reflecting, however, a commitment to professional autonomy, the Commission held that the decision about whether to breach confidentiality was to remain with the physician and was not to be imposed as a matter of law. That too was the stance of a wide spectrum of public health officials, including the Association of State and Territorial Health Officials (1988), who chose to speak of a "privilege to disclose" rather than a duty to warn. The lingering ethical question is whether such a strategy meets the moral challenge posed to clinicians confronted with patients who may threaten the lives of their partners.

Coercive Controls

The question of how to respond to individuals whose behavior represented a threat to unknowing partners inevitably provoked discussion of the public health tradition of imposing restrictions on liberty in the name of communal welfare. The specter of quarantine has haunted all such discussions, not because there was any serious consideration in the United States of the Cuban approach to AIDS—which until recently mandated the lifelong isolation of all persons infected with HIV (Bayer and Healton 1989)—but because of fears that even a more limited recognition of the authority to quarantine would lead to egregious intrusions upon privacy and invidiously imposed deprivations of freedom.

Although fierce opposition has surfaced to all efforts to bring AIDS within the scope of state quarantine statutes, more than a dozen states had done so between 1987 and 1990, typically using the occasion to modernize their disease control laws to reflect contemporary constitutional standards that detail procedural guarantees, and to require that restrictions on freedom represent the "least restrictive alternative" available to achieve a "compelling state interest."

Despite the intensity of the debate that has surrounded this issue, the only empirical study of the use of the power of isolation has found that state health departments have almost never exercised the authority granted by statute. From 1981 to 1990, only 10 cases were documented, and in virtually every case the duration of confinement has been very brief. Far more common has been the use of the public health authority to warn individuals that their behavior posed a risk. Such warnings have often been accompanied by "cease and desist orders" (Bayer and Fairchild-Carrino 1993).

The enactment of statutes criminalizing behaviors linked to the spread of AIDS has paralleled the political receptivity to laws extending the authority of public health officials to control individuals whose behavior posed a risk of HIV transmission. Such use of the criminal law, broadly endorsed by the Presidential Commission on the HIV Epidemic (1988), called upon a tradition of state enactments that made the knowing transmission of venereal disease a crime. Although they almost never were enforced, the existence of the older laws served as a rationale for new legislative initiatives. Between 1987 and 1989, 20 states enacted such statutes, most of which defined the proscribed acts as felonies despite the fact that older statutes typically treated knowing transmission as a misdemeanor. As important, aggressive prosecutors have relied on laws defining assaultive behavior and attempted murder to bring indictments even in the absence of AIDS-specific legislation.

A 1990 survey estimated that from 50 to 100 prosecutions had been initiated involving acts as diverse as spitting, biting, blood splattering, blood donation, and sexual intercourse with an unsuspecting partner (Gostin 1990). Although small in number, these cases have drawn great attention. In most there was either an acquittal or the prosecution was dropped. In the small number of cases that produced guilty verdicts, there have been some unusually harsh sentences.

Whatever the allure of such measures and of the rediscovery of traditional public health approaches in the effort to combat the spread of HIV infection, it has remained clear that the future course of the AIDS epidemic will be determined by the creation of a social and institutional milieu within which radical voluntary changes in behavior can occur and be sustained. Educational campaigns and counseling programs, most effectively undertaken by groups linked to the populations at risk, have remained the centerpiece of that preventive effort.

THE ETHICS OF RESEARCH

The HIV epidemic has provided the circumstances for the emergence of a broad and potent political movement that has sought to reshape radically the conditions under which research is undertaken. The role of the randomized clinical trial, the importance of placebo controls, the centrality of academic research institutions, the dominance of scientists over subjects, the sharp distinction between research and therapy, and the protectionist ethos of the Belmont Report have all been brought into question.

Although scholars concerned with the methodological demands of sound research and ethicists committed to the protection of research subjects have played a crucial role in the ensuing discussions, both as defenders of the received wisdom and as critics, the debate has been driven by the articulate demands of those most threatened by AIDS. Most prominent have been groups such as the People With AIDS Coalition and ACT-UP, organizations made up primarily of white, gay men. But advocates of women's, children's, and prisoners' rights have also made their voices heard. What has been so stunning, disconcerting to some and exciting to others, has been the rhythm of challenge and response. Rather than the careful exchange of academic arguments, we have been witness to the mobilization of disruptive and effective political protest.

The threat of death has hovered over the process. As Carol Levine has noted, "the shortage of proven therapeutic alternatives for AIDS and the belief that trials are, in and of themselves, beneficial have led to the claim that people have a right to be research subjects. This is the exact opposite of the tradition starting with Nuremberg—that people have a right *not* to be research subjects" (1988). It is that striking reversal that has resulted in a rejection of the model of research conducted at remote academic centers, with restrictive (protective) standards of access and strict adherence to the "gold standard" of the randomized clinical trial. Blurring the distinction between research and treatment—"A Drug Trial Is Health Care Too"—persons insistent on radical reform have sought to open wide the points of entry to new "therapeutic" agents both within and outside of clinical trials and have demanded that the paternalistic ethical warrant for the protection of the vulnerable from research be replaced by an ethical regime informed by respect for the autonomous choice of potential subjects who could weigh, for themselves, the potential risks and benefits of new experimental treatments for HIV infection. Thus, demands have been made that women be enrolled in trials in greater numbers, that prisoners and drug users be granted access, and that children be included in trials at a much earlier point than had been considered acceptable. Moreover, the revisionists have demanded a basic reconceptualization of the relationship between researchers and subjects. In place of protocols imposed from above, they have proposed a more egalitarian and democratic model in which negotiation would replace scientific authority (Dubler, Levine, and Levine 1991).

The reformulation of the ethics of research that has begun under the impact of AIDS has implications that go far beyond the epidemic of HIV disease because the emerging new concepts and standards could govern the conduct of the entire research enterprise. Protagonists, who have been locked in often acrimonious debate, foretell very different consequences of the changing social standards of research. Proponents of the new ethos hold out the prospect of a new regime that is both respectful of individual rights and the requirements of good science. George Annas, on the other hand, has warned that the blurring of the distinction between research and treatment can only harm the desperate. "It is not compassionate to hold out false hope to terminally ill patients so that they spend their last dollars on unproven 'remedies' that they might live longer" (1989).

THE ETHICS OF CARE

For almost 4 decades, health-care workers in America, as well as in other advanced industrial societies, were largely shielded from what had been the routine experience of those who had in prior eras worked with the sick: the acquisition of their patients' infections and sometimes lethal diseases. Although never as total as many had come to believe, this invincibility was psychologically ruptured by the intrusion of AIDS, beginning in 1981. AIDS forced physicians and health-care workers to consider the possibility that theirs was indeed a "dangerous trade."

Early in the history of this epidemic, anecdotal reports began to surface about hospital aides leaving food trays at the doors of those who were sick, and of nurses, physicians, and dentists refusing to treat patients with the new disease. As noted earlier, the CDC confronted such behavior by publishing in late 1985 and 1986 a series of reports in *Morbidity and Mortality Weekly Report* (*MMWR*) that sought to provide guidance for sound infection control practice and rational social policy.

Confronted with the challenge represented by the threat of patient abandonment, persons committed to stanching the emerging trend turned to history (Zuger 1987) in hopes that an unambiguous lesson on responsibility of physicians would emerge. Physicians had, after all, been called to respond when epidemics were more common, when morbidity was awesome. For those who had hoped to discover a univocal message from the chronicles of the past, the turn of history proved a disappointment. Although some physicians had stayed behind to care for their patients, many had fled. At times they did so to attend to their fleeing patrons, sometime simply to protect themselves. Perhaps most significant as a reflection of the extent to which many physicians refused to remain with those afflicted in earlier plagues was the need to make arrangements for the care of the sick through the special institution of the "plague doctor." Employed by local merchants and the political elites, these physicians took up where others had failed (Fox 1988).

If history provided no clear guidance, what of the codes of ethics that have expressed the aspirations of the guilds and associations of medical practitioners? Remarkably, such codes had been silent on the duty of physicians to treat in the time of epidemics. In this regard, the AMA code of 1847 (Zuger 1987) was unique in its forthright assertion of such a responsibility. "And when pestilence prevails, it is their duty to face the danger and to continue their labors for the alleviation of suffering, even at the jeopardy of their own lives." This provision remained in the code until 1957, when a revised and shortened statement eliminated the stipulation that must certainly have seemed an anachronism. After all, the era of epidemics had come to an end in the advanced industrial world.

But remaining in the code was a provision—first incorporated into the AMA's statement of professional responsibility of 1912—that in the absence of a strong assertion of a duty to care was to be a source of great confusion when AIDS confronted American medicine. "A physician shall," stated Section VI of the AMA's code, "in the provision of appropriate patient care, except in emergencies, be free to choose whom to serve" (Zuger 1987). Amending the blunt articulation of an unencumbered professional freedom, the AMA's Judicial Council has ruled that refusals to treat on the basis of race, religion, or creed were unethical (AMA 1980). In November 1987, in the seventh year of the AIDS epidemic, the Council ruled that "A physician may not ethically refuse to treat a patient whose condition is within the physician's current realm of competence solely because the patient is seropositive" (AMA 1987). In so doing, the AMA joined the American Nurses' Association, which had a year earlier denounced discrimination against patients with AIDS.

As philosophers attempted to struggle with this issue, they, at times, stressed the importance of a *social* responsibility to guarantee each HIV-infected individual with access to health care (for the responsibility of the health-care *professions*, as collective entities, to provide appropriate care to those in need), rather than the responsibility of each individual health-care worker to treat. In short, some argued, if somewhat reluctantly, that as long as the needs of the HIV infected were met, there might be no sound ethical grounds for insisting that each health-care worker share in the responsibility.

Others have argued for a more universal obligation. Edmund Pellegrino stated, "to refuse to care for AIDS patients, even if the danger were greater than it is, is to abnegate what is essential to being a physician" (1987). For many who have stressed a universal obligation to treat, it is clear that the relatively low risk of infection has been central. Were the risks of HIV transmission very much greater, it would have required an ethics of heroism to insist that each health-care worker bear the responsibility of ensuring adequate and appropriate health care to the infected. Given the level of risk entailed in the face of HIV infection, even among surgeons and obstetricians, those who stressed the obligation to treat argued that it was not heroism but more straightforward duty that was involved.

The issue of access to care is not, however, primarily raised by the specter of physician abandonment. Rather, it centers on the problem of the structure of the U.S. health-care system. Despite the extraordinary increase in expenditures for health care over the past 3 decades and the rise in government financing through Medicare and Medicaid, significant and growing inequities continue to plague the health-care system. Millions of people either have no health-care insurance or are inadequately protected by limited and intermittent coverage. The vulnerability of those with HIV infection must be viewed in this context.

The striking contrast between important clinical advances in the care of those with HIV infection and the social organization of U.S. medicine led the National Commission on Acquired Immunodeficiency Syndrome to warn in a December 1989 report to the President that medical breakthroughs would "mean little unless the health care system can incorporate them and make them accessible to people in need" (National Commission on AIDS 1989). The existence of a medically disenfranchised class meant that for many, access to care was almost solely through the "emergency room door of one of the few hospitals in the country that treats people with HIV infection and AIDS."

The looming crisis in health care for those with HIV disease set the stage for congressional action in mid-1990 that could scarcely have been imagined a short time earlier. Such action represented the fruit of dogged efforts on the part of AIDS activists, their allies, and some political leaders from the cities and states that had borne the disproportionate share of AIDS cases. In the winter of 1990, Senator Edward Kennedy, the exemplar of Democratic party liberalism, and Senator Orrin Hatch, a Republican whose stance on abortion often cast him in the role of a conservative, jointly sponsored legislation—the Ryan White Comprehensive AIDS Resource Emergency Act of 1990—that was to provide a major infusion of federal assistance to those localities most severely burdened by AIDS. As the government had responded to natural disasters, the Kennedy–Hatch Bill asked it to respond to the medical disaster of AIDS. "The Human Immunodeficiency Virus constitutes a crisis as devastating as an earthquake, flood or drought. Indeed, the death toll of the unfolding AIDS tragedy is already a hundredfold greater than any natural disaster to strike our nation in this century" (Senator Edward Kennedy, unpublished letter, 1990).

However important the Ryan White Act, named for a boy with AIDS who had been barred from school, it could not be a substitute for the fundamental change in the organization and financing of health care in the United States that will be required by the chronic management of the medical and social needs of all HIV-infected persons at a moment when so many other medical needs of the nation's poor remain unmet. Much will depend on the ultimate course of health care reform. Justice for people with AIDS is thus inextricably linked to justice in health care for all Americans.

AIDS AND THE WORLD

In a grim way, AIDS links the most advanced technological societies such as the United States and the poorest nations of Africa, Asia, and Latin America. The vast proportion of HIV infection in the world exists outside North America and Western Europe. In the next decade the already stark contrast will become even sharper. In the face of the social catastrophe now making itself felt, it will be critical to confront the question of what the rich nations of the world owe the poor as the latter confront the issues of prevention and treatment. The social, economic, and political realities of general assistance to the Third World are a background context that cannot be ignored as we confront the AIDS pandemic. The basic fact is that the advanced industrial world does very little to meet the needs of the Third World, in terms of food, health care, or other basic goods.

It is all too easy to imagine the development of expensive therapeutic agents that will be reserved for persons who fall ill as a result of HIV infection in the advanced industrial societies but that will not be available to those similarly situated in Third World nations. But would such a situation be morally tolerable? If and when a vaccine were developed, would it be made available to those most in need? And who would pay the cost of production and distribution for those nations too poor to bear the cost? These questions are especially pertinent now that strong epidemiological arguments are being made for using Africa for research into the efficacy of candidate vaccines.

AIDS, because of its dramatic features, underscores the limitations of our capacity to conceive of and act upon notions of shared responsibility across national boundaries. At stake, of course, is the question of justice and the global distribution of resources.

CONCLUSION

AIDS compels us to recognize what the history of earlier epidemics has demonstrated. The social response to threatening pathogens is always shaped by cultural and political forces as well as by the state of scientific knowledge. Positivists who hold out a vision of an "objective" asocial response to disease assume that if values intrude upon efforts to control epidemics, either ignorance or profound misjudgments are involved. But it is neither ignorance nor misjudgment that forces social values to the forefront in the making of public health policy. Rather, it is the inevitable consequences of the need to balance and consider competing and, sometimes, irreconcilable interests and sociopolitical commitments in the face of epidemic disease.

To recognize the extent to which efforts to control AIDS will call forth sharp ethical and social controversies is not, however, the end of the analysis. It is, in fact, just the beginning. Which values—with what impact on the lives of men, women, and children, with what implications for democratic social life, with what likely consequences for the further spread of HIV infection—should guide us? This is the question posed for us by ethics in this time of epidemic.

DISCUSSION QUESTIONS

1. What moral, social and psychological risks could be connected with testing for HIV? Are there any circumstances in which compulsory testing would be morally justifiable? What about newborn infants whose mothers are known to be HIV positive? Pregnant women who refuse to be tested? Surgeons and other professionals at risk for transmitting HIV? Patients scheduled for surgery who could expose health professionals and others to HIV?

2. May a health-care professional—physician, nurse, or dentist, for example—be allowed to refuse to treat a patient who is HIV positive if that individual is otherwise competent to treat the patient?

3. Is there ever a situation in which it would be morally justified for a health-care professional to report a diagnosis of HIV to third parties? If so, which third parties? state health departments? police? other health-care professionals? the spouse or sexual partners of the infected individual?

4. Should hospitals, public health authorities, or both be permitted to collect data on the HIV status of groups of people for research and epidemiological purposes? If so, should data be collected with identifiers so that those who are positive could be contacted, if necessary, or should the data be cleaned of all identifying information?

5. Some people believe that HIV and AIDS are punishment for behaviors believed to be sinful, unlawful, or otherwise inappropriate. How should one respond to someone who makes such a claim? Is there any morally relevant difference between someone who develops HIV infection as a result of sharing drug needles or sexually promiscuous behavior and someone who contracted the disease through contaminated blood transfusion or transmissions during birth from an HIV-infected mother?

REFERENCES

Books and Articles

Abel, R. M. "Risk Is Too High in AIDS Patient Surgery." *New York Times*, November 9, 1987: 22A.

American Civil Liberties Union, Northern California Branch. *AIDS and Civil Liberties.* San Fransisco: Northern California Branch, ACLU, 1986.

American Medical Association. Current Opinions of the Council on Ethical and Judicial Affairs, American Medical Association: Ethical Issues. Chicago: American Medical Association, 1987.

———. Current Opinions of the Council on Ethical and Judicial Affairs, American Medical Association: Ethical Issues, sections 9, 11. Chicago: American Medical Association, 1986.

———. "Prevention and Control of Acquired Immunodeficiency Syndrome." *JAMA* 258 (1987): 2097–2103.

———. *Principles of Medical Ethics.* Chicago: American Medical Association, 1980.

———. *Report of the Council on Ethical and Judicial Affairs: Ethical Issues Involved in the Growing AIDS Crisis,* Chicago: American Medical Association, 1987.

Annas, G. "Faith (healing), Hope and Charity at the FDA: The Politics of AIDS Drug Trials." *Villanova L Rev* 34 (1989): 771–797.

Arras, J. "The Fragile Web of Professional Responsibility: AIDS and the Duty to Treat." *Hastings Cent Rep* (Special Suppl) 18 (1988): 10–20.

Association of State and Territorial Health Officials. *ASTHO Guide to Public Health Practice: HTLV III Antibody Testing and Community Approaches.* Washington, DC: Public Health Foundation, 1985.

———. *Guide to Public Health Practice: HIV Partner Notification Strategies.* Washington, DC: Public Health Foundation, 1988.

Bayer, R. *Private Acts, Social Consequences: AIDS and the Politics of Public Health,* 2nd ed. New Brunswick: Rutgers University Press, 1991a.

———. "Public Health Policy and the AIDS Epidemic: An End to HIV Exceptionalism." *N Engl J Med* 324 (1991b): 1500–1504.

Bayer, R., Fairchild-Carrino, A. "AIDS and the Limits of Control: Public Health Orders, Quarantine, and Recalcitrant Behavior." *Am J Public Health* 83 (1993): 1471–1476.

Bayer, R., Healton, C. "Controlling AIDS in Cuba." *N Engl J Med* 320 (1989): 1022–1024.

Bayer, R., Levine, C., Wolf, S. M. "HIV Antibody Screening: An Ethical Framework for Evaluating Proposed Programs." *JAMA* 256 (1986): 1768–1774.

Centers for Disease Control and Prevention. "Education and Foster Care for Children Infected with Human T-Lymphotropic Virus Type III/Lymphadenopathy-Associated Virus." *MMWR* 34 (1985): 517–521.

———. "Recommendations for Assisting in the Prevention of Peri-Natal Transmission of Human T-Lymphotropic Virus Type III/Lymphadenopathy-Associated Virus and Acquired Immunodeficiency Syndrome." *MMWR* 34 (1985): 721–726, 731–732.

———. "Recommendations for Preventing Transmission of Infection with Human T-Lymphotropic Virus Type III/Lymphadenopathy-Associated Virus During Invasive Procedures." *MMWR* 35 (1986): 221–223.

———. "Recommendations for Preventing Transmission of Infection with Human T-Lymphotropic Virus Type III/Lymphadenopathy-Associated Virus in the Workplace." *MMWR* 34 (1985): 681–686, 691–695.

———. "Update: Acquired Immunodeficiency Syndrome and Human Immunodeficiency Virus Infection Among Health-Care Workers." *MMWR* 37(1988): 229–239.

Dickens, B. M. "Legal Limits of AIDS Confidentiality." *JAMA* 259 (1988): 3449–3451.

Dubler, N., Levine, C., Levine, R. "Building a New Consensus: Ethical Principles and Policies for Clinical Research on HIV/AIDS." *IRB* 13 (1991): 1–17.

Faden, R., Geller, G., Powers, M. B. *AIDS, Women and the Next Generation: Towards a Morally Acceptable Public Policy for HIV Testing of Pregnant Women and Newborns.* New York: Oxford University Press, 1991.

Faden, R., Holtzman, N., Chwalow, A. "Parental Rights, Child Welfare, and Public Health: The Case of PKU Screening." *Am J Public Health* 72 (1982): 1396–1400.

Fox, D. "The Politics of Physicians' Responsibility in Epidemics: A Note on History." *Hastings Cent Rep* (Special Suppl) 18 (1988): 5–10.

Gostin, L. "HIV-Infected Physicians and the Practice of Seriously Invasive Procedures." *Hastings Cent Rep* 19 (1989): 32–39.

———. "The AIDS Litigation Project: A National Review of Court and Human Rights Commission Decisions, Part I: The Social Impact of AIDS." *JAMA* 263 (1990): 2086–2093.

Institute of Medicine and National Academy of Sciences. *Confronting AIDS.* Washington, DC: National Academy Press, 1986.

Levine, C., Bayer, R. "The Ethics of Screening for Early Intervention in HIV Disease." *Am J Public Health* 12 (1989): 1661–1667.

Levine, C. "Has AIDS Changed the Ethics of Human Subjects Research?" *Law, Med Health Care* 16 (1988): 167–173.

National Commission on AIDS. *Annual Report.* Washington, DC: U.S. Government Printing Office, 1989.

Pellegrino, E. "Altruism, Self Interest and Medical Ethics." *JAMA* 258 (1987): 1939–1940.

Presidential Commission on the Human Immunodeficiency Virus Epidemic. *Final Report.* Washington, DC: U.S. Government Printing Office, 1986.

Report of the Presidential Commission on the Human Immunodeficiency Virus Epidemic. Washington, DC: U.S. Government Printing Office, 1988.

U.S. Public Health Service. "Guidelines for Prophylaxis Against Pneumocystis Carinii Pneumonia for Persons Infected with Human Immunodeficiency Virus Disease." *MMWR* 38 (Suppl 5) (1989): 1–9.

U.S. Surgeon General's Report on Acquired Immune Deficiency Syndrome. Washington, DC: U.S. Public Health Service, 1986.

Zuger, A., Miles, S. H. "Physicians, AIDS and Occupational Risk: Historic Traditions and Ethical Obligations." *JAMA* 258 (1987): 1924–1928.

Cases and Acts

Ryan White Comprehensive AIDS Resource Emergency Act, Pub. Law 101-381, 1990.

Tarasoff v. Regents of the State of California, 17 Cal. 3d 425, 551 2d 334, 131 Cal Rptr 14 (1976).

14

National Health-Care Reform

NORMAN DANIELS

SUMMARY

Inequities in the U.S. health-care system compromise the very purpose of health care: to protect equality of opportunity. This chapter examines several requirements of justice, articulated as design principles that emphasize morally important properties essential to a fair health-care structure. Five systems are described—the current U.S. system, the 1994 Clinton proposal, the Cooper plan, the Chafee plan, and the single-payer system—and analyzed according to the design principles.

The framework of analysis is constructed, first, around the elimination of exclusionary health-care practices. Justice here requires that no one be excluded (universal coverage principle) because of failure to purchase private insurance in a mixed system (compulsory coverage principle), because of the existence of or anticipation of risk (nonexclusion principle), or because of coverage limited to a particular employment status (portability principle). Although financial barriers to inclusion could be ameliorated by implementing a common price for insurance regardless of risk (community rating principle), nonfinancial barriers to access, such as lack of primary care providers in rural areas and inner cities, must be eliminated if the goal of equity is to be actualized. Each proposed health-care program is evaluated considering these principles.

The chapter then explores criteria for determining priorities among services covered in an equitable health-care system. Rather than limiting entire categories of service such as mental health, a just health-care program would adhere to a comprehensive benefits principle that rejects sharp categorical distinctions (mental vs. physical, preventive vs. acute). Although the prospect of rationing is appalling to many people, justice requires that proponents of a health plan fund research to explore the efficacy of certain therapies and refuse to cover services that simply enhance human function or appearance. It is essential to ensure that the grounds for establishing such

Acknowledgment: Excerpted from *Seeking Fair Treatment: From the AIDS Epidemic to National Health Care Reform* by Norman Daniels (pp. 153–181, as edited and approved by the author). Copyright © 1995 by Norman Daniels. Reprinted by permission of Oxford University Press, Inc., New York.

priorities are publicly available and fair and that the poorest groups do not bear the primary burden when access to services is restricted.

Because a wasteful system exhausts resources and leaves the vulnerable at risk, principles of justice indicate that health-care services should compete with other important social goods. Furthermore, fairness in a health-care system is fostered by the delivery of efficient health care through reduced administrative costs and limited tort litigation. A person's inability to pay must not render an individual uninsured; subsidization or a progressive tax could provide possible funding. These principles highlight the injustice of perpetuating a cost-ineffective system and failing to support persons unable to participate financially.

The chapter concludes by examining the importance of effective, informed consumer choice in a health-care system. Consumer choice would provide incentives for physicians to discuss alternative treatments with patients. An independently operated agency must make information about the performance of a health plan and its physicians readily available so that consumers may make authentic choices about treatments and physicians. Assessing each health plan's success in complying with this and other design principles of justice would clarify which features enhance justice. Such an analysis could aid in understanding the requirements of an equitable health-care system.

All of us potentially face exclusion from health insurance because of risk; loss of insurance coverage with job loss or job change; maldistribution of appropriate providers; and inadequate coverage for home care, mental health care, and other services, including drugs. A system to correct these and other problems we all risk having to confront would go a long way toward ensuring fair treatment. The most effective way to do so would be to enact comprehensive national health-care reform that meets key criteria for justice or fairness.

But what *does* a just or fair system require? What criteria of fairness should it be judged by? Specifically, in a climate of widespread determination to reform the system, what criteria should we use to assess the fairness of health-care reform proposals?

Access to appropriate, willing physicians and other providers is a requirement of justice. Society has the obligation to ensure that there are adequate practitioners to meet the health-care needs of patients, and that professional and individual practitioner obligations and prerogatives are compatible with the requirements of justice. Ordinary exclusionary practices of health-care insurers employing standard underwriting procedures violate considerations of justice. Health-care insurance must be governed by different criteria of fairness than some other forms of insurance against risk, because its primary goal is to ensure access to services that play a central role in ensuring fair equality of opportunity. Charging significantly higher premiums to those at higher risk violates requirements about the fair sharing of the burdens of meeting health-care needs. Fair treatment involves careful consideration of the kinds of services that should be included in an insurance benefit package. We should not deny access to a new technology simply because it is expensive or because it falls into a particular category of services such as long-term care rather than acute care. Rather, we should limit access to a beneficial service only if we can show it is less important to offer it—because of its "opportunity cost"—than other services we should be offering. If we are to impose fair limits on services, we must develop reasonable criteria and fair procedures for making such decisions.

INTRODUCING DESIGN PRINCIPLES

The time has now come to consider more systematically what all of us should consider fair treatment in health-care reform. Of course, there is no uniquely just health-care system. A variety of institutional designs may exhibit the crucial features and functions that principles of justice require. For example, a just system might be purely public (as in Canada) or mixed (as in Germany), or a just system might involve a national health service (as in Great Britain) or national health insurance (as in most other countries). When we fashion institutions, our goal must be to reconcile political feasibility and efficiency with the requirements of justice without violating the principles that inform those requirements. As we shall see, comparing the fairness or justice of reform proposals is a complex and multidimensional task.

To bring my views about justice to bear on the different proposals, I shall use a series of what I will call "design principles," which are intended to highlight morally important properties and functions of just health-care institutions. Design principles—although they are not themselves principles of morality—are reasonable requirements to impose, given our views about justice and health care and given our knowledge of how the delivery of health care actually works. Any list of design principles could be expanded or contracted, practically *ad libitum* (depending in part on the degree of rigor with which one wished to evaluate the institutions or proposals in question); the discussion here concerns what seem to be the most salient of the many principles one might wish to apply. Among these are *efficacy, compulsory coverage, comprehensive benefits, universal coverage, portability, non-exclusion, community rating, explicit rationing,* and *financing by ability to pay*.

What these design principles do is help specify appropriate answers to critical questions such as these: How universal is insurance coverage? How portable are insurance benefits? How comprehensive are the benefits provided? Design principles also provide a multidimensional matrix that can be used to assess the fairness or justice of a broad range of competing reform proposals (not only the ones considered here),[1] including detailed proposals that continue to emerge as the legislative process evolves at both federal and state levels. To illustrate how the matrix of design principles can help us assess the fairness of a health-care *system*, I shall apply it to some actual reform *proposals* that emerged in the U.S. health-care debate of 1994. This is risky business because the landscape of reform surreally shifts before my eyes as I write. Still, a few landmarks stand out, and, because they illustrate a spectrum of central ideas about the design of a reformed system, they will serve my purpose here.

THE LEADING REFORM PROPOSALS

In the 1994 debate, the Clinton "Health Security Act" dominated the scene and called for a combination of market forces—"managed competition"—and robust government regulation (and mandates) to guarantee universal coverage and cost controls. To its left stood the Wellstone–McDermott version of a Canadian-style "single-payer" system; its taxed-based system would have eliminated private insurance companies and joined everyone in a uniform, public health-care insurance scheme. To its right were other plans such as Senator Chafee's "Health Equity and Access Reform Today" (HEART) and Representative Cooper's plan that called for more reliance on market forces and less on government involvement. These four concrete 1994 proposals can be used as examples of major models for kinds of national plans that could be adopted. Any health-care reform that is enacted—whether it is federal or ultimately state-by-state reform—will likely embody elements of these proposals.

Before fully developing the matrix of design principles, however, I want to describe very briefly the central features of the plans to which I will apply it. This description, of course, cannot be complete because the plans are quite complex. But seeing how the matrix allows us to analyze and evaluate the fairness of the main proposals will illustrate its value in assessing

---

[1] In March 1993, I presented a paper articulating design principles for assessing health-care reform at a conference at the Dana-Farber Institute. Also that month I began participating as a member of the Ethics Working Group of the White House Health Care Task Force. The Dana-Farber paper influenced the work of the Ethics Working Group. Specifically, when Dan Brock and I formulated a set of "Ethical Principles and Values for the New Health Care System," we drew on ideas in the original draft. Further discussion within the Ethics Working Group, and especially with Dan Brock (Brown University), with whom I co-authored Brock and Daniels (1994), as well as comments by Robert Baker (Union College) and Donald Light (Rutgers), have led me to modify somewhat the design principles originally discussed in March 1993, adding a few and modifying the description of others. The articulation of this matrix of design principles is part of a larger project Donald Light and I have worked on, supported by the Robert Wood Johnson Foundation. In that work, the design principles, considerably modified, have evolved into benchmarks that can be used to score reform proposals on a numerical scale (Daniels, Light, and Caplan 1996).

actual reforms. I will comment on other features of each proposal as I apply the matrix to them in subsequent sections.

Single-Payer Systems

This sketch of leading reform proposals begins with the most radical plan, the effort to adopt a Canadian-style "single-payer" system. The Wellstone–McDermott proposal, backed by nearly 90 members of Congress, called for eliminating all private insurers. This was highly popular because many people believe health insurers have diverted a significant proportion of health-care dollars into administrative costs and profits, and thus have contributed greatly to the relatively high cost of the current health-care system in the United States. Because it eliminates the "hassle factor" involved in negotiating reimbursements for treatment from insurers with different rules and procedures, it was popular with patients as well as with many practitioners.

Instead of myriad private insurers, the single-payer proposal would make the government a public insurer that could negotiate fees and payments to hospitals, physicians, and other providers who would offer services to all citizens on presentation of a health-care card. Funding would require that a payroll tax replace the complex system of general tax revenues, employer contributions, and individual payments of premiums and out-of-pocket payments currently in place, making the funding mechanism relatively progressive (although for many whose employee benefits are now "invisible," a payroll tax seems to be a new tax).

Benefits were not fully detailed in the proposals, but the advocates of this style of reform intend to make them comprehensive, aiming for parity between mental and physical health, and between acute and chronic or long-term care. The uniform health plan would not involve "tiering." Because there would be no competing insurers trying to avoid adverse selection by high-risk patients, there would be no risk exclusions. Coverage would be completely portable. Tax revenues would constitute a global budget (i.e., a single fixed pool of resources) for health-care expenditures. Cost containment would result from several factors: the global budget would force careful consideration of investment in new technologies and apply pressure against overutilization of many services; large-scale fee and hospital-charge negotiation, under budget constraints, would markedly slow the rate of growth of these costs.

Managed-Care Plans

The Clinton "Health Security Act" attempted to seize a political middle ground between such a single-payer ("big government"), public-insurance scheme, on the one hand, and proposals that relied almost entirely on "managed" market forces (and weak or absent government mandates), on the other. One option open to the states under the Clinton proposal was for them each individually to adopt a "single-payer" system. This option seemed necessary because competition among health-care plans is feasible only in large population areas that can sustain stable, noncolluding competitors, although more than 30 percent of the population lives in areas where competition is not feasible (Kronick et al. 1993). But the primary focus of Clinton's reform incorporated an idea that was shared with various plans to its political right, namely "managed competition."

No one should confuse managed competition with *managed care*. The latter is an insurance plan that tries to control cost and quality through the selection of providers and the regulation of services. *Managed competition*, in contrast, provides for a "sponsor" to act on behalf of large numbers of insurees to negotiate favorable prices from competing, "qualified" health-care plans, many of which, incidentally, would be managed-care plans. The sponsor may be a public agency, such as the "Health Alliances" under Clinton's plan, or a large employer. Purchasers, whether individuals or employers, would buy insurance at the "managed" (that is, negotiated) rates, but they would be made conscious of costs by the way employee tax benefits for health-care premiums would be reduced or eliminated. For example, the plan Clinton proposed mandated employers to provide insurance, but at the most they would pay 80 percent of the premium of a "basic" plan, while employees would pay the remaining 20 percent, as well as any additional cost for a more generous insurance plan. Unemployed or self-employed individuals would have to buy insurance through Health Alliances; subsidies to low-income individuals would help them purchase insurance. All health plans would have to offer a "comprehensive" package of benefits that would have been defined by the Clinton legislation. (Later in this chapter, we shall look at what is meant by "comprehensive" benefits.)

Although the Clinton, Chafee, and Cooper proposals all incorporated elements of managed competition, Clinton's plan gave the "managers"—his public health alliances—a more determinative set of powers than their counterparts in the other plans would have had. In addition, the Clinton plan called for a National Health Board to be empowered to set "premium caps" that would limit the increase in premiums by tying increases to growth in the gross national product. (This regulatory mechanism has been denounced as a form of "price controls" by those touting more market-based plans.) Without question, it gave the Clinton plan a feature that resembled the single-payer budget as a form of social control over health-care expenditures.

The Clinton plan also involved more powerful mandates to ensure universal coverage—for example, its mandate to all employers. Although the Chafee plan required individuals (as opposed to employers) to purchase insurance, the phase-in of universal coverage was expected to take many years and to depend on the availability of savings produced by competition among health plans. The Cooper plan, stripping away even more of the possible government control, eliminated any mandate for universal coverage and depended very heavily on market forces to make insurance more affordable.

All the proposed plans agreed that private insurers should no longer exclude people on the basis of risk but disagreed on how to adjust reimbursements to make taking on higher-risk patients affordable. Plans also differed on how comprehensive the covered benefits should be in a "basic" plan eligible for subsidies and on who should make the determinations. Those who supported more reliance on market forces and consumer choice, of course, wanted less government regulation of benefits.

APPLYING DESIGN PRINCIPLES TO NATIONAL HEALTH-CARE REFORM PROPOSALS

What are the important design principles and how is one to apply them? It can be argued that the central, unifying purpose of health care is to promote "normal functioning"—functioning that is typical or normal for our species. By impairing normal functioning, disease and disability shrink our shares of opportunity from what is fair. Health care—be it preventive, acute, long-term, or palliative—thus protects equality of opportunity. Because we have a general social obligation to ensure that people have fair equality of opportunity, we have specific obligations to provide health-care services that promote normal function. These obligations require that there be no financial or other barriers to a level of care that promotes normal functioning, given reasonable or necessary limits on resources. The design principles here spell out the implications of this view; they capture features and functions of a health-care system that are important from the point of view of justice.

I will use these design principles to assess the answers to five central questions: Who is covered? What is covered? How are costs contained and efficiency ensured? How are costs shared? What choices do people have? (These headings disguise points of overlap, and so some of the principles will appear or come up for discussion more than once.) I will first discuss what seem to me the relevant design principles under each question, and I will then summarize my analysis of the salient points made about the principles governing each question in table form (one table per question). In the tables, I use symbols to indicate qualitative differences in the way the proposals comply (or do not) with the principles. The rationale for most of the judgments will have been provided in the text.[2]

---

[2]It should be noted that the evaluations the tables contain—as I have included them here—are only qualitative, sometimes involving judgments about the degree of compliance or improvement over the status quo; it is possible, however, to develop more refined criteria for the application of these principles and to score compliance with them numerically (for numerically scoreable "benchmarks of fairness," see Daniels, Light, and Caplan 1996). Given that my goal in this context is to illustrate how we can assess the fairness of health-care reforms, however, it is not necessary to pursue here the complications such a scoring system involves.

As the debate about health-care reform progresses, legislation may emerge that combines features from various proposals. For example, the Clinton Health Care Task Force originally recommended full parity between mental and physical health care. In early 1994, when the Health Security Act was presented, however, parity was eliminated in favor of a *promise* of parity by the year 2001. Other reform proposals weakened mental health benefits still further. But, although the matrix of design principles will help us track the implications for fairness of these changes as legislation is passed and implemented, it is not exhaustive; the matrix is a tool that begs for refinement.

Who Is Covered?

To protect equality of opportunity, health-care institutions must provide appropriate, effective services to everyone, regardless of their race, economic status, geographical location, or health risks. Several of the design principles address aspects of this question.

Ideally, no one should be excluded from coverage; the *Universal Coverage Principle* makes that a requirement. Leaving significant "gaps" in insurance coverage violates this design principle. The Cooper plan, for instance, imposed no mandate on either employers or individuals to provide or purchase insurance. The result was that, although it would be easier for some people to acquire insurance under this proposal, serious gaps would be left, and universal coverage was but a distant goal.

Insurance gaps can arise for a variety of reasons, some of which might initially seem justified. Therefore, although strictly speaking I need only one design principle governing access to insurance and services to evaluate proposals, it is useful—for analytic purposes—to look at more than one principle in order to focus attention on several of the ways universality can fail. For example, in a mixed public–private system in which the purchase of insurance is voluntary, people who "choose" not to buy coverage, although they can afford it, are responsible for their lack of coverage. If we as a society then provide needed medical services to these imprudent people, feeling an obligation to assist those in need, we encourage freeriders. Similarly, private insurers fearing adverse selection may identify and exclude high-risk insurees, even claiming they are obliged to do so because it is "actuarially unfair" and therefore unjust to force those at low risk to subsidize those at higher risk. Risk selection also traps people in jobs where they *do* have coverage; fear of losing the coverage keeps them from daring to switch jobs.

Several design principles work to close these specific gaps in access. A *Compulsory Coverage Principle* requires people to purchase private insurance in a mixed system. In a purely public, tax-financed system (such as Canada's), the principle is trivially satisfied because taxes are compulsory and coverage is therefore automatic. In a mixed public–private system, where employers or individuals must purchase insurance, the Compulsory Coverage Principle does away with freeriders. Requiring people to buy insurance makes their premiums function like a tax, but it also eliminates adverse selection, making it easier to require insurers to cover all people regardless of risk.

Clinton's 1994 Health Security Act included provisions requiring all who are uninsured to enroll in a health plan when they show up for treatment; the problem would primarily involve the unemployed and self-employed because of the universal employer-mandate. Chafee's HEART proposal, which mandated individual purchase of insurance, quite probably would make the problem of freeriders more widespread. HEART relied on the IRS and Department of Health and Human Services to track nonpurchasers through tax and medical records. The Cooper plan failed to alter the status quo, for it neither mandated coverage nor provided any mechanism for eliminating freeriders.

The *Non-Exclusion Principle* closes the gap caused by insurance underwriting and by the latitude allowed under current legislation (called ERISA) to self-insuring employers. This principle prohibits the exclusion of people from coverage because of existing conditions or anticipated health risks. (Such a principle governs private German insurers.) Those who most need insurance in our current system—people with "prior conditions" and people at high risk—are denied coverage or given only reduced coverage at higher premiums. In the popular mind, these exclusions undermine the whole point of insurance, which is to protect people by sharing risks as widely as possible.

Insurers, however, view health insurance as another commodity in the risk-management market: People buy insurance to manage their health risks (which insurers like to imply are just like any other risks), and they should be charged a price that reasonably reflects only their own risks. The "product" should remain attractive or marketable to those who know they are at less-than-average risk, and adverse selection must be avoided. Sharing risks, however intuitively appealing, is no longer a marketable idea to those with low risk, once they know their risk is low.

The public's intuitive view about sharing risks can be supported by assigning a different social function to health insurance. In buying health insurance people are not simply buying economic security at an actuarially fair price; they are ensuring themselves access to needed medical services. And this is the function assigned to health insurance by the fair-equality-of-opportunity account. Because we have a shared social obligation to protect opportunity against the effects of disease and disability, low-risk individuals cannot disavow an obligation to subsidize those at higher risk. That obligation is part of the cost of protecting opportunity for all, including in the end those who at present *appear* to be at low risk.

There is no room for actuarial fairness in a just health-care system. Not only *must* those at higher risk be given coverage, they *must not* be made to bear the extra financial burden of their risks. The burden must be shared. Specifically, the *Community Rating Principle* requires that people pay a common price for insurance regardless of their level of risk.

In a single-payer system like Canada's, the whole population forms a single risk pool. No standard underwriting practices are possible. Non-Exclusion is clearly satisfied, and Community Rating is not applicable because people pay their share of insurance costs through progressive taxes rather than through insurance premiums.

The Clinton, Chafee, and Cooper proposals also prohibited risk-based exclusions or reductions in coverage. Clinton's Health Alliances would be required to sell insurance at community rates, while adjusting reimbursement rates of health plans that take on higher risk patients. Community rating would be protected in the Clinton plan if employers who "opt out" of Health Alliances paid a surcharge to them whenever their employees form a lower risk pool than Health Alliance insurees do. The Chafee and Cooper plans were less explicit than Clinton's about how non-exclusion and community rating would be accomplished.

All of these plans, however, depended on developing a mechanism for "risk adjustment," so that health plans could be reimbursed in ways that compensate them for taking on higher-risk patients. Unfortunately, it is controversial whether the technology for risk adjustment could be developed and refined enough to enable full compliance with the principle. Some reform proposals—less comprehensive than the plans we are comparing—called for insurance-market reform, including the elimination of risk exclusion and risk rating. If universal coverage is not mandated and made feasible, however, it is very difficult to see what form the legislation could take that would enable it to accomplish its stated aims.

Protection of equality of opportunity through health insurance should not be left to the vagaries of employment status. According to the *Portability Principle*, coverage must persist outside one's home region; it must form a seamless web among all employed persons regardless of whether they are working full- or part-time, in a large or a small company, and so on. Portability promotes efficiency and security: People should not be chained to jobs because of their health status (or that of their dependents).

The Canadian Medicare card offers a paradigm of portability, ensuring all who carry it access to any provider in the country. Similarly, the McDermott–Wellstone proposal complied fully with the Portability Principle. Clinton's plan boasted of such a card, symbolizing access, but the existence of many different health plans made portability a matter for negotiation among plans and for enforcement by Health Alliances. In addition, employees of large companies (firms with more than 5,000 employees) that opt out of the Health Alliances would have to change plans and doctors if they changed or lost jobs. If the Clinton proposal allowed smaller employers to act as "corporate alliances," then portability might be compromised further. The Chafee plan was set up in a way that made it difficult to assess issues of portability: Individuals would be able to buy plans that are not tied to their employment status or employer's choices, but many employers would still provide coverage. The Cooper plan also left many of the portability problems in the

TABLE 14.1 Who Is Covered?

Design Principle	Current U.S. Plan	Cooper Plan	Chafee Plan	Clinton Plan	Single-Payer Plan
Universal Coverage	V	PC	PC	C*	C*
Compulsory Coverage	V	V	C	C	C
Non-exclusion	V	PC*	PC*	C*	C
Community Rating	V	PC⁻	PC⁺	C⁺⁺	C^DNA
Portability	V	V	PC>	PC>>	C

V = Violates or maintains status quo.
PC = Partial compliance or some improvement over status quo.
C = Compliance or significant improvement over status quo.

- Except for nonlegal residents.
- Difficult without universal coverage.
- Risk adjustment more difficult without powerful health alliances.
⁻ Unclear how ensured.
⁺ "Ideal" only if risk adjustment works.
⁺⁺ Provided large employers who opt out subsidize.
> Some gain, some do not.
>> Large employer opt-out reduces portability.
DNA Commentary does not apply.

current system unaddressed. Still, to the extent that all three reform proposals eliminated risk exclusion, at least some of the barriers to portability were to be diminished.

Justice requires that nonfinancial barriers to access also be reduced. These barriers are diverse: lack of primary-care providers in rural and inner-city areas, cultural and educational barriers to utilization, physical barriers to the disabled. No one feature of design can address them all. The Clinton plan specifically confronted the issue of increasing the number of primary-care practitioners by changing the rules about medical education. The less-comprehensive Chafee and Cooper proposals did not undertake to deal with these issues.

What Is Covered?

According to the fair-equality-of-opportunity account, we have social obligations to provide those services that most effectively and efficiently protect our fair shares of the normal opportunity range once reasonable or necessary limits on resources are taken into consideration. This includes preventive, curative, restorative, chronic, compensatory, and palliative services. But because scarcity is unavoidable—in part because health care is not the only important good people seek in a society—we cannot provide everyone with *all* beneficial services. Where we withhold services, however, we must assess their effect on protecting opportunity rather than arbitrarily limiting whole categories of service (as insurers now do with regard to preventive, mental health, and long-term-care services, for instance). The fair-equality-of-opportunity account also, of course, rejects restrictions on beneficial services that apply only to the poorest sectors of society.

The *Comprehensive Benefits Principle* comes into play here, telling us that all categories of service that meet health-care needs will be included and that the judgments we make about including some services rather than others must be based on the effects of these services on the range of opportunities we enjoy. Such judgments cut across the traditional distinctions of category—such as mental versus physical, preventive versus acute, and acute versus long-term—that have led to underprovision of many important services by both public and private insurers. In effect, comprehensive benefits are promised but are not delivered when legislative or contract language assures us that insurance provides all "medically necessary" services (Sabin, Forrow, and Daniels 1991, Sabin and Daniels 1994). Adherence to the principle would mean parity between mental and physical health and an end to the bias in favor of acute-care services that we have now.

Our current system clearly violates the Comprehensive Benefits Principle. The 1994 Clinton plan appealed to the notion of a comprehensive, mandated benefit package, but recognized the principle without achieving full compliance with it. Although it would have added many preventive services and gone some way toward establishing parity of benefits between mental and physical health, it made only incremental improvements in long-term care. The Chafee and Cooper plans left the full content of the benefit package unspecified, and the Chafee plan even left the door open to *reducing* the benefit package in unspecified ways if savings from reform were inadequate to fund subsidies needed to move the system toward universal coverage. The McDermott–Wellstone plan included a more comprehensive benefit package than the Clinton package, adding a more robust long-term-care benefit.

Our obligation to ensure access to needed health-care services extends only to providing efficacious services. We are obliged to provide what we have reasonable evidence to believe *works*. We are *not* obliged to provide unproven or unnecessary treatments. The *Efficacy Principle* emphasizes the need to fund research about health outcomes and to develop practice guidelines: We are woefully underinformed about which medical practices actually meet reasonable standards of efficacy. At the same time, we have extensive evidence that much unnecessary treatment is given; regional variations in utilization rates imply that utilization is supply- rather than need-driven (Hadorn 1992; Kolata 1994). This all means that we must develop not only information but incentives, regulation, and training for producing compliance with practice protocols. The Efficacy Principle implies that we should cover proven therapies but not experimental ones, which means we need a fair process for deciding how to draw the distinction; this principle also warrants distinguishing treatments of disease and disability from services that merely enhance function (or appearance) that is already normal for our species. This chapter does not undertake to comment on this very particular application of my account because I have done so elsewhere, and it does not in any case bear centrally on the issue at hand (Daniels 1992, Sabin and Daniels 1994).

All the reform proposals criticized the current U.S. system for not complying with the Efficacy Principle and noted the importance of measures aimed at improving compliance. The Clinton proposal, with its premium caps and the expanded powers of the Health Alliances to provide consumers with information, put more pressure on health plans to induce providers to comply with the Efficacy Principle. It also emphasized improving consumer information about outcome measures of the different health plans. Still, it did not specify just what federal support would be given to outcomes research. The Chafee proposal also called for setting up an information system adequate to telling us more about outcomes and appropriate practice guidelines. The details of the system would have had to have been developed further; however, like the Clinton plan, it failed to specify funding for outcomes research. The Cooper plan was silent on many of these matters. Finally, there is nothing about a single-payer system that makes it intrinsically better than the Clinton proposal at complying with the Efficacy Principle. In the Canadian system, as in some managed-care plans, physicians internalize restraints on ineffective utilization because they must retain credibility with other professionals who control limited resources under global budgets. But all professionals still need hard information about what does and does not work.

Some people believe that rigid adherence to the Efficacy Principle would make it unnecessary to engage in the rationing of beneficial services. Squeezing all the waste out of the system would suffice to make available resources adequate to meet other needs. This was the stance taken by the Clinton Administration when members of the Ethics Working Group of its Health Care Task Force requested that the proposal pay careful attention to the need to limit the use of beneficial services—the need to ration. Those of us on the Ethics Working Group were told that there should be no mention of rationing in our writing about the plan, that rationing would not be necessary; the Clinton Administration feared appearing to condone rationing. Despite this attempt to shield the plan from one type of criticism, advocates of other reforms attacked the Clinton plan anyway for opening the door to rationing on the grounds that its premium cap and the powers it would have given to a National Health Board to monitor the benefit package over time amounted to rationing. And so it did. These attacks were, however, highly disingenuous. The current system already rations care at many levels—by excluding people from both public and private insurance and by making many decisions about what services and technologies to cover.

All reform proposals that fail to establish a fair mechanism for addressing rationing decisions will thus continue the highly inconsistent and capricious set of decision-making processes we now employ—which themselves result in rationing. Given the rate of growth of new medical technologies—the prime force affecting the rate of cost increase in health care worldwide—we are simply going to have to be prepared to make decisions about withholding some beneficial treatments whose costs are not worth their benefits (Schwartz 1987, Newhouse 1993).

When we ration beneficial services, we make choices about whose opportunities we will protect. Calabresi and Bobbitt (1978) argue that the social cost of publicly and explicitly making such "tragic choices" is high, and that sometimes we should sacrifice the legitimacy such openness brings in favor of less visible methods. When rationing affects the fundamental life prospects of people, I believe the requirements of publicity are quite stringent. We need a publicly accountable process for making these decisions. The *Explicit Rationing Principle* says that the grounds or principles for establishing priorities among services must be publicly available and open to democratic criticism, and that rationing decisions must result from a fair process.

The fair-equality-of-opportunity principle, like other general, distributive-justice principles, falls short of telling us precisely *how* to make certain rationing choices (Daniels 1993). For example, although the equal-opportunity principle implies that we should give *some* priority to those whose opportunities are most seriously restricted, it does not tell us "how much." Similarly, it allows us to aggregate the effects on the opportunities of various individuals so that modest benefits to many people can sometimes outweigh more significant benefits to few—but, it does not tell us what principle of aggregation to employ. Again, it does not tell us how to weigh "getting the best outcome" from some service against "giving people a fair chance" at getting some benefit from it. Because we do not have principled solutions to these rationing problems, I interpret the Explicit Rationing Principle to require a fair procedure that includes *making public* the grounds for all choices.

None of the 1994 reform proposals clearly complied with the Explicit Rationing Principle. The Clinton proposal assigned the National Health Board the task of deciding what treatments to include in a comprehensive benefits package, but it did not (for reasons explained before) mention "rationing" health care or even consider how to take costs explicitly into account when thinking about coverage decisions or quality of care. Clinton's plan included a mechanism for a "grievance procedure" within health plans to address complaints that both patients and doctors made about benefits. Of course, *ex post* rather than *ex ante* fair process is better than nothing, but it still was not adequate. No other proposals specified anything that pertained to a public process for making rationing decisions. Moreover, it should be noted that single-payer systems are not immune from arranging to keep public scrutiny away from rationing decisions; the Canadian system has little provision for a public, democratic process in the decisions about limitations on services.

The *Structure of Inequality Principle* says that restrictions on access to beneficial services must not apply primarily to the worst-off or poorest groups in society. Suppose that budget limitations mean we cannot include certain (significant) beneficial services in the only plan low-income people can afford. If these benefits are then available to most other people, who can afford to buy better insurance, the structure of inequality is unacceptable. In contrast, if these benefits are available only to the richest groups in society, while the great majority—including the poor—cannot afford them, then the structure of inequality is more acceptable. Fair equality of opportunity proscribes leaving the poor well behind the rest of society, but it does not mean that strict equality is a requirement in health-care rationing. Whether the extra advantages enjoyed by the rich are acceptable will further depend on how significant those advantages are judged to be (and on whether the income distribution is itself just, overall).

Our current system fails to comply with the Structure of Inequality Principle; at the other extreme, the proposed McDermott–Wellstone single-payer system did. We have contemporary examples in other countries, as well. Consider how the Canadian system works: The best-off Canadians avoid queues and purchase some services in the United States, but the great majority of persons are all affected roughly alike by rationing decisions. Similarly, in Germany and the Netherlands, the wealthiest third of the population may enjoy more amenities in its private insurance, but the rich receive no treatments offering *significant* benefits that are unavailable through public schemes.

The Clinton proposal tried to limit violation of this principle within a managed-competition system by setting a 20 percent limit on the degree to which health plans could exceed the "benchmark" price for health plans. The goal was to limit both the degree to which more expensive plans could portray themselves as vastly superior in quality and the degree to which low-cost plans are labeled as low quality, with the result that low-income people dependent on subsidies are locked into the lowest tier of plans.

If the only differences between plans are in amenities, market segmentation would not clearly violate the Structure of Inequality Principle. Richer plans, however, could also "buy" more or better specialists, or introduce cutting-edge technologies more quickly. Where significant effects on health outcomes result, the Structure of Inequality Principle is violated; regulatory restrictions prohibiting such inequalities (e.g., restricting the range of premiums charged or offering more generous subsidies) would go some distance toward satisfying it.

The other proposals, which emphasized their appeal to market forces, did not impose any restrictions on the emergence of such tiering and inequality. To some extent, the problem was obscured by the claim that a basic, uniform benefit package would be described by an appropriate commission, both in the Chafee and Cooper plans. The basic package might have turned out to be thin; even if it was not, plans that charge more, selling themselves on

TABLE 14.2   What Is Covered?

Design Principle	Current U.S. Plan	Cooper Plan	Chafee Plan	Clinton Plan	Single-Payer Plan
Comprehensive Benefits	V	V+	PC++	PC+++	PC+++
Efficacy	V	PC	PC>	PC>	PC?
Explicit Rationing	V	V??	V??	PC??	PC??
Structure of Inequality	V	V&	V&	PC&	C

V   = Violates or maintains status quo.
PC = Partial compliance or some improvement over status quo.
C   = Compliance or significant improvement over status quo.

+   Did not provide adequate details on benefits.
++   Covers only serious mental illness; no long-term care.
+++ Clinton promised full parity of mental and physical by 2001, offered extensive preventive services and some expansion of long-term care.
>   All reform proposals talked about using outcomes research, but Clinton and Chafee proposed information systems that would support such research efforts.
?   Advocates of single-payer systems rely on the global budget, but this was short-sighted.
??   Cooper and Chafee allowed for benefits to vary by tier according to ability to pay; Clinton's Task Force was instructed to avoid public talk about rationing; rationing by queuing, as in Canada, is explicit, but there was not enough attention to fair public processes to decide what queues should exist.
&   Clinton allowed only 20 percent gap between benchmark and high-cost plans, which reduced tiering; Chafee and Cooper did not counter tiering.

quality, could develop different coverage patterns despite the apparent uniformity of benefits. Medicaid offers broad benefits, like many other insurers, for instance; but it offers (or is typically perceived to offer) a distinctly lower quality of care. Replicating the inequalities between Medicaid and the best private insurance plans would certainly violate the Structure of Inequality Principle.

How Are Costs Contained and How Is Efficiency Ensured?

Efficiency is often thought to compete with justice: Fairness can be costly, and efficiency may be unfair (to some). Nevertheless, promoting efficiency within a just system by avoiding wasteful uses of resources will enhance its fairness in crucial ways. A wasteful system puts too many health-care dollars into administrative costs, or into treatments that do not work, or into services that provide very little benefit relative to the cost involved. As a result, wasteful systems force the rationing of useful services that less-wasteful systems can afford to deliver. A wasteful system thus leaves some individuals and groups at risk, while a less-wasteful system better protects them. Justice requires us to meet our health-care obligations with as little waste as possible.

By raising the overall costs of delivering reasonable medical benefits, a wasteful system can drain resources into the health-care sector that can be better spent elsewhere. Promoting health—however important—is not our only important social goal. For example, a larger investment in education or job training might actually protect the range of opportunities open to people more than the investment we make in low-benefit medical services.

Some people object to restricting what we spend on health care, claiming that there is no one spending level that justice requires or permits. People "vote" with their dollars; if people vote in this manner for more health insurance, then that is the democracy of the market in action. To sing such a refrain is to ignore the degree to which corporations and professionals control this vote; it also ignores the fact that other social goods do not compete with health care on a level playing field in our system. We determine expenditures for many other socially important programs, such as education, crime protection, social welfare, and defense, when our representatives pass government budgets. But our largely private "votes" to buy health-care services are what determines our collective health-care expenditures, including those in entitlement programs.

Several design principles aim at reducing waste within the health-care sector and at preventing us from spending too much on health care. The *Comparability Principle* requires that demand for health-care services should compete with the demand for other comparably important social goods through mechanisms that control supply in similar ways. We express our demand for educational services, police and fire protection, national defense, public-health services, transportation, and social-welfare programs largely through our tax dollars; we weigh their relative importance through public budget decisions. In contrast, we express our demand for health-care services largely through tax-sheltered employee benefits, while professionals who act as our agents tell us what we need and spend our dollars for us. At best, these agents "pull out all the stops" and do "everything possible" for us; at worst, they manage the demand for a good they have a vested interest in promoting. Both "best" *and* "worst" inflate demand in this instance.

Two market strategies aim at improving comparability. Some conservative economists recommend "privatizing" other government functions, but they have failed to persuade us that our social obligations can be met that way. We will continue to make public budget choices, not merely private ones, for other important goods. Comparability must therefore be sought in another way. Managed competition tries to eliminate the distorting influence of public (tax) subsidies on private decisions, for example, by reducing tax-sheltering for employee benefits. But raising private "cost consciousness" in this way will not force the same discipline that we show in the public sphere, where the goods directly compete with each other. In any case, cost consciousness also erects significant barriers to access based on ability to pay. Comparability must be sought in the public sphere.

The global budgeting of health-care expenditures achieves comparability in the public sphere. The comparability principle can be operationalized by substituting a *Global Budgeting Principle* for it. The broader the scope of a global budget (that is, the more health-care expenditures it captures) and the "harder" (or more enforceable) it is, the more effectively the public can act on its choices about the importance of health care.

The Global Budgeting Principle is clearly violated by the current system, while it is satisfied by a Canadian-style, single-payer system such as the McDermott–Wellstone proposal. The Clinton plan proposed that a National Health Board set a premium cap on the growth of health-care expenditures in a given year. States would have to be accountable for staying within the cap. To control cost increases, a global budget must prevent cost shifting. This is most straightforwardly done when all existing insurance sectors—Medicaid, Medicare, Veterans, Department of Defense, Workers' Compensation, and all supplementary insurers—are integrated under one budget, and there is a specified agency accountable for translating the budget into component budgets for different elements in the health-care system. The Clinton proposal would likely have been in partial compliance with the global budgeting principle because it left some room for health expenditures not captured by a premium cap. Neither the Chafee nor the Cooper plan called for any kind of budget cap, relying instead solely on market forces to contain health-care costs.

The Global Budgeting Principle seeks comparability between health care and other social goods, but global budgeting also aims at reducing wasteful services within the health-care sector. Canada uses its global budget to force decentralized decisions about the priorities that should be followed in delivering other health-care services. Physicians who do not follow reasonable priorities, such as in pursuing CT scans or in home health services for their own patients (claiming their patients are urgent cases when they are not), are soon seen as uncooperative. Of necessity, doctors learn to internalize a sense of restraint—even though they work on a fee-for-service basis, which encourages less wasteful use of resources. Some of these effects are possible within the "global" budgets of well-run managed-care plans.

Global budgeting and competition need not be mutually exclusive: They may be combined in various ways and at different levels in a health-care system. The Clinton proposal incorporated competition among health plans within a globally budgeted system, gambling that competition would generate highly efficient delivery systems once cost shifting had been eliminated by the force of a global budget. Specifically, the proposal gambled that these gains in efficiency would outweigh the higher administrative costs of a more complex system. The proposal also gambled that competition would not push costs up if "upscale" tiers created a demand for enriching the lower tiers. But managed-care systems also reformulated ratios between specialists and primary-care generalists without invoking the heavy hand of the government. Simply introducing a single-payer system like Canada's in the United States would not bring with it parallel savings unless we also established their more favorable ratio of generalists to specialists.

In light of these remarks, we must be tentative in assessing compliance with the *Efficient Management Principle,* which seeks the delivery of effective health care with low administrative costs in a system that is easy for doctors and patients to use. The current system clearly fails to comply; its private-insurance sector has high administrative costs and imposes a serious "hassle factor" on both doctors and patients through complex reimbursement procedures and micromanagement of clinical decision making.

In contrast, the Canadian single-payer system has remarkably low administrative costs and imposes little bureaucratic burden on either patient or doctor. The Chafee and Cooper plans promised little to reduce the complexity and administrative inefficiency of the current system. Both plans in effect gambled that competition among managed-care plans would produce administrative savings, despite increased complexity—but it should be noted that little in the experience of managed care in the United States to date gives us reason to be optimistic on that score. The Clinton proposal made the same gamble, but it also sought to simplify medical reporting requirements and reimbursement processing.

If increased competition under a global budget drives many insurers out of the market, some complexity will be eliminated. Putting more information about the performance of different plans in the hands of consumers would also create pressure to simplify administration because consumer satisfaction is likely to be lower in plans that have a high hassle factor. Still, how well the Clinton proposal would have performed in this arena is a matter of speculation: The competitive forces have an unknown effect, while the complexity of the system is a familiar worry for practitioners.

Physicians accept a role as gatekeepers if they see that role as deriving from their own sense of what competent medicine requires under fair and reasonable resource constraints. Professionally generated practice guidelines, internalized through good training in environments that support those guidelines and backed up by "profiling" of physicians, are far more likely to promote efficiency than microregulation of case-by-case clinical decisions by insurance "bureaucrats." In the best HMOs, providers are involved in the process of developing practice guidelines, believe in their content, and accept the constraints of managed care with little "gaming" of the system. Whether more intense competition would support or undercut such successful management practices is quite unclear.

A focus on primary care is a key to controlling costs in the Canadian system, in many European systems, and within managed-care plans. Compliance with the *Primary Care Principle,* which calls for needs-based distribution of generalists and specialists, would mean that fewer specialists would have incentives to overutilize and overdisseminate specialized technologies.

TABLE 14.3 How Are Costs Contained and How Is Efficiency Ensured?

Design Principle	Current U.S. Plan	Cooper Plan	Chafee Plan	Clinton Plan	Single-Payer Plan
Global Budgeting (comparability)	V	V	V	PC	C
Efficient Management	V	V	PC?	PC?	C?
Primary Care	V	V>	V>	PC>	C
Negotiated Fee	V	V	V	V	C
Tort Litigation Reduction	V	PC*	PC*	PC*	PC*

V = Violates or maintains status quo.
PC = Partial compliance or some improvement over status quo.
C = Compliance or significant improvement over status quo.

? Managed competition gambles that competition will produce delivery efficiencies that offset the complexity lacking in low-administrative-cost single-payer systems.

> Managed-care plans redefine generalist–specialist ratios within the plans, but it is unclear what effect they have on overall ratios; Clinton's plan refocused training and incentives on primary care; introducing single-payer in the United States would have no short-term solution to unfavorable ratios unless explicit measures to redefine ratios were undertaken.

* All reform proposals talk about some malpractice reform. This row is a placeholder for a more detailed evaluation not provided here.

The principle is clearly violated in the United States as a whole, while it is satisfied in Canada. The Chafee and Cooper proposals relied on each health plan to define its own ratio. In theory, this would put pressure on specialists to undertake more primary-care work and would create a long-term incentive to reduce the number of specialists being trained. The Clinton proposal added to these pressures by refocusing training funds on primary-care physicians, and in so doing it more clearly aimed at compliance than the other reform proposals did (which said little or nothing about the matter).

One design principle that addresses cost containment and the allocation of personnel simultaneously is the *Negotiated Fee Principle*. Canadian provinces negotiate directly with the provincial medical association to establish a fee structure for a whole region. The fee structure keeps physician costs within the constraints of a global budget and creates incentives to alter primary-care/specialist ratios. None of the reform proposals being reviewed here, aside from single-payer, complied with this design principle, although it would have been available under the Clinton plan to states that chose a single-payer plan. The Clinton plan, like the Chafee and Cooper plans, relied mainly on negotiation with individual managed-care plans to contain fee increases and incorporate incentives to alter the composition of the health-care workforce. Whether these mechanisms would be as effective at achieving what is done through regionally negotiated fees is unknown.

Compliance with the *Tort Litigation Reduction Principle* would also reduce waste in the system, although I have no specific reform in mind. Any reform would have to reduce the defensive overutilization of services by physicians and the costs of liability insurance, while retaining a fair procedure for compensatory justice. The table here does not evaluate the reform proposals for compliance with this principle (Table 14.3), but does include the principle to indicate that it will need to be part of any final, complete assessment of the fairness of a reform proposal.

How Are Costs Shared?

Although our obligation to provide access to needed health-care services is a social one, the fair-equality-of-opportunity account itself does not have anything to say about the fair distribution of income and wealth or about fair patterns of taxation or subsidization. Earlier, when I defended the *Community Rating Principle*, I argued that those at low risk cannot disavow an obligation to subsidize the costs of those at high risk; however, this falls short of telling us how to finance our general obligation to provide health-care services—an issue that deserves at least a brief discussion.

One main option is to retain health insurance premiums and to subsidize their purchase for people who cannot afford them. Financing for such a subsidy could itself be funded through more- or less-progressive forms of taxation. By relying on the *Financing by Ability to Pay Principle*, this option captures one crucial element of fair sharing: No one shall be denied coverage because of the *lack* of ability to pay. Compared to our current system, this option involves the least redistribution of income even though families will vary enormously in their ability to pay for health insurance premiums.

The second main option is to finance purchase of insurance through a more progressive tax, a move that itself divides into more- and less-progressive alternatives, depending on which kind of tax is chosen. A fixed-percentage payroll tax would be more progressive than a premium-based contribution, but it would be less progressive than a graduated income tax (especially one that included, as taxable, unearned income). For the purpose here—where I am concerned primarily with introducing the *idea* of these design principles—it will suffice to assume that the more progressive the tax base, the more fairly costs are shared (a more exhaustive account would, of course, have to defend this assumption); accordingly, Table 14.4 is constructed on the strength of that assumption. Table 14.4 also repeats the assessment of the Community Rating Principle because that principle also captures a critical feature of the fair sharing of costs.

TABLE 14.4   How Are Costs Shared?

Design Principle	Current U.S. Plan	Cooper Plan	Chafee Plan	Clinton Plan	Single-Payer Plan
Financing by Ability to Pay	V	$PC^?$	$PC^{??}$	$PC^{???}$	$C^{\&}$
Community Rating	V	PC^-	PC^+	C^{++}	C^{DNA}

V = Violates or maintains status quo.
PC = Partial compliance or some improvement over status quo.
C = Compliance or significant improvement over status quo.

?   Increased subsidization for people who could not buy insurance; plan was somewhat more progressive than current system.
?? No progressive taxation in the plan; improvement was to come from a more generous subsidy to individuals with incomes well above federal poverty level, but funds for subsidies had to come from savings elsewhere in the system.
??? Regressive tobacco tax was proposed, plus a mandate for employer contributions, with subsidies for small employers; no new progressive tax base was proposed.
&   Payroll tax was proposed.
-   Unclear how ensured.
+   "Ideal" only if risk adjustment were to work.
++ Provided large employers who opt out subsidize.
DNA Commentary does not apply.

What Choices Do Consumers Have?

A health-care system defines a set of choices for both consumers (patients, purchasers of insurance) and practitioners. The fair-equality-of-opportunity account says little about choice: To say that whatever arrangements best promote equal opportunity without violating anyone's basic liberties are acceptable does not suffice; more must be said about choice from the perspective of justice and fair treatment. Specifically, I urge a *Consumer Choice Principle*, which requires that a health-care system facilitate making effective and informed choices about providers, health-care plans, and treatments. Choice in each of these areas is affected by the range of options open to us, the information we have about them, and the number of people who can exercise these choices; there may *be* no "best" proposal for promoting consumer choice because enhancing choice in one area may require trade-offs with choices in another. Consumer choice is important for the health of the system, not just for individuals: Informed, effective choice is a powerful engine of reform, driving concerns about quality and cost.

Today it is widely recognized that patients have the right to give informed, voluntary consent to the treatments they undergo. Although this is sometimes cast simply as a right to refuse certain treatments, it has broader implications for the process of deciding about treatments. Specifically, physicians must invest the time to discuss alternative, *available* treatments with patients so they can make informed choices that reflect their own values and preferences. Reimbursements to plans and providers must therefore provide incentives to give time for such discussions. Moreover, good information about outcomes must be available or the physician cannot properly inform patients; this kind of information, too, has costs associated with it.

The choice of health plans is complex because plans differ in the services they cover, in the quality of their services, in their amenities, and in their price. In the current system, consumers have poor information about the performance of health plans; they may have some information about coverage (although it is often not detailed), and they may have access to information about costs (although it is often confusing because of co-payment and deductible requirements). To empower consumer choices about health plans, a significant investment must be made in providing information about both outcomes and consumer satisfaction in various treatment areas. Without such information, consumer choice in health care is far less informed than the choices made by those same consumers when they buy cars or plumbing fixtures (which at least are reviewed in *Consumer Reports*). Provision of the information cannot be left to the health plans: There must be an independent agency responsible for making information about plan performance readily available (and helping to ensure that it can be understood). The effective range of choices open to people is also important. If "tiering" occurs because health plans compete on price and there are significant premium differences among health plans, the choice range for low-income individuals will be reduced.

For most people, "choice" means choice of physician. Proponents of managed competition argue that people in the United States overvalue having a choice of physicians and that these choices are generally not well informed. For example, people typically turn for recommendations to friends or relatives who have little hard information even about their own physicians. The alternative may not be to replace choice of physician with choice of health-care plan, but rather to provide better information about the performance of physicians. In any case, it will be particularly important to devise a system that does not require interfering with the satisfactory, long-term relationships with physicians that many people have—and fear losing. Perhaps, especially for people with disabilities or other special medical problems, this is a critical issue, but a good relationship with a specialist *or* a primary-care physician cannot always be easily replicated.

Evaluating the various proposals for their effect on Consumer Choice is particularly difficult because there are so many different dimensions of choice. The current health-care system in the United States clearly fails to protect (or in some instances even to offer) consumer choice in several important ways. Although some people can (at great cost) retain their choice of physician, many others lose those choices because of the power employers have to select and impose health plans (which in turn restrict physician choice). For many people, whether they realize it or not, the status quo is actually on course to reduce significantly their choice of physician. In addition, there is little provision at

TABLE 14.5   What Choices Do Consumers Have?

Consumer Choice Principle		Current U.S. Plan	Cooper Plan	Chafee Plan	Clinton Plan	Single-Payer Plan
Physicians	R	PC*	PC*	PC*	PC*	C
	I	V	V	V	V	V
Plans	R	PC**	PC**	PC**	PC**	DNA
	I	V	V	PC?	C	DNA
Treatments	R	PC⁻	PC⁻	PC⁻	PC⁺	C
	I	PC⁻	PC⁻	PC⁻	PC⁺	PC

R = Range of choices.
I = Steps taken to provide adequate information.
V = Violates or maintains status quo.
PC = Partial compliance or some improvement over status quo.
C = Compliance.

*   Partial compliance varies; current system has little choice for uninsured, decreasing choice for many, considerable choice for some; Cooper has decreasing choice as managed care increases, which leaves employers with control of plan choices in many cases; Chafee reduces employer provision; some buying through alliances could leave some employees with more choice; Clinton plan promises every health alliance retains plan giving full physician choice, but decreases in choice for those in managed care; decreased control by employer increases choices.

**   Current system has myriad plans in some areas, few in others, control of range by employers, recent growth of preferred provider organizations (some with options to increase choice of specialist); Cooper did not change current forces except that more individuals would have some choice of plan because of more subsidy for insurance; Chafee reduced somewhat employer choice of plans and increased individual choice, but not by design; Clinton's plan reduced employer choice of plans significantly (except for large employers) and mandated Health Alliances to offer options including full-choice plan; Clinton plan could have led to fewer overall plans.

?   Unclear whether extra effort to provide good consumer information.

⁻/⁺   Negative/Positive interference with doctor–patient decisions by insurers, except for Clinton promise to simplify microregulation; improved information on what works in Clinton plan and possibly also in Chafee plan.

DNA   Commentary does not apply.

present for adequate information about physicians, plans, *or* treatments. We may be better at informing patients about treatments than many other countries, but we know no more than others about what works.

The Cooper plan would have put the power of choice in the hands of employers rather than consumers in many cases; it also did not address the problem of information. Aside from providing some more people with coverage—people who now have no choice of plan or physician—there is no clear gain over the status quo. The Chafee plan mandated individuals to purchase insurance; to the extent that some or many employers would stop providing insurance, there might have been an unanticipated gain in individual choice. The availability of a comprehensive information system could be used to increase choice of plans, but the Chafee proposal did not pursue this idea as far as the Clinton plan, which emphasized developing "report cards" to provide information about plan performance. Although the Clinton plan, like the Chafee and Cooper plans, would have driven more people into managed care, costing some people their existing choice of physicians, the plan reduced employer control over choice of plans except for very large employers. Moreover, the Clinton proposal mandated that all alliances—corporate and public—had to offer an indemnity plan with full choice of physicians. (The cost of the plan might have put these choices out of reach of most people, however.)

A single-payer system could leave people with a much broader choice of physicians, even if it eliminated the choice of plans. Proponents of the Canadian system argue that no one cares about choice of *plans* as long as a choice of physician and hospital is still available. Information about the performance of physicians and hospitals is no better in Canada than it is here, however, and thus we are faced with the choice between the known satisfaction expressed about the choice available in the Canadian system and the promise of benefits that could result if we give ourselves effective choices among competing health plans.

CONCLUSION

Comprehensive health-care reform is the single most important step we can take to enhance fair treatment. In the debate about health-care reform, fairness is usually not a prominent issue: We hear instead about costs, efficiency, and political feasibility. This chapter develops a framework—a matrix—for assessing the fairness or justice of competing reform proposals. Drawing on my fair-equality-of-opportunity account of justice and health care, I have discussed a set of design principles that articulate features and functions of a just health-care system.

The application of this matrix to leading reform proposals yields the conclusion that the Canadian-style, single-payer plan complies better with the design principles than the proposed alternatives did, although all plans offer some improvement over the status quo. The Clinton proposal, which would have given states a choice of a single-payer or a modified version of managed competition, did almost as well; the Chafee and Cooper plans fell off sharply in their fair treatment of everyone in the system. The crucial issue of political feasibility—which has not been discussed here at all—of course has to be faced at some point. Clearly, many design features of the Clinton plan were aimed at making it politically more acceptable than a pure single-payer plan might be. Whether Clinton underestimated the public acceptability of the single-payer plan is hard to assess. He may even have underestimated the power of the lobbies representing insurers and other vested interests, and he may have given away too much to start with to advocates of more modest plans. I will leave further exploration of these matters to others, however, because *my* goal is ethical rather than political analysis.

DISCUSSION QUESTIONS

1. What is the difference between evaluating health-care plans on the basis of fairness and on the basis of efficiency? Which plans discussed in this chapter are likely to be the most efficient in producing health-care benefits? Which are the most fair?

2. What ethical problems are raised by having two-tier or multiple-tier health-care plans? Would a second tier of health-care insurance be more acceptable if it provided coverage for services beyond those included in a fair basic tier? What services could morally be excluded from a basic tier that might be covered by a second tier? Could any of the following be limited to a second tier of coverage: experimental chemotherapy for cancer, continuing life support for anencephalic infants (without enough brain capacity to permit them ever to be conscious), ventilators or medically supplied nutrition for patients who are permanently unconscious, surgery to improve vision, dental care, cosmetic surgery? Can you identify other treatments that could justifiably be limited to a second tier?

3. What are the ethical implications of having a single-payer system rather than multiple insurance companies? Would it be ethical to have a single-payer system but also offer different packages of coverage (perhaps all arranged to provide equal costs)?

4. How should abortion, in vitro fertilization, sterilization, infertility treatment, hospice treatment for the terminally ill, alternative therapies, and other morally controversial treatments be covered in health-care insurance to be fair to all parties?

5. If people engage in voluntary behaviors that pose risks to their health, should basic insurance cover resultant medical care needs? If so, should those engaging in these behaviors be expected to pay larger premiums to cover their expected greater needs? If not, how would you propose to care for such patients when they have medical needs? How would you cover illnesses related to alcoholism, smoking, high-risk occupations, skiing, mountain climbing, or professional sports?

REFERENCES

Calabresi, G., Bobbitt, P. *Tragic Choices.* New York: W. W. Norton, 1978.

Daniels, N. "Growth Hormone Therapy for Short Stature: Can We Support the Treatment/Enhancement Distinction." *Growth & Growth Hormone* 8 (May, suppl. 1) (1992): 46–48.

Daniels, N. "Rationing Fairly: Programmatic Considerations." *Bioethics* 7(2–3) (1993): 224–233.

Daniels, N., Light, D., Caplan, R. *Benchmarks of Fairness for Health Care Reform.* New York: Oxford University Press, 1996.

Hadorn, D. C. "Necessary Care Guidelines." In D. C. Hadorn, Ed., *Basic Benefits and Clinical Guidelines.* Boulder, CO: Westview Press, 1992.

Kolata, G. "Their Treatment, Their Lives, Their Decisions." *New York Times Magazine* (April 24) (1994): 66, 100, 105.

Kronick, R., et al. "The Marketplace in Health Care Reform: The Demographic Limits of Managed Competition." *N Engl J Med* (14 January 1993): 148–153.

Newhouse, J. P. "An Iconoclastic View of Health Cost Containment." *Health Affairs* (suppl.) 12 (1993): 152–171.

Sabin, J., and Daniels, N. "Determining 'Medical Necessity' in Mental Health Practice: A Study of Clinical Reasoning and a Proposal for Insurance Policy." *Hastings Cent Rep* 24(6) (1994): 5–13.

Sabin, J. E., Forrow, L., Daniels, N. "Clarifying the Concept of Medical Necessity." Group Health Association of America. *Group Health Insur Proc* (1991): 693–708.

Schwartz, W. B. "The Inevitable Failure of Current Cost Control Strategies: Why They Can Provide Only Temporary Relief." *JAMA* 257 (1987): 220–224.

Glossary

Anencephalic	literally, the condition of having no encephalon or brain (normally applied to infants with no cerebrum)
Anorexia nervosa	an eating disorder characterized by persistent, health-threatening loss of appetite
Antinomianism	the position that ethical action is determined independent of law or rules (cf. situationalism, rules of practice, legalism)
A priori	derived from self-evident proposition
Autonomy	the governing of one's self according to one's own system of morals and beliefs
Beneficence	the state of doing or producing good (cf. non-maleficence)
Best interest standard	judgment based on an idea of what would be most beneficial to a patient (cf. substituted judgment)
Ceteris paribus	other things being equal; if all other conditions are the same
Chemotherapy	a form of treatment that consists of the use of chemicals to control disease
Consequentialism	the normative theory that the rightness or wrongness of actions is determined by anticipated or known consequences (cf. deontologism)
Covenant	a solemn agreement between two or more parties
De facto	in reality, actual (cf. de jure)
De jure	by right, by law (cf. de facto)
Deontologism	a theory according to which actions are judged right or wrong based on inherent right-making characteristics or principles rather than on their consequences
Double Effect, the Doctrine of	the theory that an evil effect is morally acceptable provided a proportional good effect will accrue, evil is not intended, the evil effect is not the means to the good, and the action is not intrinsically evil

Dyspepsia	indigestion
Egalitarian	a social philosophy that advocates human equality
Euthanasia	the merciful hastening of death, often limited to willful and merciful actions to kill one who is injured or terminally ill
Fatuity	something foolish
Fidelity	the state of being faithful
Germ line	the cells which constitute gametes or reproductive cells
Gesisah	the state of being that immediately precedes death and during which, according to the Jewish faith, one ought not to intervene to interfere with the dying process
Histocompatible	the condition in which tissues will not react to produce a rejection during transplantation
Human Immuno-deficiency virus (HIV)	a retrovirus responsible for acquired immuno-deficiency syndrome (AIDS)
Hypochondriasis	morbid concern about one's health
Immunodeficiency	the state of substandard expression of the immune system
Immunosuppression	the state of inhibiting the expression of the immune system
Intubation	the insertion of a tube into an organ
Legalism	the position that ethical action consists of strict conformity to law or rules (cf. antinomianism, rules of practice, situationalism)
Macroallocation	the distribution of resources on a large scale
Maternal serum alpha-fetoprotein	a protein secreted during gestation that predicts fetal abnormalities such as spina bifida
Metaethics	the branch of ethics having to do with the meaning and justification of ethical terms and norms
Metaphysical	the principles underlying a particular subject or system of beliefs
Microallocation	distribution of resources on a small scale
Nonmaleficence	the state of not doing harm or evil (cf. beneficence)
Nontherapeutic	something which does not serve the purposes of benefitting an individual patient
Normative	the branch of ethics having to do with standards of right or wrong (cf. metaethics)
Normativism	the doctrine that moral standards or norms determine the rightness or wrongness of actions
Null hypothesis	in scientific research, the hypothesis that there exists no difference in the effect of two or more treatments

Parentalism	the system of action in which one person treats another the way a parent treats a child, striving to promote the other's good even against the other's wishes (cf. autonomy, paternalism)
Pareto improvement	additions to aggregate good brought about by exchanges between pairs of individuals in which each believes his or her welfare increases
Pareto optimality	the system of distribution whereby pairs of individuals are permitted to make exchanges until no pairs are willing to make further exchanges, thus leaving all parties as well off as possible without violating the interests of any party
Paternalism	the system of action in which one person treats another the way a father treats a child, striving to promote the other's good even against the other's wishes (cf. parentalism)
Persistent vegetative state	a state of brain pathology in which the brain stem is intact but there is no content to consciousness; characterized by a state of profound dementia which is associated with a loss of awareness and ability to interact with the environment
Prima facie	all things being the same "at first sight"
Pythagorean	of or relating to the theories and beliefs of the Greek philosopher Pythagorus
Randomized clinical trial (RCT)	a scientific research design in which treatment varies for two or more groups selected at random
Renal dialysis	treatment by the use of an artificial kidney machine
Rules of practice	the position that rules govern practices such that actions are normally judged by rules (cf. antinomianism, situationalism, legalism)
Schizophrenia	a psychotic disorder characterized by personality disintegration and distortion in the perception of reality
Secular ethics	theories of what is good and bad, or right or wrong, based on criteria other than religious doctrine
Seropositivity	the state of positive results of a study of antigen-antibody reactions in vitro
Situationalism	the position that ethical action must be judged in each situation, guided by, but not directly determined by, rules (cf. antinomianism, rules of practice, situationalism)
Somatic	all cells other than germ-line cells
Substituted judgment standard	the standard of judgment based on an estimation of what an individual would have chosen

Surrogate	someone serving as a substitute decision maker
Taxonomy	a system of classification
Teleological	explaining phenomena by their design, purpose, or final causes
Therapeutic	relating to therapy
Therapy	the provision of remedies in the treatment of disorders or illnesses
Utilitarian	the view that an action is deemed morally acceptable because it produces the greatest balance of good over evil, taking into account all individuals affected
Utility	the state of being useful or producing good
Vertigo	dizziness; confusion
Virtue	a persistent trait of good character

Index